HANDBOOK OF COMMONLY PRESCRIBED DRUGS

(with Therapeutic, Toxic & Lethal Levels)

Eighteenth Edition

G. John DiGregorio, M.D., Ph.D.
National Medical Services
Willow Grove, Pennsylvania
and
Professor of Pharmacology and Medicine
Drexel University School of Medicine
Philadelphia, Pennsylvania

Edward J. Barbieri, Ph.D.
Toxicologist
National Medical Services
Willow Grove, Pennsylvania

2003

HANDBOOK OF COMMONLY PRESCRIBED DRUGS
(With Therapeutic, Toxic & Lethal Levels)

Eighteenth Edition

PREFACE

The **Eighteenth Edition** of the **HANDBOOK OF COMMONLY PRESCRIBED DRUGS (With Therapeutic, Toxic & Lethal Levels),** has maintained the new section that was initiated with the last edition that has information on serum, plasma and blood levels of many drugs. As previously, not all of the drugs listed in the handbook have this information included; rather, we have focused on those compounds in which we have found and verified published values. We have received positive feedback that clinicians who have used this handbook found this information helpful and have utilized the material as a quick reference to blood levels for more effective treatment of their patients and observed toxic effects.

It is important to emphasize that the information on therapeutic, toxic and lethal levels contained herein are only reference guidelines. Depending upon the specific reference source, these levels may be found to vary. Factors such as the patient population, dosage, route(s) of administration, time of the measurement, and the analytical procedure used all influence the reported levels of drugs. We have used a few well-read reference sources to compile this information (cited at the end of the section) and we are cognizant that many other highly regarded references are available.

As in all previous editions, the drugs listed, the preparations which are available, and the therapeutic dosages have been edited to reflect the most recent information that could be found. Many new therapeutic agents and new dosage forms are always presented and listed below are some of the new individual therapeutic agents that have been added to this edition:

Adefovir Dipivoxil (HEPSERA) — a new antiviral drug indicated for the treatment of chronic hepatitis B

Brompheniramine Tannate (BROVEX, BROVEX CT) — an antihistamine usually found only in combination products is now being used as a single drug

Desloratadine (CLARINEX) — the dextro- isomer of the popular nonsedating antihistamine, loratatdine (CLARITIN)

Dexmethylphenidate (FOCALIN)) — the dextro- isomer (and the more active form) of methylphenidate

Diclofenac Sodium (SOLARAZE) — a new topical form of the drug for treating actinic keratoses

Eplerenone (INSPRA) — a new antihypertensive drug that acts as a selective aldosterone receptor antagonist

Ertapenem (INVANZ) and Moxifloxacin Hydrochloride (AVELOX) — two new antibacterial drugs, a carbapenem-type and a fluoroquinolone, respectively, used for a variety of systemic infections

Escitalopram Oxalate (LEXAPRO) — the levo- isomer of the antidepressant, citalopram (CELEXA)

Ezetimibe (ZETIA) — a new oral drug for treating hyperlipidemias

Frovatriptan Succinate (FROVA) — a new tryptophan detivative indicated for use as an oral antimigraine drug

Nicotine (NICOTROL STEP 1, Step 2 and Step 3) — new stepwise trandermal nicotine preparations

Olmesartan Medoxomil (BENICAR) — a new angiotensin II receptor antagonist for use as an antihypertensive drug

Peginterferon alfa-2a (PEGASYS) — a new interferon for the treatment of chronic hepatitis C infection

Pimecrolimus (ELIDEL) — a new topical immunomodulator

Tenofovir Disoproxil Fumarate (VIREAD) — a nucleotide analogue reverse trandscriptase inhibitor antiviral drug used to treat HIV-1 infection

Valdecoxib (BEXTRA) — a new oral COX-2 inhibitor used as an antiinflammatory agent for treating arthritides and as an analgesic for the pain of primary dysmenorrhea

---

In addition to numerous preparation changes of OTC products, some of the new prescription combination products that have been added include:

ADDERALL 5 mg to 30 mg — new amphetamine / dextroamphetamine combinations for the treatment of narcolepsy

ADVICOR 500/20, 750/20 and 1000/20 — new niacin / lovastatin combinations for the treatment of hyperlipidemias

APRI — a new combination monophasic oral contraceptive preparation

AUGMENTIN XR — an extended-release form of this widely used antibacterial combination product

AVANDAMET — three combinations of rosiglitazone maleate (1, 2 and 4 mg) with 500 mg of metformin hydrochloride for treating patients with type II diabetes

EXCEDRIN QUICK TABS — quick-dissolving tablets of this aspirin-free analgesic has now come to the OTC market

NUVA-RING — a new intrauterine contraceptive in a vaginal ring form containing a new progesterone, etonogestrel

ORTHO EVRA — the first transdermal contraceptive to be marketed

ORTHO TRI-CYCLEN LO — a low-estrogenic form of the combination triphasic contraceptive, ORTHO TRI-CYCLIN

TUSSIZONE-12 RF — a new long-acting antihistamine-antitussive combination preparation with chlorheniramine tannate and carbetapentane tannate

---

This past year many drugs have received FDA approval for new indications and a few examples of these products which are now included in the text are:

Celecoxib (CELEBREX) — approved for use in the treatment of acute pain and primary dysmenorrhea

Gabapentin (NEURONTIN) — this antiepileptic drug been approved for use in the treatment of postherpetic neuralgia

Gatifloxacin Sesquihydrate (TEQUIN) — the indications for use of this drug have been expanded

Irbesartan (AVAPRO) — this angiotensin II receptor inhibitor is now indicated for treating nephropathy in type II diabetic patients

Paroxetine Hydrochloride (PAXIL) — the indications for this drug have been expanded to include treatment of post-traumatic stress disorder

Rofecoxib (VIOXX) — the indications for this COX-2 inhibitor now includes the treatment of rheumatoid arthritis

Tacrolimus (PROGRAF) — the indications for this immunosuppressant have been expanded to include use in kidney transplantation

Valacyclovir HCl (VALTREX) — expanded indications now include treatment of Herpes labialis infections

Valsartan (DIOVAN) — a new indication was added for the treament of heart failure

Zoledronic Acid (ZOMETA) — now indicated for use in multople myeloma and metastatic bone lesions from solid tumors

Examples of a few new dosage forms of existing drugs that were marketed in the United States this past year and that have been added to this edition include:

Brimonidine Tartrate (ALPHAGAN P) — a new ophthalmic dosage form

Budesonide, Micronized (ENTOCORT EC) — a corticosteroid now available as capsules

Fluticasone Propionate (FLOVENT DISKUS) — preparations have been added to this database

Lovastatin (ALTOCOR) — a new preparation of this antihyperlipidemic drug as extended-release tablets

Methylphenidate Hydrochloride (RITALIN LA) — new extended-release capsule preparations of this drug

Paroxetine Hydrochloride (PAXIL CR) — a controlled-release preparation of this drug for treatment of depression and panic disorder

Ziprasidone Mesylate (GEODON FOR INJECTION) — this antipsychotic is now available in an injectable form

This handbook has been published in order to provide medical personnel with a concise reference source for drug names, the preparations available, and common dosages in adults in a tabular format. Although the pocket size of the handbook has been exceptionally popular (with well over 1,000,000 copies in circulation of over the 18 years of publication), because of the ever-expanding number of drugs, preparations and indications it is getting large so that it becomes more difficult to fit it into a jacket or laboratory coat pocket and carried. Therefore, we have developed an even smaller version to be carried throughout the hospital, emergency room, and classroom. The original size still is perfect for the desk in your office.

We attempt to present the most common trade names, adult dosages and blood levels of drugs, and should be used only as a guideline to these. This handbook should not be considered as an official therapeutic document. If there is a discrepancy in therapeutic category; preparations; dosages; or therapeutic, toxic or lethal blood levels of any drug, the reader is advised to obtain official and more complete information from the pharmaceutical manufacturer.

As always, we are most grateful for your continued interest and support. Any comments that you have that will continue to improve the product is always welcome.

G. John DiGregorio, M.D., Ph.D.
Edward J. Barbieri, Ph.D.

TABLE OF CONTENTS

THERAPEUTIC CATEGORY LISTING[a]

a   This section lists, by Therapeutic Category, drugs found in the **SELECTED INDIVIDUAL DRUG PREPARATIONS** (pp. 29 to 220) and the **SELECTED COMBINATION DRUG PREPARATIONS** (pp. 221 to 267) sections only. Refer to the **INDEX** for a more complete listing of drugs.

Drug names in UPPER CASE represent TRADE NAMES; the TRADE NAMES without generic names preceeding them are COMBINATION PRODUCTS.

The symbol (*) prior to the generic name of a drug indicates that there is information on therapeutic, toxic and/or lethal blood concentrations of the drug in the **DRUG LEVELS** section (pp. 269 to 307).

2

3

4

5

7

9

10

11

12

13

17

18

26

Notes

SELECTED

INDIVIDUAL

DRUG

PREPARATIONS

C-II: Controlled Substance, Schedule II
C-III: Controlled Substance, Schedule III
C-IV: Controlled Substance, Schedule IV

(*):   indicates that there is information on therapeutic, toxic and/or lethal blood concentrations of the drug in the **DRUG LEVELS** section (pp. 269 to 306).

GENERIC NAME	COMMON TRADE NAMES	THERAPEUTIC CATEGORY	PREPARATIONS	COMMON ADULT DOSAGE
Abacavir Sulfate	ZIAGEN	Antiviral	**Oral Solution:** 20 mg/mL **Tab:** 300 mg	300 mg bid po in combination with other antiretroviral agents.
Acarbose	PRECOSE	Hypoglycemic Agent	**Tab:** 50, 100 mg	**Initial:** 25 mg tid po at the start (with the first bite) of each main meal. **Maintenance:** Adjust the dosage at 4 - 8 week intervals. The dosage may be increased to 50 mg tid po; in some the dosage may be raised to 100 mg tid po. Maximums: 50 mg tid for patients ≤ 60 kg; 100 mg tid for patients > 60 kg.
Acebutolol Hydrochloride (*)	SECTRAL	Antihypertensive, Antiarrhythmic	**Cpsl:** 200, 400 mg	**Hypertension:** Initially, 400 mg once daily po. An optimal response is usually achieved with 400 - 800 mg daily. **Ventricular Arrhythmias:** Initially, 200 mg bid po; increase dosage gradually until an optimal clinical response is obtained, generally at 600 - 1200 mg daily.
Acetaminophen (*)	ANACIN, ASPIRIN FREE	Non-Opioid Analgesic, Antipyretic	**Cplt, Tab & Gelcap:** 500 mg	1000 mg tid or qid po.
	PANADOL, MAXIMUM STRENGTH		**Cplt & Tab:** 500 mg	1000 mg q 4 h po.
	TYLENOL, REGULAR STRENGTH		**Cplt & Tab:** 325 mg	325 - 650 mg tid or qid po.
	TYLENOL, EXTRA-STRENGTH		**Cplt, Tab, Gelcap & Geltab:** 500 mg **Liquid:** 500 mg/15 mL (7% alcohol)	1000 mg tid or qid po. 30 mL (1000 mg) q 4 - 6 h po.
	TYLENOL SORE THROAT ADULT LIQUID		**Liquid:** 500 mg/15 mL	30 mL (1000 mg) q 4 - 6 h po.
	TYLENOL ARTHRITIS EXTENDED RELIEF		**Extended-Rel. Cplt:** 650 mg	1300 mg q 8 h po.

30

Generic	Brand	Class	Forms	Dosage
	FEVERALL, JUNIOR STRENGTH		Rectal Suppos: 325 mg	Insert 2 rectally q 4 - 6 h.
	ACETAMINOPHEN UNISERTS		Rectal Suppos: 650 mg	Insert 1 rectally q 4 - 6 h.
Acetazolamide (*)	DIAMOX	Diuretic, Antiepileptic, Anti-Glaucoma Agent	Tab: 250, 500 mg Inj: 500 mg	**Diuresis in CHF:** 250 - 375 mg once daily in the morning po or IV. Best results occur when given on alternate days, or for 2 days alternating with a day of rest. **Drug-induced Edema:** 250 - 375 mg once daily po or IV for 1 or 2 days. **Epilepsy:** 8 - 30 mg/kg/day in divided doses po (optimum range: 375 to 1000 mg daily). **Glaucoma:** 250 - 1000 mg per day usually in divided doses po.
	DIAMOX SEQUELS	Anti-Glaucoma Agent	Sustained-Rel. Cpsl: 500 mg	Glaucoma: 500 mg bid po.
Acetic Acid	VOSOL	Antibacterial (Topical), Antifungal (Topical)	Otic Solution: 2%	Carefully remove all cerumen and debris. Insert a wick saturated with the solution into the ear canal. Keep in for at least 24 h and keep moist by adding 3 - 5 drops of solution q 4 - 6 h.
Acetohexamide (*)	DYMELOR	Hypoglycemic Agent	Tab: 250, 500 mg	250 - 1500 mg once daily po.
Acetylcysteine Sodium	MUCOMYST, MUCOSIL	Mucolytic	Solution: 10, 20%	**Nebulization (tracheostomy, mask or mouth piece):** 3 - 5 mL (of 20% solution) or 6 - 10 mL (of 10% solution) tid to qid. **Direct Instillation:** 1 - 2 mL (of 10 or 20% solution) q 1 - 4 h.
Acetylsalicylic Acid [see Aspirin]				
Acitretin	SORIATANE	Anti-Psoriasis Agent	Cpsl: 10, 25 mg	25 - 50 mg once daily po with main meal. May cease when psoriatic lesions resolve.

GENERIC NAME	COMMON TRADE NAMES	THERAPEUTIC CATEGORY	PREPARATIONS	COMMON ADULT DOSAGE
Acyclovir (*)	ZOVIRAX	Antiviral	Cpsl: 200 mg Susp: 200 mg/5 mL Tab: 400, 800 mg	**Herpes simplex:** **Initial Genital Herpes:** 200 mg q 4 h (5 times daily) po for 10 days. **Chronic Suppressive Therapy for Recurrent Disease:** 400 mg bid po for up to 1 year. **Intermittent Therapy:** 200 mg q 4 h (5 times daily for 5 days. **Herpes zoster, Acute Treatment:** 800 mg q 4 h (5 times daily) po for 7 to 10 days. **Chickenpox:** 20 mg/kg (not to exceed 800 mg) qid po for 5 days.
		Antiviral (Topical)	Oint: 5%	Apply sufficient quantity to adequately cover all lesions q 3 h, 6 times daily for 7 days.
Acyclovir Sodium (*)	ZOVIRAX	Antiviral	Powd for Inj: 500, 1000 mg	**Mucosal and Cutaneous *Herpes simplex* Infections in Immunocompromised Patients:** 5 mg/kg infused IV at a constant rate over 1 h, q 8 h (15 mg/kg/day) for 7 days. **Herpes simplex Encephalitis:** 10 mg/kg infused IV at a constant rate over at least 1 h, q 8 h for 10 days. **Varicella zoster in Immunocompromised Patients:** 10 mg/kg infused IV at a constant rate over at 1 h, q 8 h for 7 days.
Adapalene	DIFFERIN	Anti-Acne Agent	Cream, Gel & Sol: 0.1%	After washing, apply a thin film once daily to the affected areas in the evening before bed.
Adefovir Dipivoxil	HEPSERA	Antiviral	Tab: 10 mg	**Chronic Hepatitis B:** 10 mg once daily po.
Adenosine	ADENOCARD	Antiarrhythmic	Inj: 3 mg/mL	Initial dose is 6 mg (rapid IV bolus given over a 1 - 2 second period). If the first dose does not stop the arrhythmia within 1 - 2 minutes, 12 mg should be given (by rapid IV bolus). The 12 mg dose may be repeated a second time if required.

Alatrofloxacin Mesylate [see Trovafloxacin Mesylate (TROVAN)]

Albendazole	ALBENZA	Anthelmintic	Tab: 200 mg	**Hydatid Disease:** Administer in a 28-day cycle followed by a 14-day albendazole-free interval, for a total of 3 cycles. **< 60 kg:** 15 mg/kg/day po in divided doses (bid) with meals (Maximum: 800 mg/day). **≥ 60 kg:** 400 mg bid po with meals. **Neurocysticercosis:** Administer for 8 - 30 days. **< 60 kg:** 15 mg/kg/day po in divided doses (bid) with meals (Maximum: 800 mg/day). **≥ 60 kg:** 400 mg bid po with meals.
Albuterol	PROVENTIL, VENTOLIN	Bronchodilator	Aerosol: 90 µg/spray	**Bronchospasm:** 2 inhalations q 4 - 6 h. **Prevention of Exercise-Induced Bronchospasm:** 2 inhalations 15 minutes prior to exercise.
Albuterol Sulfate (*)	PROVENTIL, VENTOLIN NEBULES	Bronchodilator	**Solution for Inhalation:** 0.083% (1 mg/mL, equal to 0.83 mg/mL of albuterol base)	2.5 mg tid - qid by nebulization. This solution requires no dilution prior to administration.
	PROVENTIL, VENTOLIN		**Solution for Inhalation:** 0.5% (6 mg/mL, equal to 5 mg/mL of albuterol base)	2.5 mg tid - qid by nebulization. Dilute 0.5 mL of the 0.5% solution with 2.5 mL of sterile normal saline before administration.
			Syrup: 2 mg (as the base)/5 mL **Tab:** 2, 4 mg (as the base)	2 - 4 mg tid or qid po. For those who do not respond to 2 mg qid, the dose may be cautiously increased stepwise, but not to exceed 8 mg qid as tolerated.
	VENTOLIN ROTACAPS		**Cpsl for Inhalation:** 200 µg	200 µg inhaled q 4 - 6 h using a Rotahaler inhalation device. In some, 400 µg inhaled q 4 - 6 h may be required.
	PROVENTIL REPETABS		**Extended-Rel. Tab:** 4 mg	4 - 8 mg q 12 h po.
	VOLMAX		**Extended-Rel. Tab:** 4, 8 mg	8 mg q 12 h po.

33

GENERIC NAME	COMMON TRADE NAMES	THERAPEUTIC CATEGORY	PREPARATIONS	COMMON ADULT DOSAGE
Alclometasone Dipropionate	ACLOVATE	Corticosteroid (Topical)	Cream & Oint: 0.05%	Apply a thin film to affected skin areas bid to tid; massage gently until the medication disappears.
Alendronate Sodium	FOSAMAX	Bone Stabilizer	Tab: 5, 10, 35, 70, 40 mg	Take at least 30 min. before the first food, beverage, or medication of the day. **Osteoporosis in Postmenopausal Women:** **Treatment:** 10 mg once daily po or 70 mg once weekly po. **Prevention:** 5 mg once daily po or 35 mg once weekly po. **Osteoporosis in Men:** 10 mg once daily po. **Glucocorticoid-Induced Osteoporosis:** 5 mg once daily po. For postmenopausal women not receiving estrogen - 10 mg once daily po. **Paget's Disease:** 40 mg once daily po for 6 months.
Alfentanil Hydrochloride (*) (C-II)	ALFENTA	Opioid Analgesic	Inj: 500 μg/mL	**Duration of Anesthesia:** **Under 30 min:** 8 - 20 μg/kg IV, followed by increments of 3 - 5 μg/kg IV q 5 - 20 minutes or 0.5 - 1 μg/kg/min IV. **30 - 60 min:** 20 - 50 μg/kg IV, followed by increments of 5 - 15 μg/kg IV q 5 - 20 minutes.
Alitretinoin	PANRETIN	Antineoplastic (Topical)	Gel: 0.1%	Initially, apply bid to Kaposi's Sarcoma cutaneous lesions. Application frequency can be gradually increased to tid or qid. Apply sufficient gel to cover lesion; allow the gel to dry for 3 - 5 min. before covering with clothing.
Allopurinol (*)	ZYLOPRIM	Antigout Agent	Tab: 100, 300 mg	**Mild Gout:** 200 - 300 mg daily po. **Moderately Severe Gout:** 400 - 600 mg daily po.

Generic	Brand	Class	Form	Dosage
Allopurinol Sodium	ALOPRIM	Antineoplastic Adjunct (Cytoprotective Agent)	Powd for Inj: 500 mg	200 - 400 mg/m²/day by IV infusion. Can be given as a single injection or in equally divided infusions at 6-, 8-, or 12-h intervals. Maximum: 600 mg/day.
Almotriptan Maleate	AXERT	Antimigraine Agent	Tab: 6.25, 12.5 mg	6.25 - 12.5 mg po. If the headache returns, the dose may be repeated after 2 h. Do not exceed 2 doses within 24 h.
Alprazolam (*) (C-IV)	XANAX	Antianxiety Agent	Tab: 0.25, 0.5, 1, 2 mg	0.25 - 0.5 mg tid po.
Alteplase, Recombinant	ACTIVASE	Thrombolytic	Powd for Inj: 50, 100 mg	**Acute Myocardial Infarction: 3-Hour Infusion:** 100 mg IV given as: 60 mg in the first hour (of which 6 - 10 mg is given as an IV bolus over the first 1 - 2 min), 20 mg over the second hour and 20 mg over the third hour. **Accelerated Infusion:** **> 67 kg:** 100 mg as a 15 mg IV bolus, followed by 50 mg infused over the next 30 min and then 35 mg infused over the next 60 min. **≤ 67 kg:** 15 mg IV bolus, followed by 0.75 mg/kg infused over the next 30 min not to exceed 50 mg and then 0.5 mg/kg over the next 60 min not to exceed 35 mg. **Acute Ischemic Stroke:** 0.9 mg/kg (maximum: 90 mg) IV (infused over 60 min) with 10% of the total dose administered as an IV bolus (over 1 min). **Pulmonary Embolism:** 100 mg by IV infusion over 2 hours.
Altretamine	HEXALEN	Antineoplastic	Cpsl: 50 mg	260 mg/m²/day po in 4 divided doses after meals and hs. Administer either for 14 or 21 consecutive days in a 28 day cycle.

GENERIC NAME	COMMON TRADE NAMES	THERAPEUTIC CATEGORY	PREPARATIONS	COMMON ADULT DOSAGE
Aluminum Hydroxide Gel	ALTERNAGEL	Antacid	Liquid: 600 mg/5 mL	5 - 10 mL po, prn, between meals & hs.
	ALU-CAP ALU-TAB		Cpsl: 475 mg Tab: 600 mg	3 capsules tid po. 3 tablets tid po.
Amantadine Hydrochloride (*)	SYMMETREL	Antiparkinsonian, Antiviral	Tab: 100 mg Syrup: 50 mg/5 mL	**Parkinsonism:** 100 mg bid po. **Influenza Virus:** 200 mg once daily po or 100 mg bid po.
Ambenonium Chloride	MYTELASE	Cholinomimetic	Tab: 10 mg	5 - 25 mg tid to qid po. Start with 5 mg and gradually increase dosage.
Amcinonide	CYCLOCORT	Corticosteroid (Topical)	Cream & Oint: 0.1% Lotion: 0.1%	Apply to affected areas bid to tid. Rub into affected areas bid.
Amikacin Sulfate (*)	AMIKIN	Antibacterial	Inj (per mL): 50, 250 mg	**Usual Dosage:** 15 mg/kg/day IM or by IV infusion (over 30 - 60 min) divided in 2 or 3 equal doses at equal intervals. **Uncomplicated UTI:** 250 mg bid IM or by IV infusion (over 30 - 60 min).
Amiloride Hydrochloride	MIDAMOR	Diuretic	Tab: 5 mg	5 mg once daily po with food. The dosage may be increased to 10 mg daily if needed.
Aminocaproic Acid (*)	AMICAR	Systemic Hemostatic	Syrup: 250 mg/mL Tab: 500 mg Inj: 250 mg/mL	5 g po during the first hour, followed by 1 to 1.25 g po per hour for about 8 h or until bleeding has been controlled. 4 - 5 g by IV infusion during the first hour, followed by a continuing infusion at the rate of 1 g/h in 50 mL of diluent for about 8 h or until bleeding has been controlled.
Aminosalicylic Acid (*)	PASER	Tuberculostatic	Delayed-Rel. Granules: 4 g per packet	4 g (1 packet) tid po. Sprinkle on applesauce or yogurt or swirl in a glass of tomato juice or orange juice to suspend the granules.

Amiodarone Hydrochloride (*)

CORDARONE

Antiarrhythmic

Tab: 200 mg

Loading Doses: 800 - 1600 mg/day po for 1 to 3 weeks (sometimes longer) until therapeutic response occurs. Administer in divided doses with meals if daily dose ≥ 1000 mg, or when gastrointestinal upset occurs. For life-threatening arrhythmias, administer loading doses in a hospital.
Dosage Adjustment and Daily Maintenance Dose: For approximately 1 month, 600 - 800 mg po; then 400 mg daily po.

CORDARONE INTRAVENOUS

Inj: 50 mg/mL

First 24 Hours:
Loading Infusions: 150 mg IV over the FIRST 10 minutes (15 mg/min) (concentration = 1.5 mg/mL), followed by 360 mg IV over the NEXT 6 hours (1 mg/min) (concentration = 1.8 mg/mL).
Maintenance Infusion: 540 mg IV over the REMAINING 18 hours (0.5 mg/min).
After the First 24 Hours: The maintenance infusion rate of 0.5 mg/min (720 mg/24 h) should be continued at a concentration of 1 - 6 mg/mL.

Amitriptyline Hydrochloride (*)

ELAVIL

Antidepressant

Tab: 10, 25, 50, 75, 100, 150 mg

Outpatients: Initially, 75 mg daily po in divided doses; may be increased to 150 mg daily po in divided doses if needed; increases are preferably made in the late afternoon or hs. Alternatively, begin with 50 to 100 mg po hs; may increase by 25 or 50 mg prn hs to a total dose of 150 mg per day. The usual maintenance dose is 50 - 100 mg daily po.
Hospitalized Patients: Initially, these patients may require up to 100 mg daily po; may be raised to 200 mg daily if necessary. Usual maintenance dose is 50 - 100 mg daily po.
Adolescent Patients: 10 mg tid po, with 20 mg hs, may be satisfactory.

[Continued on the next page]

37

GENERIC NAME	COMMON TRADE NAMES	THERAPEUTIC CATEGORY	PREPARATIONS	COMMON ADULT DOSAGE
Amitriptyline Hydrochloride [Continued]	ELAVIL		Inj: 10 mg/mL	Initially, 20 - 30 mg qid IM. Amitriptyline tablets should replace the injection as soon as possible.
Amlexanox	APHTHASOL	Antiinflammatory (Topical)	Oral Paste: 5%	**Aphthous Ulcers (Canker Sores):** Apply 1/4 inch to each ulcer qid (preferably following oral hygiene after breakfast, lunch, dinner, and at bedtime). Continue until ulcer heals.
Amlodipine Besylate (*)	NORVASC	Antihypertensive, Antianginal	Tab: 2.5, 5, 10 mg	**Hypertension:** 2.5 - 5 mg once daily po. **Angina:** 5 - 10 mg once daily po.
Amoxapine (*)	ASENDIN	Antidepressant	Tab: 25, 50, 100, 150 mg	Initially, 50 mg bid or tid po. Depending upon tolerance, dosage may be increased to 100 mg bid or tid po by the end of the first week. When an effective dosage is established, the drug may be given in a single dose (not to exceed 300 mg) hs.
Amoxicillin (*)	AMOXIL	Antibacterial	Cpsl: 250, 500 mg Tab: 500, 875 mg Chewable Tab: 125, 200, 250 mg Powd for Susp (per 5 mL): 125, 200, 250, 400 mg	**Infections of the Lower Respiratory Tract:** 500 mg q 8 h po or 875 mg q 12 h po. **Gonorrheal Infections, Acute Uncomplicated:** 3 g (+ 1 g of probenecid) as a single po dose. **Other Susceptible Infections:** **Mild to Moderate:** 250 mg q 8 h po or 500 mg q 12 h po. **Severe:** 500 mg q 8 h po or 875 mg q 12 h po.
	WYMOX		Cpsl: 250, 500 mg Powd for Susp (per 5 mL): 125, 250 mg	Same dosages as for AMOXIL above.
Amphotericin B (*)	FUNGIZONE	Antifungal (Topical)	Cream, Lotion & Oint: 3%	Apply topically bid - qid.
	FUNGIZONE ORAL SUSPENSION	Antifungal	Susp: 100 mg/mL	1 mL qid po. If possible, administer between meals.

Drug	Brand	Class	Supplied	Dosage
Amphotericin B Cholesteryl (*)	AMPHOTEC	Antifungal	Powd for Inj: 50, 100 mg	Initially, 3 - 4 mg/kg/day by slow IV infusion (rate 1 mg/kg/h) diluted in 5% Dextrose for Injection. A test dose immediately before the first dose is advisable when beginning all new courses of treatment.
Amphotericin B Desoxycholate (*)	FUNGIZONE INTRAVENOUS	Antifungal	Powd for Inj: 50 mg	Initially, 0.25 mg/kg/day by slow IV infusion (given over 6 h); dose may be increased gradually as tolerance permits. A 1 mg test dose (by slow IV infusion) is advisable to determine patient tolerance.
Amphotericin B Lipid Complex (*)	ABELCET	Antifungal	Powd for Inj: 100 mg	Aspergillosis: 5 mg/kg daily as a single IV infusion at 2.5 mg/kg/h.
Amphotericin B Liposomal (*)	AMBISOME	Antifungal	Powd for Inj: 50 mg	Empirical Therapy: Initially, 3.0 mg/kg/day by slow IV infusion (given over 2 h); the dose should be individualized as tolerance permits. Systemic Fungal Infections: Initially, 3.0 - 5.0 mg/kg/day by slow IV infusion (given over 2 h); the dose should be individualized as tolerance permits. Cryptococcal Meningitis in HIV Infections: 6 mg/kg/day using a controlled infusion device over 60 - 120 minutes.
Ampicillin Anhydrous (*)	OMNIPEN	Antibacterial	Cpsl: 250, 500 mg Powd for Susp (per 5 mL): 125, 250 mg	Respiratory Tract and Soft Tissue Infections: 250 mg q 6 h po. Genitourinary or Gastrointestinal Tract Infect. other than Gonorrhea: 500 mg q 6 h po. Gonorrhea: 3.5 g (plus 1.0 g of probenecid) as a single po dose.

GENERIC NAME	COMMON TRADE NAMES	THERAPEUTIC CATEGORY	PREPARATIONS	COMMON ADULT DOSAGE
Ampicillin Sodium (*)	OMNIPEN-N	Antibacterial	Powd for Inj: 125, 250, 500 mg; 1, 2 g	**Respiratory Tract and Soft Tissue Infections:** Under 40 kg: 25 - 50 mg/kg/day in equally divided doses at 6 - 8 h intervals IM or IV. Over 40 kg: 250 - 500 mg q 6 h IM or IV. **Genitourinary or Gastrointestinal Tract Infections including Gonorrhea in Females:** Under 40 kg: 50 mg/kg/day in equally divided doses at 6 - 8 h intervals IM or IV. Over 40 kg: 500 mg q 6 h IM or IV. **Urethritis in Males due to *N. gonorrhoeae*:** Two doses of 500 mg each IM or IV at an interval of 8 - 12 h. Repeat if necessary. **Bacterial Meningitis:** 150 - 200 mg/kg/day in equally divided doses q 3 - 4 h. Treatment may be initiated with IV drip and continued with IM injections. **Septicemia:** 150 - 200 mg/kg/day. Start with IV administration for at least 3 days and continue with IM injections q 3 - 4 h.
Ampicillin Trihydrate (*)	PRINCIPEN	Antibacterial	Cpsl: 250, 500 mg Powd for Susp (per 5 mL): 125, 250 mg	Same dosages as for OMNIPEN above.
Amprenavir	AGENERASE	Antiviral	Solution: 15 mg/mL Cpsl: 50, 150 mg	1200 mg (eight 150 mg cpsls) bid po in combination with other antiretroviral agents. Drug may be taken with or without food, but high-fat meals should be avoided.
Amrinone Lactate [renamed: see Inamrinone Lactate]				
Anastrozole	ARIMIDEX	Antineoplastic	Tab: 1 mg	**Breast Cancer:** 1 mg once daily po.
Anistreplase	EMINASE	Thrombolytic	Powd for Inj: 30 units	30 units IV (over 2 to 5 minutes).

Anthralin	ANTHRA-DERM DRITHOCREME	Anti-Psoriasis Agent (Topical)	**Oint:** 0.1, 0.25, 0.5, 1.0% **Cream:** 0.1, 0.25, 0.5, 1.0%	Begin with the 0.1% concentration and after at least 1 week gradually increase until the desired effect is obtained. Apply a thin layer to psoriatic areas once daily; rub in gently.
	DRITHO-SCALP		**Cream:** 0.25, 0.5%	Begin with the 0.25% concentration; apply to the psoriatic lesions only once daily and rub in well. After at least 1 week, may increase dosage with the 0.5% strength.
Aprotinin	TRASYLOL	Systemic Hemostatic	**Inj:** 10,000 KIU (Kallikrein Inhibitor Units)/mL (equivalent to 1.4 mg/mL)	Two dosage regimens (A and B) are suggested. Regimen A appears to be more effective in patients given aspirin preoperatively. The experience with Regimen B (reduced dosage) is limited (see table below).

Dosage Regimen	IV Test Dose (given at least 10 minutes before the loading dose is administered)	IV Loading Dose (given slowly over 20 - 30 minutes after induction of anesthesia but prior to sternotomy)	IV Pump Prime Dose	Constant IV Infusion Dose (continued until surgery is complete and patient leaves the operating room)
A	1 mL (10,000 KIU)	200 mL (2 million KIU)	200 mL (2 million KIU)	50 mL/h (500,000 KIU/h)
B	1 mL (10,000 KIU)	100 mL (1 million KIU)	100 mL (1 million KIU)	25 mL/h (250,000 KIU/h)

Asparaginase	ELSPAR	Antineoplastic	**Powd for Inj:** 10,000 IUnits	200 IU/kg/day IV (over a 30 minute period) for 28 days.
Aspirin (*)	BAYER CHILDREN'S ASPIRIN ASPIRIN REGIMEN BAYER	Non-Opioid Analgesic, Antipyretic, Antiinflammatory	**Chewable Tab:** 81 mg **Enteric Coated Tab:** 81 mg **Enteric Coated Cplt:** 325 mg	**Usual Dosage:** 325 - 650 mg q 4 h po, prn. **Analgesic or Antiinflammatory:** the OTC maximum dosage is 4000 per day po in divided doses.

[Continued on the next page]

41

GENERIC NAME	COMMON TRADE NAMES	THERAPEUTIC CATEGORY	PREPARATIONS	COMMON ADULT DOSAGE
Aspirin [Continued]	BAYER ASPIRIN BAYER ASPIRIN, EXTRA STRENGTH	Drug for Suspected Acute MI	Cplt, Gelcap & Tab: 325 mg Cplt, Gelcap & Tab: 500 mg	**Transient Ischemic Attacks in Men:** 1300 mg daily po in divided doses (650 mg bid or 325 mg qid). **Suspected Acute Myocardial Infarction:** 160 to 162.5 mg po, as soon as the infarct is suspected & then daily for at least 30 days.
	BAYER 8-HOUR ASPIRIN		Cplt: 650 mg	
	ST. JOSEPH ADULT CHEWABLE ASPIRIN		Chewable Cplt: 81 mg	
	ECOTRIN	Non-Opioid Analgesic, Antiinflammatory	Enteric Coated Tab: 81, 325, 500 mg	Same dosages as for ASPIRIN REGIMEN BAYER above.
	ECOTRIN, BAYER ASPIRIN EXTRA-STRENGTH ARTHRITIS PAIN FORMULA	Non-Opioid Analgesic, Antiinflammatory	Enteric Coated Cplt: 500 mg	Same dosages as for ASPIRIN REGIMEN BAYER above.
	EASPRIN	Non-Opioid Analgesic, Antiinflammatory	Enteric Coated Tab: 975 mg	1 tab tid to qid po.
	HALFPRIN	Drug for Suspected Acute MI	Tab: 162 mg	162 mg po, taken as soon as the first infarct is suspected & then daily for at least 30 days.
Atenolol (*)	TENORMIN	Antihypertensive, Antianginal, Post-MI Drug	Tab: 25, 50, 100 mg	**Hypertension & Angina:** Initially, 50 mg once daily po; dosage may be increased to 100 mg daily if necessary. **Acute Myocardial Infarction:** In patients who tolerate the full IV dose (10 mg), give 50 mg po 10 minutes after the last IV dose, followed by 50 mg po 12 h later. Thereafter, 100 mg daily po or 50 mg bid po for 6 - 9 days or until discharged from the hospital.
	TENORMIN I.V.	Post-MI Drug	Inj: 5 mg/10 mL	**Acute Myocardial Infarction:** 5 mg IV (over 5 to 10 minutes), followed by 5 mg IV 10 minutes later.

Generic	Brand	Class	Forms	Dosage
Atorvastatin Calcium	LIPITOR	Antihyperlipidemic	**Tab:** 10, 20, 40, 80 mg	**Heterozygous, Types IIa & IIb Hyperlipidemia:** Initially, 10 or 20 mg once daily po. If more than a 45% reduction in LDL cholesterol is needed, may start at 40 mg once daily po. The dosage range is 10 - 80 mg once daily. **Homozygous Familial Hypercholesterolemia:** 10 - 80 mg once daily po.
Atovaquone (*)	MEPRON	Antiprotozoal	**Susp:** 750 mg/5 mL	**Usual Dosage:** 750 mg bid po with food for 21 days. *Pneumocystis carinii* **Pneumonia Prophylaxis:** 1500 mg once daily po with food.
Atracurium Besylate (*)	TRACRIUM INJECTION	Neuromuscular Blocker	**Inj:** 10 mg/mL	0.4 - 0.5 mg/kg IV bolus when used alone; 0.25 - 0.35 mg/kg IV bolus when used under steady state with certain general anesthetics. Doses of 0.08 - 0.10 mg/kg for maintenance during prolonged surgery.
Atropine Sulfate (*)		Anticholinergic	**Tab:** 0.4, 0.6 mg **Inj:** 0.05 to 1.0 mg/mL	0.4 - 0.6 mg po. 0.4 - 0.6 mg IV, IM or SC.
	ISOPTO ATROPINE	Mydriatic - Cycloplegic	**Ophth Solution:** 0.5, 1% **Ophth Solution:** 2%	1 - 2 drops in eye(s) up to qid.
			Ophth Oint: 1%	Apply to eye(s) up to bid.
Attapulgite	DIASORB	Antidiarrheal	**Liquid:** 750 mg/5 mL **Tab:** 750 mg	20 mL or 4 tablets (3000 mg) po at the first sign of diarrhea, and repeat after each subsequent bowel movement. Maximum: 60 mL or 12 tablets per 24 hours.
	KAOPECTATE		**Liquid:** 750 mg/15 mL **Cpt:** 750 mg	30 mL or 2 caplets (1500 mg) po at the first sign of diarrhea and after each subsequent loose bowel movement. Maximum: 7 doses per 24 hours.
Auranofin (*)	RIDAURA	Antirheumatic	**Cpsl:** 3 mg	3 mg bid po or 6 mg daily po.

43

GENERIC NAME	COMMON TRADE NAMES	THERAPEUTIC CATEGORY	PREPARATIONS	COMMON ADULT DOSAGE
Aurothioglucose	SOLGANAL	Antiarthritic	Inj: 50 mg/mL	First dose: 10 mg IM; second and third doses: 25 mg IM; fourth and subsequent doses: 50 mg IM. The interval between doses is 1 week. The 50 mg dose is continued at weekly intervals until 0.8 - 1.0 g has been given. If the patient has improved and shows no sign of toxicity, the 50 mg dose may be continued for many months longer, at 3 - 4 week intervals.
Azathioprine	IMURAN	Immunosuppressant	Tab: 50 mg	
Azathioprine Sodium	IMURAN	Immunosuppressant	Powd for Inj: 100 mg	Renal Homotransplantation: Initial dose is usually 3 - 5 mg/kg daily po or IV, beginning at the time of transplant. Usually given as a single daily dose. Therapy is often initiated with the IV administration of the sodium salt and continued with the tablets after the postoperative period. Dose reduction to maintenance levels of 1 - 3 mg/kg is usually possible. Rheumatoid Arthritis: Initially, 1 mg/kg (50 to 100 mg) as a single daily dose or on a bid schedule. May increase dose at 6 - 8 weeks and thereafter by steps at 4-week intervals. Dose increments should be 0.5 mg/kg daily, up to a maximum dose of 2.5 mg/kg/day.
Azelaic Acid	AZELEX, FINEVIN	Anti-Acne Agent	Cream: 20%	Gently massage a thin film into affected areas bid, in the morning and evening.
Azelastine Hydrochloride	ASTELIN	Antihistamine	Nasal Spray: 137 μg/spray	2 sprays in each nostril bid.
	OPTIVAR	Antihistamine (Topical)	Ophth Solution: 0.5 mg/mL (0.05%)	Instill 1 drop into each affected eye bid.

Azithromycin Dihydrate (*)	ZITHROMAX	Antibacterial	Tab: 250, 500, 600 mg Powd for Susp (per 5 mL): 100, 200 mg Powd for Susp: 1 g packets	**Usual Dosage:** 500 mg po as a single dose on the first day followed by 250 mg once daily on days 2 through 5. Administer Suspension on an empty stomach; tablets may be taken with or without food. **Non-gonococcal Urethritis and Cervicitis due to C. trachomatis:** 1 g po as a single dose. Administer Suspension on an empty stomach; tablets may be taken with or without food. **Gonococcal Urethritis and Cervicitis due to N. gonorrhea:** 2 g po as a single dose. **Genital Ulcer Disease due to H. ducreyi (Chancroid):** 1 g po as a single dose. **Disseminated M. avium Complex (MAC):** **Prevention:** 1200 mg po once weekly. **Treatment:** 600 mg po once daily po in combination with ethambutol (15 mg/kg).
Aztreonam (*)	AZACTAM	Antibacterial	Powd for Inj: 0.5, 1, 2 g Inj (per 100 mL): 0.5, 1, 2 g	**Urinary Tract Infections:** 0.5 - 1.0 g q 8 or 12 h by IV infusion or IM. **Moderately Severe Systemic Infections:** 1 - 2 g q 8 or 12 h by IV infusion. **Severe Systemic or Life-Threatening Infections:** 2 g q 6 or 8 h by IV infusion.
Bacitracin		Antibacterial (Topical)	Ophth Oint: 500 units/g Oint: 500 units/g	Apply to affected eye(s) 1 or more times daily. Apply topically to the affected areas 1 - 3 times daily.
Baclofen (*)	LIORESAL	Skeletal Muscle Relaxant	Tab: 10, 20 mg	5 mg tid po for 3 days; increase by 5 mg tid every 3 days (maximum 80 mg daily (20 mg qid)) until optimum effect is achieved.
Balsalazide Disodium	COLAZAL	Bowel Antiinflammatory Agent	Cpsl: 750 mg	Three 750 mg cpsl tid po (total dose 6.75 g) for 8 weeks.

45

GENERIC NAME	COMMON TRADE NAMES	THERAPEUTIC CATEGORY	PREPARATIONS	COMMON ADULT DOSAGE
Barley Malt Extract	MALTSUPEX	Bulk Laxative	**Liquid:** 16 grams/15 mL	30 mL bid po for 3 or 4 days, or until relief is noted; then 15 - 30mL daily po hs for maintenance, prn. Take a full glass (8 fl. oz.) of liquid with each dose.
			Powder: 8 grams/scoop	Up to 4 scoops bid po for 3 or 4 days, or until relief is noted; then 2 - 4 scoops daily po hs for maintenance, prn. Take a full glass (8 fl. oz.) of liquid with each dose.
			Tab: 750 mg	Initially 4 tablets qid po with meals and hs. Adjust dosage according to response. Drink a full glass of liquid (8 fl. oz.) with each dose.
Beclomethasone Dipropionate	QVAR	Corticosteroid	**Aerosol:** 40, 80 μg/spray	2 inhalations bid.
	BECONASE, VANCENASE		**Nasal Aerosol:** 42 μg/spray	1 spray in each nostril bid - qid.
	BECONASE AQ, VANCENASE AQ		**Nasal Spray:** 0.042% (42 μg/spray)	1 or 2 inhalations in each nostril bid.
	VANCENASE AQ DOUBLE STRENGTH		**Nasal Spray:** 0.084% (84 μg/spray)	1 or 2 inhalations in each nostril once daily.
Benazepril Hydrochloride	LOTENSIN	Antihypertensive	**Tab:** 5, 10, 20, 40 mg	Initially, 10 mg once daily po. Maintenance dosage is 20 - 40 mg daily as a single dose or in two equally divided doses.
Bendroflumethiazide	NATURETIN	Diuretic, Antihypertensive	**Tab:** 5, 10 mg	**Diuresis:** 5 mg once daily po, preferably given in the morning. To initiate therapy, doses up to 20 mg may be given once daily or divided into two doses. For maintenance, 2.5 - 5 mg once daily should suffice. **Hypertension:** Initially, 5 - 20 mg daily po. Maintenance doses range from 2.5 - 15 mg daily.

Benzocaine	AMERICAINE	Local Anesthetic	Lubricant Gel: 20%	Apply evenly to exterior of tube or instrument prior to use.
			Spray: 20%	Apply liberally to affected areas not more than tid to qid.
	ANBESOL MAXIMUM STRENGTH		Liquid & Gel: 20%	Apply topically to the affected area on or around the lips, or within the mouth.
Benzonatate (*)	TESSALON	Antitussive	Cpsl: 100, 200 mg	100 - 200 mg tid po. Swallow whole; do not suck or chew.
Benzoyl Peroxide	BREVOXYL-4 BREVOXYL-8	Anti-Acne Agent	Gel: 4% Gel: 8%	Cleanse affected area. Apply topically once or twice daily.
	BENZAC, BENZAGEL, PANOXYL BENZAC W, PANOXYL AQ		Gel: 5, 10% Water Base Gel: 2.5, 5, 10%	Cleanse affected area. Apply topically once or twice daily. Cleanse affected area. Apply topically once or twice daily.
	BENZAC W WASH		Liquid: 5, 10%	Wash face with product once or twice daily.
	DESQUAM-X		Gel: 5, 10% Water Base Gel: 5, 10%	Cleanse affected areas. Rub gently into all affected areas once or twice daily. Wash affected areas with product once or twice daily. Rinse well.
	PANOXYL		Bar: 5, 10%	Wash entire area with fingertips for 1 or 2 minutes bid to tid. Rinse well.
Benzphetamine Hydrochloride (*) (C-III)	DIDREX	Anorexiant	Tab: 50 mg	Initially, 25 - 50 mg once daily po with subsequent increase to tid according to the response. A single daily dose is preferably given in mid-morning or mid-afternoon.

GENERIC NAME	COMMON TRADE NAMES	THERAPEUTIC CATEGORY	PREPARATIONS	COMMON ADULT DOSAGE
Benzthiazide	EXNA	Diuretic, Antihypertensive	**Tab:** 50 mg	**Diuresis:** Initially, 50 - 200 mg daily po for several days, or until dry weight is attained. With 100 mg or more daily, it is preferable to administer in two doses following AM & PM meals. For maintenance, 50 - 150 mg daily po depending on patient's response. **Hypertension:** Initially, 50 - 100 mg daily po as a single dose or in two divided doses. For maintenance, adjust according to the patient's response. Max: 50 mg qid po.
Benztropine Mesylate (*)	COGENTIN	Antiparkinsonian	**Tab:** 0.5, 1, 2 mg **Inj:** 1 mg/mL	0.5 - 2 mg daily or bid po. 0.5 - 2 mg daily or bid IM.
Bepridil Hydrochloride (*)	VASCOR	Antianginal	**Tab:** 200, 300 mg	200 mg once daily po. After 10 days, the dosage may be raised; most patients are maintained at 300 mg daily.
Betamethasone Dipropionate, Regular	DIPROSONE, MAXIVATE	Corticosteroid (Topical)	**Cream & Oint:** 0.05% (in a standard vehicle)	Apply a thin film to affected areas once or twice daily.
			Lotion: 0.05%	Massage a few drops into affected areas bid.
	DIPROSONE		**Topical Aerosol:** 0.1%	Apply sparingly to affected skin areas tid.
Betamethasone Dipropionate, Augmented	DIPROLENE	Corticosteroid (Topical)	**Gel & Oint:** 0.05% (in an optimized vehicle) **Lotion:** 0.05%	Apply a thin film to affected areas once or twice daily. Massage a few drops into affected areas once or twice daily.
	DIPROLENE AF		**Cream:** 0.05%	Apply a thin film to affected areas once or twice daily.

Betamethasone Valerate	VALISONE	Corticosteroid (Topical)	Cream: 0.1% Lotion & Oint: 0.1%	Apply topically 1 - 3 times daily. Apply topically 1 - 3 times daily.
	VALISONE REDUCED STRENGTH		Cream: 0.01%	Apply a thin film to affected areas 1 - 3 times daily.
	LUXIQ		Foam: 0.12%	Invert can and dispense a small amount of foam onto a clean saucer or other cool surface. Pick up a small amount of foam and massage into affected scalp areas until foam disappears; repeat until the entire affected area of scalp is treated. Use bid (AM and PM) for up to 2 weeks.
Betaxolol Hydrochloride (*)	BETOPTIC BETOPTIC S	Anti-Glaucoma Agent	Ophth Solution: 0.5% Ophth Suspension: 0.25%	1 - 2 drops into affected eye(s) bid. 1 - 2 drops into affected eye(s) bid.
	KERLONE	Antihypertensive	Tab: 10, 20 mg	10 mg once daily po. If the desired response is not achieved, the dose can be doubled in 7 to 14 days.
Bethanechol Chloride	URECHOLINE	Cholinomimetic	Tab: 5, 10, 25, 50 mg Inj: 5 mg/mL	10 - 50 mg tid or qid po. 2.5 - 5 mg tid or qid SC.
	DUVOID		Tab: 10, 25, 50 mg	10 - 50 mg tid or qid po.
Bicalutamide	CASODEX	Antineoplastic	Tab: 50 mg	50 mg once daily po (morning or evening) in combination with an LHRH analog.
Bimatoprost	LUMIGAN	Anti-Glaucoma Agent	Ophth Solution: 0.03%	1 drop into the affected eye(s) once daily in the evening.
Biperiden Hydrochloride (*)	AKINETON	Antiparkinsonian	Tab: 2 mg	2 mg tid - qid po.
Biperiden Lactate (*)	AKINETON	Antiparkinsonian	Inj: 5 mg/mL	2 mg 30 minutes IM or IV until symptoms resolve, not to exceed 4 doses in 24 hours.

49

GENERIC NAME	COMMON TRADE NAMES	THERAPEUTIC CATEGORY	PREPARATIONS	COMMON ADULT DOSAGE
Bisacodyl	CORRECTOL	Irritant Laxative	Enteric-Coated Tab & Cplt: 5 mg	5 - 15 mg po once daily.
	DULCOLAX		Enteric-Coated Tab: 5 mg Rectal Suppos: 10 mg	10 - 15 mg po once daily. Insert 1 rectally once daily.
	FLEET BISACODYL ENEMA		Rectal Susp: 10 mg/30 mL	Administer 30 mL rectally.
Bismuth Subsalicylate	PEPTO-BISMOL	Antidiarrheal	Chewable Tab: 262 mg Cplt: 262 mg Liquid: 262 mg/15 mL	2 tablets or caplets (or 30 mL of Liquid) po; repeat every 30 - 60 minutes prn, to a maximum of 8 doses in a 24 hour period.
	PEPTO-BISMOL MAXIMUM STRENGTH		Liquid: 525 mg/15 mL	30 mL po; repeat every 60 minutes prn, to a maximum of 4 doses in a 24 hour period.
Bisoprolol Fumarate	ZEBETA	Antihypertensive	Tab: 5, 10 mg	Initially 5 mg once daily po. The dose may be increased to 10 mg once daily and then to 20 mg once daily, if necessary.
Bitolterol Mesylate	TORNALATE	Bronchodilator	Solution for Inhalation: 0.2% (2.0 mg/mL)	Intermittent Aerosol Flow Nebulizer (Patient Activated Nebulizer): 0.25 to 0.75 mL (0.5 to 1.5 mg) over 10 - 15 minutes tid. Continuous Aerosol Flow Nebulizer: 0.75 to 1.75 mL (1.5 to 3.5 mg) over 10 - 15 minutes tid.
Bleomycin Sulfate	BLENOXANE	Antineoplastic	Powd for Inj: 15, 30 units	0.25 - 0.50 units/kg (10 - 20 units/m^2) IV, IM or SC once or twice weekly.

Drug	Category	Form	Dosage
Bretylium Tosylate (*)	Antiarrhythmic	Inj: 50 mg/mL	**Life-Threatening Ventricular Arrhythmias:** Administer undiluted at 5 mg/kg by rapid IV. If the arrhythmia persists, the dosage may be increased to 10 mg/kg and repeated as necessary. **Other Ventricular Arrhythmias:** **IV:** Administer a diluted solution at 5 - 10 mg/kg by IV infusion over a period greater than 8 minutes. For maintenance, the same dosage may be administered q 6 h. **IM:** Administer undiluted at 5 - 10 mg/kg. Subsequent doses may be given at 1 - 2 hour intervals if the arrhythmia persists.
Brimonidine Tartrate	Anti-Glaucoma Agent	Ophth Solution: 0.2%	1 drop into the affected eye(s) tid, approximately 8 h apart.
		Ophth Solution: 0.15%	1 drop into the affected eye(s) tid, approximately 8 h apart.
Brinzolamide	Anti-Glaucoma Agent	Ophth Suspension: 1%	1 drop into the affected eye(s) tid.
Bromocriptine Mesylate	Antiparkinsonian	Tab: 2.5 mg Cpsl: 5 mg	Initially, 1.25 mg bid po with meals. If necessary, the dosage may be increased every 14 - 28 days by 2.5 mg per day.
Brompheniramine Tannate	Antihistamine	Susp: 12 mg/5 mL	12 - 24 mg q 12 h po.
BROVEX			
BROVEX CT		Chewable Tab: 12 mg	Chew 1 - 2 tabs (12 - 24 mg) q 12 h po.
Budesonide	Corticosteroid (Topical)	Aerosol: 32 µg/spray	256 µg daily, given as either 2 sprays in each nostril in the morning and evening or 4 sprays in each nostril in the morning.
RHINOCORT			
RHINOCORT AQUA		Nasal Spray: 32 µg/spray	Initially, 1 spray in each nostril (64 µg) once daily. May increase to 2 sprays (128 µg) or 4 sprays (256 µg) in each nostril once daily.
PULMICORT TURBUHALER		Aerosol: 200 µg/spray	200 - 400 µg bid by oral inhalation.

GENERIC NAME	COMMON TRADE NAMES	THERAPEUTIC CATEGORY	PREPARATIONS	COMMON ADULT DOSAGE
Budesonide, Micronized	ENTOCORT EC	Corticosteroid	Cpsl: 3 mg	Swallow 9 mg po once daily in the AM for up to 8 weeks. Do not chew or break capsule.
Bumetanide	BUMEX	Diuretic	Tab: 0.5, 1, 2 mg	0.5 - 2 mg daily po.
Buprenorphine Hydrochloride (*) (C-V)	BUPRENEX	Opioid Analgesic	Inj: 0.3 mg/mL	0.3 mg by deep IM or slow IV (over at least 2 minutes) at up to 6-hour intervals. Repeat once, if required, in 30 - 60 minutes.
Bupropion Hydrochloride (*)	WELLBUTRIN	Antidepressant	Tab: 75, 100 mg	100 mg bid po. Dosage may be increased to 100 mg tid po no sooner than 3 days after beginning therapy.
	WELLBUTRIN SR	Antidepressant	Sustained-Rel. Tab: 100, 150, 200 mg	Initially, 150 mg daily po in the AM. Dosage may be increased to 150 mg bid po (at least 8 h apart) as early as 4 days after beginning therapy.
	ZYBAN	Smoking Deterrent	Sustained-Rel. Tab: 150 mg	Initially, 150 daily po for the first 3 days, followed by 300 mg/day po in divided doses given at least 8 h apart. Continue treatment for 7 - 12 weeks.
Buspirone Hydrochloride (*)	BUSPAR	Antianxiety Agent	Tab: 5, 10, 15 mg	7.5 mg bid po. Dosage may be increased 5 mg daily at 2 to 3 day intervals. Maximum: 60 mg per day.
Busulfan	MYLERAN	Antineoplastic	Tab: 2 mg	Daily dosage range is 4 - 8 mg po. Dosing on a weight basis is approximately 60 μg/kg daily or 1.8 mg/m^2 daily.
Butabarbital Sodium (C-III)	BUTISOL SODIUM	Sedative / Hypnotic	Elixir: 30 mg/5 mL (7% alcohol) Tab: 15, 30, 50, 100 mg	Preoperative Sedation: 50 - 100 mg po, 60 to 90 minutes before surgery. Daytime Sedation: 15 - 30 mg tid to qid po. Bedtime Hypnosis: 50 - 100 mg hs po.
Butamben Picrate	BUTESIN PICRATE	Local Anesthetic	Oint: 1%	Spread thinly on painful or denuded lesions of the skin, if these are small. Apply a loose bandage to protect the clothing.

Butenafine Hydrochloride	LOTRIMIN ULTRA, MENTAX	Antifungal	Cream: 1%	Apply to cover the affected area and the immediately surrounding skin once daily for 2 - 4 weeks.
Butoconazole Nitrate	MYCELEX-3	Antifungal	Vaginal Cream: 2%	1 applicatorful intravaginally hs for 3 days. Treatment can be extended for another 3 days if necessary.
Butorphanol Tartrate (*) (C-IV)	STADOL	Opioid Analgesic	Inj (per mL): 1, 2 mg	IM: 2 mg. May be repeated q 3 - 4 h prn. IV: 1 mg. May be repeated q 3 - 4 h prn.
	STADOL NS		Nasal Spray: 10 mg/mL	1 spray in one nostril. If pain is not relieved in 60 - 90 minutes, an additional 1 spray may be given. The initial 2 dose sequence may be repeated in 3 - 4 h prn.
Caffeine (*)	NO DOZ MAXIMUM STRENGTH	CNS Stimulant	Tab: 200 mg	100 - 200 mg q 3 - 4 h po prn.
Calcifediol	CALDEROL	Vitamin D Analog	Cpsl: 20, 50 μg	300 - 350 μg weekly po, administered on a daily or alternate-day schedule. Most patients respond to doses of 50 - 100 μg daily or 100 - 200 μg on alternate days.
Calcipotriene	DOVONEX	Anti-Psoriasis Agent (Topical)	Cream: 0.005% Oint: 0.005% Scalp Solution: 0.005%	Apply a thin layer to the affected skin bid and rub in gently and completely. Apply a thin layer to the affected skin once or twice daily and rub in gently and completely. Apply only to scalp lesions and rub in gently and completely, taking care to prevent the solution spreading onto the forehead.
Calcitonin-Salmon	CALCIMAR, MIACALCIN	Antiosteoporotic, Hypocalcemic	Inj: 200 IUnits/mL	**Paget's Disease:** 100 IU daily SC or IM. In many patients, 50 IU daily or every other day SC or IM is satisfactory. **Hypercalcemia:** Initially, 4 IU/kg q 12 h SC or IM. After 1 or 2 days the dosage may be increased to 8 IU/kg q 12 h SC or IM. **Postmenopausal Osteoporosis:** 100 IU daily SC or IM with calcium supplementation.

GENERIC NAME	COMMON TRADE NAMES	THERAPEUTIC CATEGORY	PREPARATIONS	COMMON ADULT DOSAGE
Calcitriol (*)	ROCALTROL	Vitamin D Analog	Cpsl: 0.25, 0.5 µg Solution: 1.0 µg/mL	**Dialysis Patients:** 0.25 µg daily po. Dosage may be increased by 0.25 µg per day at 4 to 8 week intervals. Most patients respond to doses between 0.5 and 1 µg daily. **Predialysis Patients:** 0.25 µg daily po. Dosage may be increased to 0.5 µg daily if needed. **Hypoparathyroidism:** 0.25 µg daily po given in the AM. The dosage may be increased at 2 to 4 week intervals. Most patients respond to doses between 0.5 and 2 µg daily.
Calcium Carbonate (*)	CALTRATE 600	Calcium Supplement	**Tab:** 1500 mg (600 mg as elemental calcium)	1 or 2 tab daily po.
	OS-CAL 500	Calcium Supplement	**Chewable Tab:** 1250 mg (500 mg as elemental calcium)	1250 mg bid or tid po with meals.
	TUMS	Calcium Supplement, Antacid	**Chewable Tab:** 500 mg (200 mg as elemental calcium)	**Calcium Supplement:** Chew 2 tablets bid. **Antacid:** Chew 2 - 4 tablets q h prn. Do not take more than 16 tablets in 24 h.
	TUMS E-X		**Chewable Tab:** 750 mg (300 mg as elemental calcium)	**Calcium Supplement:** Chew 2 tablets bid. **Antacid:** Chew 2 - 4 tablets q h prn. Do not take more than 10 tablets in 24 h.
	TUMS ULTRA		**Chewable Tab:** 1000 mg (400 mg as elemental calcium)	**Calcium Supplement:** Chew 2 tablets bid. **Antacid:** Chew 2 - 3 tablets q h prn. Do not take more than 8 tablets in 24 h.
	TITRALAC TITRALAC EXTRA STRENGTH	Antacid	**Chewable Tab:** 420 mg **Cheable Tab:** 750 mg	Chew 2 tab q 2 - 3 h. Chew 1 - 2 tab q 2 - 3 h.
	ROLAIDS, CALCIUM RICH/ SODIUM FREE	Antacid	**Chewable Tab:** 550 mg	Chew 1 or 2 tab prn, up to a maximum of 14 tab per day.

Generic	Brand	Category	Form/Strength	Directions
	MYLANTA SOOTHING LOZENGES	Antacid	Lozenges: 600 mg	Allow 1 lozenge to dissolve in the mouth. If necessary, follow with a second. Repeat prn, up to 12 lozenges per day.
	ALKA-MINTS	Antacid	Chewable Tab: 850 mg	Chew 1 or 2 tablets q 2 h.
	MAALOX CAPLETS	Antacid	Cplt: 1000 mg	1000 mg po prn. Do not take more than 8 caplets in 24 h.
Calcium Polycarbophil	MITROLAN	Bulk Laxative	Chewable Tab: 625 mg	Chew and swallow 2 tablets qid or prn. A full glass of liquid (8 oz.) should be taken with each dose.
	FIBERCON		Tab: 625 mg	Swallow 2 tablets up to qid. A full glass of liquid (8 oz.) should be taken with each dose.
Candesartan Cilexetil	ATACAND	Antihypertensive	Tab: 4, 8, 16, 32 mg	Initially, 16 mg once daily po. May be given once daily or bid po with total doses ranging from 8 to 32 mg.
Capecitabine	XELODA	Antineoplastic	Tab: 150, 500 mg	2500 mg/m² daily po with food for 2 weeks, followed by a 1-week rest period given as 3 week cycles. Give the drug in 2 daily doses (approx. 12 h apart) at the end of a meal.
Capreomycin Sulfate	CAPASTAT SULFATE	Tuberculostatic	Powd for Inj: 1 g	1 g daily (not to exceed 20 mg/kg/day) IM or IV for 60 - 120 days, followed by 1 g IM or IV 2 or 3 times weekly.
Capsaicin	ZOSTRIX	Analgesic (Topical)	Cream: 0.025%	Apply to affected area tid or qid.
	ZOSTRIX-HP		Cream: 0.075%	Apply to affected area tid or qid.
	DOLORAC		Cream: 0.25%	Apply a thin film to the affected area bid.

GENERIC NAME	COMMON TRADE NAMES	THERAPEUTIC CATEGORY	PREPARATIONS	COMMON ADULT DOSAGE
Captopril (*)	CAPOTEN	Antihypertensive, Heart Failure Drug, Post-MI Drug	**Tab:** 12.5, 25, 50, 100 mg	**Hypertension:** Initially, 25 mg bid or tid po. Dosage may be increased after 1 - 2 weeks to 50 mg bid or tid. **Heart Failure:** Initially, 25 mg tid po. After a dose of 50 mg tid is reached, further increases in dosage should be delayed for at least 2 weeks. Most patients have a satisfactory response at 50 or 100 mg tid. **Diabetic Nephropathy:** 25 mg tid po. **Left Ventricular Dysfunction after an MI:** Initiate therapy as early as 3 days following an MI. After a single 6.25 mg po dose, give 12.5 mg tid, then increase to 25 mg tid during the next several days and to a target of 50 mg tid over the next several weeks.
Carbachol	ISOPTO CARBACHOL	Anti-Glaucoma Agent	**Ophth Solution:** 0.75, 1.5, 2.25, 3%	1 - 2 drops into eye(s) up to tid.
Carbamazepine (*)	TEGRETOL	Antiepileptic	**Susp:** 100 mg/5 mL **Chewable Tab:** 100 mg **Tab:** 200 mg	**Initial:** 100 mg qid po (Susp) or 200 mg bid po (Tabs or XR Tabs). Increase at weekly intervals by adding up to 200 mg per day using a tid or qid regimen (Susp or Tabs) or a bid regimen (XR Tabs). **Maximum:** 1000 mg daily (ages 12 to 15); 1200 mg daily (ages over 15). **Maintenance:** Adjust to minimum effective levels; usually 800 - 1200 mg daily po.
	TEGRETOL-XR		**Extended-Rel. Tab:** 100, 200, 400 mg	
Carbamide Peroxide	GLY-OXIDE	Antiseptic	**Liquid:** 10%	Apply several drops onto the affected mouth area; spit out after 2 minutes. Use up to qid pc & hs.

56

Carbenicillin Indanyl Sodium	GEOCILLIN	Antibacterial	Tab: 382 mg	**Urinary Tract Infections:** *E. coli, Proteus species,* and *Enterobacter*: 382 - 764 mg qid po. *Pseudomonas and Enterococcus*: 764 mg qid po. **Prostatitis:** 764 mg qid po.
Carboplatin (*)	PARAPLATIN	Antineoplastic	Powd for Inj: 50, 150, 450 mg	360 mg/m^2 on day 1 every 4 weeks IV. Single intermittent doses should not be repeated until the neutrophil count is at least 2,000 and the platelet count is at least 100,000.
Carisoprodol (*)	SOMA	Skeletal Muscle Relaxant	Tab: 350 mg	350 mg tid and hs po.
Carmustine	BiCNU	Antineoplastic	Powd for Inj: 100 mg	150 - 200 mg/m^2 IV q 6 weeks (given as a single dose or divided into daily injections on 2 successive days). A repeat course of drug should not be given until the leukocyte count is above 4,000/mm^3 and platelet count is above 100,000/mm^3.
Carteolol Hydrochloride	CARTROL	Antihypertensive	Tab: 2.5, 5 mg	Initially, 2.5 mg once daily po. Dosage may be gradually raised to 5 mg and 10 mg daily po.
	OCUPRESS	Anti-Glaucoma Agent	Ophth Solution: 1%	1 drop into affected eye(s) bid.
Carvedilol	COREG	Antihypertensive, Heart Failure Drug	Tab: 3.125, 6.25, 12.5, 25 mg	**Hypertension:** Initially, 6.25 mg bid po. After 7 - 14 days, the dosage may be increased to 12.5 mg bid po. After another 7 - 14 days, the dosage can be increased to 25 mg bid, if tolerated and required. **Congestive Heart Failure (in Conjunction with Digitalis, Diuretics, and ACE Inhibitors):** Initially 3.125 mg bid po for 2 weeks. If tolerated, the dosage may be increased to 6.25, 12.5, and 25 mg bid po oversuccessive intervals of at least 2 weeks to the highest level tolerated. The max. dosage is 25 mg bid for patients weighing < 85 kg (187 lb) and 50 mg bid for patients weighing > 85 kg.

GENERIC NAME	COMMON TRADE NAMES	THERAPEUTIC CATEGORY	PREPARATIONS	COMMON ADULT DOSAGE
Cascara Sagrada		Irritant Laxative	Tab: 325 mg	325 mg po hs.
Castor Oil (Plain)		Irritant Laxative	Liquid: (pure)	15 - 30 mL po.
Castor Oil, Emulsified	NEOLOID	Irritant Laxative	Liquid: 36.4% w/w	30 - 60 mL po.
	FLEET FLAVORED CASTOR OIL EMULSION		Liquid: 67% v/v (10 mL of castor oil/15 mL)	**Laxative:** 45 mL po. **Purgative:** 90 mL po.
Cefaclor (*)	CECLOR	Antibacterial	Powd for Susp (per 5 mL): 125, 187, 250, 375 mg Cpsl: 250, 500 mg	**Usual Dosage:** 250 mg q 8 h po. For more severe infections or those caused by less susceptible organisms, the dosage may be doubled. **Secondary Bacterial Infections of Acute Bronchitis or Acute Bacterial Exacerabations of Chronic Bronchitis:** 500 mg q 12 h po for 7 days. **Pharyngitis or Tonsillitis:** 375 mg q 12 h po for 10 days. **Skin and Skin Structure Infections, Uncompl.:** 375 mg q 12 h po for 7 to 10 days.
	CECLOR CD		Extended-Rel. Tab: 375, 500 mg	375 - 500 mg q 12 h po for 7 - 10 days.
Cefadroxil Monohydrate (*)	DURICEF	Antibacterial	Powd for Susp (per 5 mL): 125, 250, 500 mg Cpsl: 500 mg Tab: 1 g	**Urinary Tract Infections:** **Lower, Uncomplicated:** 1 - 2 g daily po in single or divided doses (bid). **Other:** 2 g daily po in divided doses (bid). **Skin and Skin Structure Infections:** 1 g daily po in single or divided doses (bid). **Pharyngitis and Tonsillitis:** 1 g daily po in single or divided doses (bid) for 10 days.

Drug	Trade Name	Category	Dosage Form	Indications / Dosing
Cefazolin Sodium (*)	ANCEF, KEFZOL	Antibacterial	Powd for Inj: 500 mg, 1 g	**Moderate to Severe Infections:** 500 mg - 1 g q 6 - 8 h IM or IV. **Mild Infections caused by susceptible Gram Positive Cocci:** 250 - 500 mg q 8 h IM or IV. **Urinary Tract Infect., Acute, Uncomplicated:** 1 g q 12 h IM or IV. **Pneumococcal Pneumonia:** 500 mg q 12 h IM or IV. **Severe, Life-Threatening Infections (e.g., Septicemia):** 1 - 1.5 g q 6 h IM or IV.
Cefdinir (*)	OMNICEF	Antibacterial	Cpsl: 300 mg	**Community-Acquired Pneumonia and Skin and Skin Structure Infections, Uncomplicated:** 300 mg q 12 h po for 10 days. **Acute Exacerbations of Chronic Bronchitis & Acute Maxillary Sinusitis:** 300 mg q 12 h po or 600 mg q 24 h po for 10 days. **Pharyngitis / Tonsillitis:** 300 mg q 12 h po for 5 - 10 days or 600 mg q 24 h po for 10 days.
Cefditoren Pivoxil	SPECTRACEF	Antibacterial	Tab: 200 mg (base)	**Acute Bacterial Exacerbation of Chronic Bronchitis:** 400 mg bid po for 10 days. **Pharyngitis/Tonsillitis and Skin & Skin Structure Infections (Uncomplicated):** 200 mg bid po for 10 days.
Cefepime Hydrochloride (*)	MAXIPIME	Antibacterial	Powd for Inj: 0.5, 1, 2 g	**Urinary Tract Infections: Mild to Moderate:** 0.5 - 1 g IM or IV (over 30 min.) q 12 h for 7 - 10 days. **Severe:** 2 g IV (over 30 min.) q 12 h for 10 days. **Pneumonia:** 1 - 2 g IV (over 30 min.) q 12 h for 10 days. **Skin & Skin Structure Infections:** 2 g IV (over 30 min.) q 12 h for 10 days. **Empiric Therapy for Febrile Neutropenic Patients:** 2 g IV (over 30 min.) q 8 h for 7 days or until resolution of neutropenia.

GENERIC NAME	COMMON TRADE NAMES	THERAPEUTIC CATEGORY	PREPARATIONS	COMMON ADULT DOSAGE
Cefixime (*)	SUPRAX	Antibacterial	Tab: 200, 400 mg Powd for Susp: 100 mg/5 mL	**Usual Dosage:** 400 mg once daily or 200 mg q 12 h po. **Gonorrhea, Uncomplicated:** 400 mg once daily po.
Cefonicid Sodium (*)	MONOCID	Antibacterial	Powd for Inj: 0.5, 1 g	**Usual Dosage:** 1 g daily IV or deep IM. **Urinary Tract Infections:** 0.5 g q 24 h IV or deep IM. **Mild to Moderate Infections:** 1 g q 24 h IV or deep IM. **Severe or Life-Threatening Infections:** 2 g q 24 h IV or deep IM in different large muscle masses. **Surgical Prophylaxis:** 1 g per day IV or deep IM preoperatively.
Cefoperazone Sodium (*)	CEFOBID	Antibacterial	Powd for Inj: 1, 2 g	2 - 4 g daily in equally divided doses q 12 h IM or IV. In severe infections or infections caused by less susceptible organisms, the daily dosage may be increased.
Cefotaxime Sodium (*)	CLAFORAN	Antibacterial	Powd for Inj: 0.5, 1, 2 g Inj (per 50 mL): 1, 2 g	**Gonococcal Urethritis & Cervicitis (Males and Females:** 500 mg IM as a single dose. **Gonorrhea, Rectal:** **Females:** 500 mg IM as a single dose. **Males:** 1 g IM as a single dose. **Uncomplicated Infections:** 1 g q 12 h IM or IV. **Moderate to Severe Infections:** 1 - 2 g q 8 h IM or IV. **Infections Commonly Needing Antibiotics in Higher Dosage (e.g., Septicemia:** 2 g q 6 - 8 h IV. **Life-Threatening Infections:** 2 g q 4 h IV.

Cefotetan Disodium (*)	CEFOTAN	Antibacterial	**Powd for Inj:** 1, 2 g **Inj (per 50 mL):** 1, 2 g	**Urinary Tract Infections:** 500 mg q 12 h IM or IV; or 1 - 2 g q 12 - 24 h IM or IV. **Skin and Skin Structure Infections:** **Mild to Moderate:** 2 g q 24 h IV or 1 g q 12 h IV or IM **Severe:** 2 g q 12 h IV. **Other Sites:** 1 - 2 g q 12 h IV or IM. **Severe Infections:** 2 g q 12 h IV. **Life-Threatening Infections:** 3 g q 12 h IV.
Cefoxitin Sodium (*)	MEFOXIN	Antibacterial	**Inj (per 50 mL):** 1, 2 g **Powd for Inj:** 1, 2 g	**Uncomplicated Infections (e.g., Pneumonia, Urinary Tract or Cutaneous Infections):** 1 g q 6 - 8 h IV. **Moderate to Severe Infections:** 1 g q 4 h IV or 2 g q 6 - 8 h IV. **Infections Commonly Needing Higher Dosage (e.g., Gas Gangrene):** 2 g q 4 h IV or 3 g q 6 h IV.
Cefpodoxime Proxetil (*)	VANTIN	Antibacterial	**Gran for Susp (per 5 mL):** 50, 100 mg **Tab:** 100, 200 mg	**Pharyngitis & Tonsillitis:** 100 mg q 12 h for 5 - 10 days. **Urinary Tract Infections, Uncomplicated:** 100 mg q 12 h po for 7 days. **Pneumonia:** 200 mg q 12 h po for 14 days. **Bacterial Exacerbation of Chronic Bronchitis:** 200 mg q 12 h po for 10 days. **Skin & Skin Structure Infections:** 400 mg q 12 h po for 7 - 14 days. **Gonococcal Infections:** 200 mg po as a single dose.
Cefprozil (*)	CEFZIL	Antibacterial	**Powd for Susp (per 5 mL):** 125, 250 mg **Tab:** 250, 500 mg	**Pharyngitis & Tonsillitis:** 500 mg q 24 h po for 10 days. **Acute Sinusitis:** 250 - 500 mg q 12 h po for 10 days. **Lower Respiratory Tract Infections:** 500 mg q 12 h po for 10 days. **Skin & Skin Structure Infections, Uncompl.:** 250 mg q 12 h po for 10 days or 500 mg q 12 - 24 h po for 10 days.

61

GENERIC NAME	COMMON TRADE NAMES	THERAPEUTIC CATEGORY	PREPARATIONS	COMMON ADULT DOSAGE

Ceftazidime (*)	FORTAZ, TAZIDIME
	
	TAZICEF
		Antibacterial	Powd for Inj: 0.5, 1, 2 g
			
			Powd for Inj: 1, 2 g
				Usual Dosage: 1 g q 8 - 12 h IV or IM.
				Urinary Tract Infections:
				  Uncomplicated: 250 mg q 12 h IV or IM.
				  Complicated: 500 mg q 8 - 12 h IV or IM.
				Bone & Joint Infections: 2 g q 12 h IV.
				Pneumonia, Skin & Skin Structure Infections: 500 mg - 1 g q 8 h IV or IM.
				Meningitis, Serious Gynecologic & Intra-Abdominal Infections, and Severe Life-Threatening Infections: 2 g q 8 h IV.

Ceftizoxime Sodium (*)	FORTAZ	Antibacterial	Inj (per 50 mL): 1, 2 g	Same dosages as for FORTAZ above.
Cefibuten (*)	CEDAX	Antibacterial	Cpsl: 400 mg Powd for Susp (per 5 mL): 90, 180 mg	400 mg once daily po at least 2 h before or 1 h after a meal for 10 days.
Ceftizoxime Sodium (*)	CEFIZOX	Antibacterial	Inj (per 20, 50, or 100 mL): 1, 2 g	**Usual Dosage:** 1 - 2 g q 8 - 12 h IM or IV. **Urinary Tract Infections:** 500 mg q 12 h IM or IV. **Pelvic Inflammatory Disease:** 2 g q 8 h IV. **Other Sites:** 1 g q 8 - 12 h IM or IV. **Severe or Refractory Infections:** 1 g q 8 h IM or IV; or 2 g q 8 - 12 h IM (divided dose in different large muscle masses) or IV. **Life-Threatening Infections:** 3 - 4 g q 8 h IV.
Ceftriaxone Sodium (*)	ROCEPHIN	Antibacterial	Powd for Inj: 250, 500 mg; 1, 2 g	**Usual Dosage:** 1 - 2 g once daily (or in equally divided doses bid) IM or IV. **Gonococcal Infections. Uncomplicated:** 250 mg IM, one dose. **Meningitis:** 100 mg/kg/day in divided doses q 12 h IM or IV, with or without a loading dose of 75 mg/kg. **Surgical Prophylaxis:** 1 gram IV as a single dose 30 min - 2 h before surgery.

62

Cefuroxime Axetil (*)	Antibacterial	CEFTIN	**Tab:** 125, 250, 500 mg **Powd for Susp (per 5 mL):** 125, 250 mg	**Pharyngitis & Tonsillitis:** 250 mg bid po for 10 days. **Urinary Tract Infections, Uncomplicated:** 125 - 250 mg bid po for 7 - 10 days. **Acute Bacterial Exacerbations of Chronic Bronchitis and Secondary Bacterial Infections of Acute Bronchitis:** 250 - 500 mg bid po for 10 days. **Skin or Skin Struct. Infections, Uncomplicated:** 250 - 500 mg bid po for 10 days. **Gonorrhea, Uncomplicated:** 1 g po as a single dose. **Early Lyme Disease:** 500 mg bid po for 20 days.
Cefuroxime Sodium (*)	Antibacterial	KEFUROX, ZINACEF	**Powd for Inj:** 0.75, 1.5 g	**Usual Dosage:** 750 mg - 1.5 g q 8 h for 5 - 10 days IM or IV. **Bone & Joint Infections:** 1.5 g q 8 h IM or IV. **Life-Threatening Infections or Infections due to Less Susceptible Organisms:** 1.5 g q 6 h IV may be required. **Meningitis:** Up to 3.0 g q 8 h IM or IV. **Gonorrhea:** 1.5 g IM, single dose given at 2 different sites with 1.0 g of probenecid po.
Celecoxib	Antiinflammatory, Non-Opioid Analgesic	CELEBREX	**Cpsl:** 100, 200, 400 mg	**Osteoarthritis:** 200 mg once daily po or 100 mg bid po. **Rheumatoid Arthritis:** 100 - 200 mg bid po. **Acute Pain & Primary Dysmenorrhea:** Initially 400 mg po, followed by an additional 200 mg on the first day. On subsequent days, 200 mg bid po prn.
Cephalexin (*)	Antibacterial	KEFLEX	**Powd for Susp (per 5 mL):** 125, 250 mg **Cpsl:** 250, 500 mg	**Usual Dosage:** 250 mg q 6 h po. **Streptococcal Pharyngitis, Skin and Skin Structure Infections and Cystitis:** 500 mg may be used q 12 h po. For cystitis, continue therapy for 7 - 14 days.

GENERIC NAME	COMMON TRADE NAMES	THERAPEUTIC CATEGORY	PREPARATIONS	COMMON ADULT DOSAGE
Cephalexin Hydrochloride (*)	KEFTAB	Antibacterial	Tab: 500 mg	Same dosage as for KEFLEX above.
Cephapirin Sodium (*)	CEFADYL	Antibacterial	Powd for Inj: 1 g	**Usual Dosage:** 500 mg - 1 g q 4 - 6 h IV or IM. **Serious or Life-Threatening Infections:** Up to 12 g daily IV or IM. Use IV for high doses.
Cephradine (*)	VELOSEF	Antibacterial	Powd for Susp (per 5 mL): 125, 250 mg Cpsl: 250, 500 mg	**Respiratory Tract, Skin and Skin Structure Infections:** 250 mg q 6 h po or 500 mg q 12 h po. **Lobar Pneumonia:** 500 mg q 6 h po or 1 g q 12 h po. **Urinary Tract Infections:** 500 mg q 12 h po. In more serious urinary tract infections (including prostatitis), 500 mg q 6 h po or 1 g q 12 h po.
Cetirizine Hydrochloride (*)	ZYRTEC	Antihistamine	Syrup: 5 mg/5 mL Tab: 5, 10 mg	5 - 10 mg once daily po depending on the severity of symptoms.
Chloral Hydrate (*) (C-IV)		Sedative / Hypnotic	Cpsl: 500 mg Syrup: 500 mg/10 mL	**Sedative:** 250 mg tid po, pc. **Hypnotic:** 500 mg - 1 g po, 15 - 30 minutes before bedtime or 30 min. before surgery.
Chloramphenicol (*)		Antibacterial	Cpsl: 250 mg	50 mg/kg/day in divided doses at 6 h intervals po.
	CHLOROPTIC	Antibacterial (Topical)	Ophth Solution: 0.5% Ophth Oint: 1%	2 drops in the affected eye(s) q 3 h. Continue administration day & night for 48 h, after which the dosing interval may be increased. Apply to affected eye(s) q 3 h day & night for 48 h, as above.
Chloramphenicol Sod. Succinate (*)	CHLOROMYCETIN SODIUM SUCCINATE	Antibacterial	Powd for Inj: 100 mg/mL (when reconstituted)	50 mg/kg/day in divided doses at 6 h intervals IV.

Drug	Brand	Category	Forms	Dosage
Chlordiazepoxide Hydrochloride (*) (C:IV)	LIBRIUM	Antianxiety Agent	Cpsl: 5, 10, 25 mg Powd for Inj: 100 mg	5 - 25 mg tid or qid po. 50 - 100 mg IM or IV initially; then 25 - 50 mg tid or qid, if necessary.
Chloroquine Hydrochloride (*)	ARALEN HCL	Antimalarial	Inj: 50 mg salt (= to 40 mg of chloroquine base)/mL	160 - 200 mg of chloroquine base IM initially; repeat in 6 h if necessary.
Chloroquine Phosphate (*)	ARALEN PHOSPHATE	Antimalarial	Tab: 500 mg salt (= to 300 mg of chloroquine base)	**Suppression:** 300 mg of chloroquine base once weekly po, on the same day each week. **Acute Attacks:** Initially, 600 mg of chloroquine base po, followed by 300 mg after 6 - 8 h and a single dose of 300 mg on each of two consecutive days.
Chlorothiazide (*)	DIURIL	Diuretic, Antihypertensive	Susp: 250 mg/5 mL (0.5% alcohol) Tab: 250, 500 mg	**Diuresis:** 0.5 - 1.0 g once daily or bid po. **Hypertension:** 0.5 - 1.0 g po as a single dose or in divided doses.
Chlorothiazide Sodium (*)	DIURIL	Diuretic	Powd for Inj: 500 mg	0.5 - 1.0 g once daily or bid IV.
Chloroxine	CAPITROL	Antibacterial (Topical)	Shampoo: 2%	Massage thoroughly onto wet scalp. Leave lather on for 3 min., then rinse. Repeat the application once. Use twice per week.
Chlorpheniramine Maleate (*)	CHLOR-TRIMETON ALLERGY 4 HOUR	Antihistamine	Tab: 4 mg	4 mg q 4 - 6 h po.
	CHLOR-TRIMETON ALLERGY 8 HOUR		Extended-Rel. Tab: 8 mg	8 mg q 12 h po.
	CHLOR-TRIMETON ALLERGY 12 HOUR		Extended-Rel. Tab: 12 mg	12 mg q 12 h po.
	EFIDAC 24		Extended-Rel. Tab: 16 mg	16 mg q 24 h po.

GENERIC NAME	COMMON TRADE NAMES	THERAPEUTIC CATEGORY	PREPARATIONS	COMMON ADULT DOSAGE
Chlorpromazine (*)	THORAZINE	Antiemetic	Suppos: 25, 100 mg	50 - 100 mg rectally q 6 - 8 h.
Chlorpromazine Hydrochloride (*)	THORAZINE	Antipsychotic, Antiemetic	Syrup: 10 mg/5 mL Liquid Conc: 30, 100 mg/mL Tab: 10, 25, 50, 100, 200 mg Sustained-Rel. Cpsl: 30, 75, 150 mg	**Psychoses (Hospitalized Patients, Less Acutely Disturbed):** 25 mg tid po. Increase gradually until the effective dose is reached, usually 400 mg daily. **Psychoses (Outpatients):** **Usual Dosage:** 10 mg tid or qid po; or 25 mg bid to tid po. **More Severe Cases:** 25 mg tid po. After 1 to 2 days, daily dosage may be raised by 20 - 50 mg at semiweekly intervals until patient becomes calm and cooperative. **Prompt Control of Severe Symptoms:** 25 mg IM. If necessary, repeat in 1 h. Subsequent doses should be oral, 25 - 50 mg tid. **Nausea & Vomiting:** 10 - 25 mg q 4 - 6 h po. **Presurgical Apprehension:** 25 - 50 mg po 2 - 3 h before the operation. **Intractable Hiccups:** 25 - 50 mg tid or qid po. If symptoms persist for 2 - 3 days, use injection [see dosage below].
			Inj: 25 mg/mL	**Psychoses (Hospitalized Patients, Acutely Disturbed or Manic):** 25 mg IM. If necessary, give additional 25 - 50 mg in 1 h. Increase subsequent IM doses gradually over several days (up to 400 mg q 4 - 6 h in severe cases) until patient is controlled. **Psychoses (Outpatients; Prompt Control of Severe Symptoms):** 25 mg IM. If necessary, repeat in 1 h. Subsequent doses should be oral, 25 - 50 mg tid. **Nausea & Vomiting:** **Usual Dosage:** 25 mg IM. If no hypotension occurs, 25 - 50 mg q 3 - 4 h prn, until vomiting stops; then switch to oral dosage [above].

66

Drug	Brand	Class	Form	Dosage
				During Surgery: 12.5 mg IM. Repeat in 30 min. if necessary and if no hypotension occurs. May give 2 mg IV per fractional injection at 2 min. intervals. Dilute to 1 mg/mL and do not exceed 25 mg. **Presurgical Apprehension:** 12.5 - 25 mg IM 1 - 2 h before the operation. **Intractable Hiccups:** If symptoms persist for 2 or 3 days after oral dosing, give 25 - 50 mg IM. Should symptoms persist, use <u>slow</u> IV infusion with patient flat in bed: 25 - 50 mg in 500 - 1000 mL of saline.
Chlorpropamide (*)	DIABINESE	Hypoglycemic Agent	Tab: 100, 250 mg	**Initial:** 250 mg daily po. After 5 - 7 days, dosage may be adjusted upward or downward by increments of not more than 50 - 125 mg at intervals of 3 - 5 days. **Maintenance:** ≤ 100 - 250 mg daily po.
Chlorthalidone	HYGROTON	Diuretic, Antihypertensive	Tab: 25, 50, 100 mg	**Edema:** Initially, 50 - 100 mg daily po or 100 mg on alternate days. Maintenance doses may be lower than initial doses. **Hypertension:** Initially, 25 mg daily po. May increase the dosage to 50 mg daily po and then to 100 mg daily po if necessary.
	THALITONE	Diuretic, Antihypertensive	Tab: 15, 25 mg	**Edema:** Initially, 30 - 60 mg daily po or 60 mg on alternate days. Maintenance doses may be lower than initial doses. **Hypertension:** Initially, 15 mg daily po. May increase the dosage to 30 mg daily po and then to 45 - 50 mg daily po if necessary.
Chlorzoxazone	PARAFON FORTE DSC	Skeletal Muscle Relaxant	Cplt: 500 mg	500 mg tid or qid po.

GENERIC NAME	COMMON TRADE NAMES	THERAPEUTIC CATEGORY	PREPARATIONS	COMMON ADULT DOSAGE
Cholestyramine	QUESTRAN, LoCHOLEST		Powder: 4 g drug/9 g powder	9 g of powder 1 - 3 times daily po.
	QUESTRAN LIGHT LoCHOLEST LIGHT		Powder: 4 g drug/6.4 g powder 4 g drug/5.7 g powder	6.4 g of powder 1 - 3 times daily po. 5.7 g of powder 1 - 3 times daily po.
Ciclopirox	PENLAC NAIL LACQUER	Antifungal (Topical)	Solution: 8%	Apply evenly to entire nail and surrounding 5 mm of skin of affected nails once daily, preferably hs or 8 h before washing. If possible, apply to nail bed, hyponychium, and under surface of nail plate when it is free of the nail plate. Apply over previous coat(s), then remove with alcohol once per week.
Ciclopirox Olamine	LOPROX	Antifungal (Topical)	Cream, Gel & Lotion: 1% (equal to 0.77% base)	Gently massage into affected and surrounding skin areas bid, in the AM and PM.
Cidofovir (*)	VISTIDE	Antiviral	Inj: 75 mg/mL	Induction: 5 mg/kg by IV infusion (see below) once weekly for 2 consecutive weeks. Maintenance: 5 mg/kg by IV infusion (see below) q 2 weeks. Cidofovir must be diluted in 100 mL of 0.9% NaCl solution prior to administration. The IV infusion is given at a constant rate over 1 h. Oral probenecid must be given with each dose: 2 g given 3 h prior to cidofovir and 1 g given at 2 h and 8 h after completion of the 1 h IV infusion (total probenecid dose = 4 g).
Cilostazol	PLETAL	Drug for Intermittant Claudication	Tab: 50, 100 mg	100 mg bid po taken ≥ 30 min before or 2 h after breakfast and dinner.

68

Cimetidine (*)	TAGAMET HB 200	Histamine H_2-Blocker	**Tab:** 100 mg	**Heartburn, Acid Indigestion & Sour Stomach:** 200 mg po with water up to bid.
	TAGAMET	Histamine H_2-Blocker, Anti-Ulcer Agent	**Liquid:** 300 mg/5 mL (2.8% alcohol) **Tab:** 200, 300, 400, 800 mg	**Duodenal Ulcer:** **Active:** 800 mg hs po; or 300 mg qid po with meals & hs; or 400 mg bid po in the AM and PM. **Maintenance:** 400 mg hs po. **Active Benign Gastric Ulcer:** 800 mg hs po; or 300 mg qid po with meals & hs.
				Erosive Gastroesophageal Reflux Disease: 800 mg bid po; or 400 mg qid po for 12 weeks. **Pathological Hypersecretory Conditions:** 300 mg qid po with meals & hs.
			Inj: 300 mg/2 mL	**Pathological Hypersecretory Conditions or Intractable Ulcers:** 300 mg q 6 - 8 h IM or IV (infused over 15 - 20 minutes). For a Continuous IV infusion: 37.5 mg/h (900 mg daily); may be preceded by a 150 mg loading dose by IV infusion (over 15 - 20 minutes).
Cinoxacin	CINOBAC	Urinary Tract Anti-infective	**Cpsl:** 250, 500 mg	1 g daily po, in 2 or 4 divided doses for 7 - 14 days.
Ciprofloxacin (*)	CIPRO I.V.	Antibacterial	**Inj:** 200, 400 mg	**Urinary Tract Infections:** **Mild/Moderate:** 200 mg q 12 h by IV infusion (over 60 minutes) for 7 - 14 days. **Severe/Complicated:** 400 mg q 12 h by IV infusion (over 60 minutes) for 7 - 14 days. **Lower Respiratory Tract, Bone & Joint, and Skin & Skin Structure Infections:** **Mild/Moderate:** 400 mg q 12 h by IV infusion (over 60 minutes) for 7 - 14 days (Bone & Joint = 4 to 6 weeks of therapy). **Severe/Complicated:** 400 mg q 8 h by IV infusion (over 60 minutes) for 7 - 14 days (Bone & Joint = 4 to 6 weeks of therapy).

[Continued on the next page]

69

GENERIC NAME	COMMON TRADE NAMES	THERAPEUTIC CATEGORY	PREPARATIONS	COMMON ADULT DOSAGE
profloxacin [Continued]				**Acute Sinusitis:** 400 mg q 12 h by IV infusion (over 60 minutes) for 10 days. **Chronic Bacterial Prostatitis:** 400 mg q 12 h by IV infusion (over 60 minutes) for 28 days. **Intra-Abdominal Infections:** 400 mg q 12 h by IV infusion (over 60 min) for 7 - 14 days. **Inhalational Anthrax (Post-Exposure):** 400 mg q 12 h by IV infusion (over 60 minutes) for 60 days. **Nosocomial Pneumonia:** 400 mg q 8 h by IV infusion (over 60 minutes).
Ciprofloxacin Hydrochloride (*)	CIPRO	Antibacterial	Tab: 100, 250, 500, 750 mg	**Urinary Tract Infections:** **Acute, Uncomplicated:** 100 mg q 12 h po for 3 days. **Mild/Moderate:** 250 mg q 12 h po for 7 - 14 days. **Severe/Complicated:** 500 mg q 12 h po for 7 - 14 days. **Lower Respiratory Tract and Skin & Skin Structure Infections:** **Mild/Moderate:** 500 mg q 12 h po for 7 - 14 days. **Severe/Complicated:** 750 mg q 12 h for 7 to 14 days. **Bone & Joint Infections:** **Mild/Moderate:** 500 mg q 12 h po for 4 - 6 weeks. **Severe/Complicated:** 750 mg q 12 h po for 4 - 6 weeks. **Infectious Diarrhea:** 500 mg q 12 h po for 5 - 7 days. **Bacterial Prostatitis, Chronic:** 500 mg q 12 h po for 28 days. **Typhoid Fever & Acute Sinusitis:** 500 mg q 12 h po for 10 days. **Gonococcal Infections, Uncomplicated:** 250 mg po (as a single dose).

	CILOXAN	Antibacterial (Topical)	**Ophth Solution:** 0.3%	**Corneal Ulcers:** 2 drops in affected eye(s) q 15 min. for the 1st 6 hours, then 2 drops q 30 min. for the rest of the 1st day. Second day: 2 drops q 1 h; 3rd - 14th day: 2 drops q 4 h. **Conjunctivitis:** 1 - 2 drops in affected eye(s) q 2 h while awake for 2 days, then 1 - 2 drops q 4 h while awake for the next 5 days.
			Ophth Oint: 0.3% (as the base)	Place 1/2 in strip into the conjunctival sac tid for 2 days, then bid for 5 days.
Cisplatin (*)	PLATINOL PLATINOL AQ	Antineoplastic	**Powd for Inj:** 10, 50 mg **Inj:** 1 mg/mL	**Metastatic Testicular Tumors:** 20 mg/m² IV daily for 5 days. **Metastatic Ovarian Tumors:** 100 mg/m² IV once every 4 weeks. **Advanced Bladder Cancer:** 50 - 70 mg/m² IV q 3 - 4 weeks.
Citalopram Hydrobromide (*)	CELEXA	Antidepressant	**Tab:** 10, 20, 40 mg (as the base) **Solution:** 2 mg/mL (as the base)	20 mg once daily po in the AM or PM. Dose increases should usually occur in increments of 20 mg at intervals of no less than 1 week. Maximum: 40 mg daily.
Clarithromycin (*)	BIAXIN	Antibacterial	**Granules for Susp (per 5 mL):** 125, 250 mg **Tab:** 250, 500 mg	**Usual Dosage:** 250 - 500 mg q 12 h po for 7 - 14 days. **Mycobacterium avium Complex (MAC):** 500 mg bid po. **Active Duodenal Ulcer Associated with Helicobacter pylori Infection:** 500 mg tid po for days 1 - 14 plus omeprazole 40 mg po each AM or ranitidine bismuth citrate 400 mg bid for days 1 - 14.
	BIAXIN XL		**Extended-Rel. Tab:** 500 mg	**Usual Dosage:** 1000 mg once daily po with food for 7 - 14 days. **Bronchitis:** 1000 mg once daily po with food for 7 days. **Sinusitis:** 1000 mg once daily po with food for 14 days.

71

GENERIC NAME	COMMON TRADE NAMES	THERAPEUTIC CATEGORY	PREPARATIONS	COMMON ADULT DOSAGE
Clemastine Fumarate	TAVIST	Antihistamine	Syrup: 0.67 mg/5 mL (5.5% alcohol)	**Allergic Rhinitis:** 10 mL bid po. **Urticaria and Angioedema:** 20 mL bid po.
	TAVIST ALLERGY TAVIST		Tab: 1.34 mg Tab: 2.68 mg	1.34 mg q 12 h po. 2.68 mg bid or tid po.
Clindamycin Hydrochloride (*)	CLEOCIN HCL	Antibacterial	Cpsl: 75, 150, 300 mg	**Serious Infections:** 150 - 300 mg q 6 h po. **More Severe Infections:** 300 - 450 mg q 6 h po.
Clindamycin Palmitate HCl (*)	CLEOCIN PEDIATRIC	Antibacterial	Powd for Susp: 75 mg/5 mL	Same dosages as for CLEOCIN HCL above.
Clindamycin Phosphate (*)	CLEOCIN PHOSPHATE	Antibacterial	Inj: 150 mg/mL	**Serious Infections:** 600 - 1200 mg/day IV or IM in 2, 3 or 4 equal doses. **More Severe Infections:** 1200 - 2700 mg/day IV or IM in 2, 3 or 4 equal doses. **Life-Threatening Infections:** Up to 4800 mg/day IV.
	CLEOCIN	Antibacterial (Topical)	Vaginal Cream: 2%	Insert 1 applicatorful intravaginally, preferably hs, for 7 consecutive days.
	CLEOCIN VAGINAL OVULES	Antibacterial (Topical)	Vaginal Suppos.: 100 mg	Insert 1 suppos. intravaginally, preferably hs, for 3 consecutive days.
	CLEOCIN-T	Anti-Acne Agent	Topical Solution, Gel &: Lotion: 10 mg/mL	Apply a thin film to affected areas bid.
Clobetasol Propionate	TEMOVATE	Corticosteroid (Topical)	Cream, Oint & Gel: 0.05% Scalp Application: 0.05%	Apply topically to affected areas bid. Apply to affected scalp areas bid, AM and PM.
	OLUX		Foam: 0.05%	Apply to affected areas bid, AM and PM.
Clocortolone Pivalate	CLODERM	Corticosteroid (Topical)	Cream: 0.1%	Apply sparingly to the affected area tid. Rub in gently.
Clofazimine (*)	LAMPRENE	Leprostatic	Cpsl: 50, 100 mg	100 mg daily with meals po.

Clomiphene Citrate	CLOMID, SEROPHENE	Ovulation Stimulant	**Tab:** 50 mg	50 mg daily for 5 days po.
Clomipramine Hydrochloride (*)	ANAFRANIL	Antidepressant	**Cpsl:** 25, 50, 75 mg	Initiate with 25 mg daily po with meals and gradually increase, as tolerated, to 100 mg a day during the first 2 weeks. Thereafter, the dosage may be increased gradually over the next several weeks, up to a maximum of 250 mg daily. After titration, the total daily dose may be given once daily hs.
Clonazepam (*) (C-IV)	KLONOPIN	Antiepileptic, Drug for Panic Disorder	**Tab:** 0.5, 1, 2 mg	**Seizure Disorders:** Initially, 0.5 mg tid po. Dosage may be increased in increments of 0.5 - 1 mg every 3 days; maximum 20 mg per day. **Panic Disorder:** Initially, 0.25 mg bid po. An increase to the target dose of 1 mg daily may be made after 3 days.
Clonidine	CATAPRES-TTS	Antihypertensive	**Transdermal:** rate = 0.1, 0.2, 0.3 mg/24 hr	Apply to hairless area of intact skin on the upper arm or torso, once every 7 days.
Clonidine Hydrochloride (*)	CATAPRES	Antihypertensive	**Tab:** 0.1, 0.2, 0.3 mg	Initially, 0.1 mg bid po (AM and hs). Further increments of 0.1 mg may be made until the desired response is achieved.
	DURACLON	Non-Opioid Analgesic	**Inj:** 100 μg/mL	30 μg/hr by continuous epidural infusion.
Clopidogrel Bisulfate	PLAVIX	Platelet Aggregation Inhibitor	**Tab:** 75 mg	**Recent MI, Recent Stroke, or Established Peripheral Arterial Disease:** 75 mg once daily po. **Acute Coronary Syndrome:** Initiate therapy with a single 300 mg loading dose; continue with 75 mg once daily po.

GENERIC NAME	COMMON TRADE NAMES	THERAPEUTIC CATEGORY	PREPARATIONS	COMMON ADULT DOSAGE
Clorazepate Dipotassium (*) (C-IV)	TRANXENE-T TAB	Antianxiety Agent, Antiepileptic, Drug for Alcohol Withdrawal	Tab: 3.75, 7.5, 15 mg	**Anxiety:** 15 - 60 mg daily in divided doses po; or 15 mg hs po. **Epilepsy:** The maximum recommended initial dose is 7.5 mg tid po. Dosage should be increased no more than 7.5 mg every week and should not exceed 90 mg per day. **Acute Alcohol Withdrawal:** Day 1 (1st 24 h): 30 mg po initially, followed by 30 - 60 mg po in divided doses. Day 2 (2nd 24 h): 45 - 90 mg po in divided doses. Day 3 (3rd 24 h): 22.5 - 45 mg po in divided doses. Day 4: 15 - 30 mg po in divided doses. Thereafter: gradually reduce the dose to 7.5 to 15 mg daily po.
	TRANXENE-SD	Antianxiety Agent	Gradual-Rel. Tab: 11.25, 22.5 mg	**Anxiety:** 11.25 or 22.5 mg as a single po dose q 24 h. Used as an alternative for patients stabilized on TRANXENE.
Clotrimazole	LOTRIMIN AF MYCELEX	Antifungal (Topical)	Cream, Lotion & Solution: 1% Cream: 1%	Massage into affected and surrounding skin areas bid, AM and PM.
			Troche: 10 mg	**Treatment:** Slowly dissolve 1 in the mouth 5 times daily for 14 consecutive days. **Prophylaxis:** Slowly dissolve 1 in the mouth 3 times daily for the duration of therapy.
	GYNE-LOTRIMIN 7, MYCELEX-7		Vaginal Cream: 1% Vaginal Insert: 100 mg	One applicatorful daily intravaginally for 7 consecutive days, preferably hs. Place 1 insert daily intravaginally for 7 consecutive days, preferably hs.
	GYNE-LOTRIMIN 3		Vaginal Cream: 2% Vaginal Suppos: 200 mg	One applicatorful daily intravaginally for 3 consecutive days, preferably hs. Insert 1 suppos. daily intravaginally for 3 consecutive days, preferably hs.

74

Cloxacillin Sodium (*)		Antibacterial	Cpsl: 250, 500 mg Powd for Solution: 125 mg/5 mL	**Mild to Moderate Infections:** 250 mg q 6 h po. **Severe Infections:** 500 mg q 6 h po.
Clozapine (*)	CLOZARIL	Antipsychotic	Tab: 25, 100 mg	Initially, 12.5 mg once or twice daily po; then, continue with daily dosage increments of 25 - 50 mg/day (if well-tolerated) to a target dose of 300 - 450 mg/day by the end of 2 weeks. Subsequent dosage increments should be made no more than 1 - 2 times a week in increments not to exceed 100 mg.
Codeine Phosphate (*) (C-II)		Opioid Analgesic	Inj (per mL): 30, 60 mg	15 - 60 mg q 4 - 6 h IM, SC or IV.
Codeine Sulfate (C-II)		Opioid Analgesic, Antitussive	Tab: 15, 30, 60 mg	**Analgesia:** 15 - 60 mg q 4 - 6 h po. **Antitussive:** 10 - 20 mg q 4 - 6 h po.
Colchicine (*)		Antigout Agent	Tab: 0.5, 0.6 mg	**Acute:** 1.0 - 1.2 mg po stat; then 0.5 - 1.2 mg q 1 - 2 h po, until pain is relieved, or nausea, vomiting or diarrhea occurs. **Prophylaxis:** 0.5 or 0.6 mg daily for 3 - 4 days a week.
			Inj: 1 mg/2 mL	**Acute:** 2 mg stat IV; then 0.5 mg q 6 h IV up to a maximum of 4 mg in 24 h. **Prophylaxis:** 0.5 - 1 mg once daily or bid IV.
Colesevelam Hydrochloride	WELCHOL	Antihyperlipidemic	Tab: 625 mg	3 tabs bid po with meals or 6 tabs once daily po with a meal. May increase to 7 tabs depending on the desired effect.

GENERIC NAME	COMMON TRADE NAMES	THERAPEUTIC CATEGORY	PREPARATIONS	COMMON ADULT DOSAGE
Colestipol Hydrochloride	COLESTID	Antihyperlipidemic	**Tab:** 1 g	Initially, 2 g once or twice daily po. Dosage increases of 2 g once or twice daily po should occur at 1 - 2 month intervals. Dosage range: 2 - 16 g/day po given once daily or in divided doses.
			Granules for Oral Susp: 5 g packettes and 300, 500 g bottles (Unflavored); 7.5 g packettes and 450 g bottles (Orange Flavor)	Initially, 5 g daily or bid po with a daily increment of 5 g at 1 - 2 month intervals. Usual dose: 5 - 30 g/day po given once daily or in divided doses.
Colistimethate Sodium	COLY-MYCIN M PARENTERAL	Antibacterial	**Powd for Inj:** 150 mg (= to colistin base)	2.5 - 5.0 mg/kg per day in 2 - 4 divided doses IV or IM.
Cromolyn Sodium	GASTROCROM	Antiallergic (Oral)	**Conc. Solution:** 100 mg/5 mL	200 mg qid po, 30 minutes ac & hs.
	INTAL	Drug for Asthma	**Solution for Nebulization:** 20 mg/2 mL **Inhaler:** 800 µg/spray	20 mg qid nebulized. 2 sprays qid inhaled.
	NASALCROM	Antiallergic (Nasal)	**Nasal Solution:** 40 mg/mL	1 spray in each nostril 3 - 6 times daily.
	CROLOM	Antiallergic (Ophthalmic)	**Ophth Solution:** 4%	1 or 2 drops in each eye 4 - 6 times daily at regular intervals.
Crotamiton	EURAX	Scabicide, Antipruritic	**Cream & Lotion:** 10%	**Scabies:** Massage into the skin from the chin to the toes including folds and creases. Reapply 24 hours later. A cleansing bath should be taken 48 h after the last application. **Pruritus:** Massage gently into affected areas until medication is completely absorbed. Repeat prn.

Cyanocobalamin	NASCOBAL	Vitamin	**Metered-Dose Gel:** 500 µg per actuation	500 µg (1 actuation) intranasally once a week.
				Deficiency: 25 - 250 µg daily po.
Cyclizine Hydrochloride (*)	MAREZINE	Antiemetic	**Tab:** 50 mg	50 mg q 4 - 6 h po, staring 30 minutes prior to travel.
Cyclobenzaprine Hydrochloride (*)	FLEXERIL	Skeletal Muscle Relaxant	**Tab:** 10 mg	10 mg tid po.
Cyclophosphamide	CYTOXAN	Antineoplastic	**Tab:** 25, 50 mg **Powd for Inj:** 100, 200, 500 mg; 1, 2 g	1 - 5 mg/kg/day po. 40 - 50 mg/kg IV in divided doses over a period of 2 - 5 days; or 10 - 15 mg/kg IV q 7 - 10 days; or 3 - 5 mg/kg IV twice weekly.
Cyclosporine (*)	SANDIMMUNE	Immunosuppressant	**Cpsl:** 25, 50, 100 mg **Solution:** 100 mg/mL (12.5% alcohol) **Inj:** 50 mg/mL	15 mg/kg IV, 4 to 12 hours prior to transplantation. Continue dose postoperatively for 1 - 2 weeks, then taper by 5% per week to a maintenance level of 5 - 10 mg/kg/day. 5 - 6 mg/kg/day IV, 4 to 12 hours prior to transplantation. Give as a dilute solution (50 mg in 20 to 100 mL) and administer as a slow infusion over 2 - 6 hrs. Continue this single dose postoperatively until patient can tolerate oral dosage forms.
Cyproheptadine Hydrochloride		Antihistamine, Antipruritic	**Syrup:** 2 mg/5 mL (5% alcohol) **Tab:** 4 mg	4 mg tid po.
Cytarabine, Conventional (*)	CYTOSAR-U	Antineoplastic	**Powd for Inj:** 100, 500 mg; 1, 2 g	100 mg/m² /day by continuous IV infusion or 100 mg/m² IV q 12 h.
Cytarabine, Liposomal	DEPO-CYT	Antineoplastic	**Inj:** 10 mg/mL	50 mg intrathecally (intraventricular or lumbar puncture) q 14 days for 2 to 4 doses.

77

GENERIC NAME	COMMON TRADE NAMES	THERAPEUTIC CATEGORY	PREPARATIONS	COMMON ADULT DOSAGE
Dacarbazine	DTIC-DOME	Antineoplastic	Inj: 10 mg/mL	**Malignant Melanoma:** 2 - 4.5 mg/kg/day IV for 10 days; may repeat q 4 weeks. Alternate dosage: 250 mg/m^2/day IV for 5 days; may repeat q 3 weeks. **Hodgkin's Disease:** 150 mg/m^2/day IV for 5 days, in combination with other effective drugs; may repeat q 4 weeks. Alternate dosage: 375 mg/m^2 on day 1, in combination with other drugs; repeat q 15 days.
Dalteparin Sodium	FRAGMIN	Anticoagulant	Solution (per 0.2 mL): 2,500 (16 mg); 5,000 (32 mg) anti-X$_a$ Units	**Patients Undergoing Abdominal Surgery with Risk of Thromboembolic Complications:** 2,500 Units once daily SC, starting 1 - 2 h prior to surgery and repeated once daily 5 - 10 days postoperatively. In patients with high risk of thromboembolic complications, use 5,000 Units SC in the evening before surgery and repeated once daily for 5 - 10 days postoperatively. **Hip Replacement Surgery:** 2,500 Units SC within 2 h before surgery and 2,500 Units in the evening of the day of surgery (≥ 6 h after the first dose). On the first post-operative day administer 5,000 Units SC once daily for 5 - 10 days. **Unstable Angina/Non-Q-Wave MI:** 120 Units/kg (but not more than 10,000 Units) SC q 12 h with concurrent oral aspirin (75 to 165 mg per day) therapy. Continue until the patient is clinically stabilized (usually 5 - 8 days).
Danaparoid Sodium	ORGARAN	Anticoagulant	Inj: 750 anti-Xa Units per 0.6 mL	750 anti-Xa Units bid SC starting 1 - 4 h pre-operatively; then not sooner than 2 h after surgery. Continue therapy throughout post-operative care until the risk of deep vein thrombosis has diminished (e.g., 7-10 days).

Danazol	DANOCRINE	Gonadotropin Inhibitor	Cpsl: 50, 100, 200 mg	**Endometriosis:** 100 - 200 mg bid po (mild disease) or 400 mg bid po (moderate to severe). Continue therapy for 3 - 6 months. **Fibrotic Breast Disease:** 50 - 200 mg bid po. Therapy should begin during menstruation. **Hereditary Angioedema:** 200 mg bid or tid po. After a favorable initial response, determine continuing dosage by reducing the dosage by 50% or less at intervals of 1 - 3 months or longer. If an attack occurs, increase dosage by up to 200 mg/day.
Dantrolene Sodium	DANTRIUM	Skeletal Muscle Relaxant	Cpsl: 25, 50, 100 mg	**Chronic Spasticity:** 25 mg once daily po for 7 days; then 25 mg tid for 7 days; then 50 mg tid for 7 days; then 100 mg tid. Therapy in some patients may require qid dosing. **Malignant Hyperthermia:** **Preoperatively:** 4 - 8 mg/kg/day po in 3 - 4 divided doses for 1 or 2 days prior to surgery, with the last dose given approx. 3 - 4 h before scheduled surgery. **Post Crisis Follow Up:** 4 - 8 mg/kg/day po in 4 divided doses for 1 - 3 days.
	DANTRIUM INTRAVENOUS		Powd for Inj: 20 mg	**Malignant Hyperthermia:** **Acute Therapy:** Administer by continuous rapid IV push beginning at a minimum dose of 1 mg/kg, and continuing until the symptoms subside or the max. cumulative dose of 10 mg/kg has been reached. **Preoperatively:** 2.5 mg/kg IV starting approx. 1.25 hours before anticipated anesthesia and infused over 1 h. **Post Crisis Follow Up:** Individualize dose.
Dapsone (*)	DAPSONE USP	Leprostatic	Tab: 25, 100 mg	100 mg daily po alone or in combination with other leprostatic drugs.
Delavirdine Mesylate	RESCRIPTOR	Antiviral	Tab: 100, 200 mg	400 mg tid po. Disperse the dose in 3 fl. oz. of water prior to consumption.

79

GENERIC NAME	COMMON TRADE NAMES	THERAPEUTIC CATEGORY	PREPARATIONS	COMMON ADULT DOSAGE
Demecarium Bromide	HUMORSOL	Anti-Glaucoma Agent	**Ophth Solution:** 0.125, 0.25%	1 - 2 drops in the affected eye. Usual dosage can vary from as much as 1 - 2 drops bid to as little as 1 - 2 drops twice a week; for most patients 0.125% used bid is preferred.
Demeclocycline Hydrochloride	DECLOMYCIN	Antibacterial	**Tab:** 150, 300 mg	150 mg qid po or 300 mg bid po.
Desipramine Hydrochloride (*)	NORPRAMIN	Antidepressant	**Tab:** 10, 25, 50, 75, 100, 150 mg	100 - 200 mg daily po in a single dose or in divided doses.
Desloratadine	CLARINEX	Antihistamine	**Tab:** 5 mg	5 mg po once daily.
Desmopressin Acetate	DDAVP NASAL SPRAY	Posterior Pituitary Hormone, Anti-Enuretic Agent	**Nasal Spray:** 0.1 mg/mL (delivers 0.1 mL [10 µg] per spray)	**Central Cranial Diabetes Insipidus:** 0.1 - 0.4 mL daily as a single dose or in 2 - 3 divided doses intranasally.
	DDAVP RHINAL TUBE		**Nasal Solution:** 0.1 mg/mL (with rhinal tube applicators)	**Primary Nocturnal Enuresis:** 0.2 mL intranasally hs. Dosage adjustment up to 0.4 mL may be made if necessary.
	DDAVP TABLETS		**Tab:** 0.1, 0.2 mg	**Central Cranial Diabetes Insipidus:** Initially, 0.05 mg bid po. Dosage adjustments may be made such that the total daily dosage is in the range of 0.1 - 1.2 mg divided tid or bid.
	DDAVP INJECTION		**Inj:** 4, 15 µg/mL	**Diabetes Insipidus:** 0.25 - 0.5 mL (1 - 2 µg) bid SC or IV (4 µg/mL injection only). **Hemophilia A and von Willebrand's Disease (Type I):** 0.3 µg/kg diluted in 50 mL of sterile physiological saline; infuse IV slowly over 15 to 30 minutes. If used preoperatively, give 30 minutes prior to the procedure.
	STIMATE	Posterior Pituitary Hormone	**Nasal Spray:** 1.5 mg/mL (delivers 0.1 mL [150 µg] per spray)	**Hemophilia A and von Willebrand's Disease (Type I):** 1 spray per nostril (300 µg) in patients weighing ≥ 50 kg; 1 spray only in patients weighing < 50 kg. If used preoperatively, give 2 h prior to procedure.

Desonide	DESOWEN TRIDESILON	Corticosteroid (Topical)	**Cream, Oint & Lotion:** 0.05% **Cream & Oint:** 0.05%	Apply to the affected areas bid to tid. Apply to the affected areas bid to qid.
Desoximetasone	TOPICORT	Corticosteroid (Topical)	**Cream:** 0.05, 0.25% **Oint:** 0.25% **Gel:** 0.05%	Apply a thin film to the affected areas bid. Rub in gently.
Dexamethasone	DECADRON	Corticosteroid	**Elixir:** 0.5 mg/5 mL (5% alcohol) **Tab:** 0.5, 0.75, 4 mg	Initial dosage varies from 0.75 - 9 mg daily po, depending on the disease being treated. This should be maintained or adjusted until the patient's response is satisfactory.
	MAXIDEX	Corticosteroid (Topical)	**Ophth Susp:** 0.1%	1 - 2 drops in affected eye(s). In severe disease, may use hourly; taper to discontinuation as the inflammation subsides. In mild disease, may use up to 4 - 6 times daily.
Dexamethasone Acetate		Corticosteroid	**Inj:** 8 mg/mL	**Intramuscular Inj:** 8 - 16 mg q 1 - 3 weeks. **Intralesional Inj:** 0.8 - 1.6 mg per inj. site. **Intra-articular & Soft Tissue Inj:** 4 - 16 mg q 1 - 3 weeks.
Dexamethasone Sodium Phosphate	DECADRON PHOSPHATE	Corticosteroid	**Inj:** 4 mg/mL **Inj:** 24 mg/mL [for IV use only]	**IV and IM Inj:** Initial dosage varies from 0.5 - 9 mg daily depending on the disease being treated. This dosage should be maintained or adjusted until the patient's response is satisfactory. **Intra-articular, Intralesional, and Soft Tissue Injection:** Varies from 0.2 - 6 mg given from once q 3 - 5 days to once q 2 - 3 weeks.
	DECADRON PHOSPHATE		**Ophth Solution:** 0.1%	**Eye:** 1 - 2 drops into eye(s) q 1 h during the day & q 2 h at night, initially. When a favorable response occurs, reduce to 1 drop into eye(s) q 4 h. Later, 1 drop tid - qid. **Ear:** 3 - 4 drops into aural canal bid - tid. When a favorable response occurs, reduce dosage gradually and eventually discontinue.

[Continued on the next page]

81

GENERIC NAME	COMMON TRADE NAMES	THERAPEUTIC CATEGORY	PREPARATIONS	COMMON ADULT DOSAGE
Dexamethasone Sodium Phosphate [Continued]	DECADRON PHOSPHATE, MAXIDEX		Ophth Oint: 0.05%	Apply to eye(s) tid or qid. When a favorable response occurs, reduce daily applications to 2, and later to 1 as maintenance therapy.
	DEXACORT TURBINAIRE		Topical Cream: 0.1%	Apply a thin film to affected area tid or qid.
			Nasal Aerosol: 84 μg/spray	2 sprays in each nostril bid or tid.
Dexchlorpheniramine Maleate		Antihistamine	Extended-Rel. Tab: 4, 6 mg	4 or 6 mg po hs or q 8 - 10 h during the day.
Dexmethylphenidate (C-II)	FOCALIN	CNS Stimulant	Tab: 2.5, 5, 10 mg	**Patients New to Methylphenidate:** 2.5 mg bid po. Dosage may be adjusted in 2.5 - 5.0 mg increments (in at least weekly intervals) to a maximum of 10 mg bid. **Patients Currently Using Methylphenidate:** Half the current po dose of methylphenidate.
Dextroamphetamine Sulfate (*) (C-II)	DEXEDRINE	CNS Stimulant	Tab: 5 mg Sustained-Rel. Cpsl: 5, 10, 15 mg	**Narcolepsy:** 5 - 60 mg per day in divided doses, depending on the patient response.
Dextromethorphan Hydrobromide (*)	ROBITUSSIN PEDIATRIC COUGH SUPPRESSANT	Antitussive	Liquid: 7.5 mg/5 mL	20 mL q 6 - 8 h po.
	BENYLIN PEDIATRIC COUGH SUPPRESSANT		Liquid: 7.5 mg/5 mL	20 mL (30 mg) q 6 - 8 h po.
	BENYLIN ADULT FORMULA		Liquid: 15 mg/5 mL	10 mL (30 mg) q 6 - 8 h po.
	ROBITUSSIN MAXIMUM STRENGTH COUGH SUPPRESSANT		Liquid: 15 mg/5 mL	10 mL (30 mg) q 6 - 8 h po.
Dextromethorphan Polistirex	DELSYM	Antitussive	Syrup: equal to 30 mg of dextromethorphan HBr/5 mL (0.26% alcohol)	10 mL (60 mg) q 12 h po.

Generic	Brand	Form/Strength	Category	Dosage
Diazepam (*) (C-IV)	VALIUM	Tab: 2, 5, 10 mg Inj: 5 mg/mL	Antianxiety Agent, Anticonvulsant, Skel. Muscle Relax., Drug for Alcohol Withdrawal	**Anxiety & Adjunct in Convulsive Disorders:** 2 - 10 mg bid to qid po. **Muscle Spasms:** 2 - 10 mg tid to qid po. **Anxiety (Moderate):** 2 - 5 mg IM or IV. Repeat in 3 - 4 h, if necessary. **Anxiety (Severe) and Muscle Spasms:** 5 - 10 mg IM or IV. Repeat in 3 - 4 h, if necessary. **Preoperative Medication:** 10 mg IM (preferred route) before surgery. **Status Epilepticus and Severe Recurrent Convulsive Seizures:** 5 - 10 mg IV. Repeat at 10 - 15 minute intervals, if necessary, up to a maximum dose of 30 mg. **Acute Alcohol Withdrawal:** Initially 10 mg IM or IV, then 5 - 10 mg in 3 - 4 h, if needed. **Endoscopic Procedures:** Titrate IV dosage to desired sedative response. Generally 10 mg or less is adequate, but up to 20 mg IV may be given.
	DIASTAT	Rectal Gel (Adult): 10, 15, 20 mg	Antiepileptic	Administer 0.2 mg/kg rectally. Calculate the recommended dose by rounding up to the next available unit dose. A second dose, when required, may be given 4 - 12 h after the first dose. Do not treat more than 5 episodes/month or more than 1 episode q 5 days.
Diazoxide (*)	PROGLYCEM	Susp: 50 mg/mL Cpsl: 50 mg	Hyperglycemic Agent	3 - 8 mg/kg po. divided into 2 or 3 equal doses q 8 - 12 h.
	HYPERSTAT I.V.	Inj: 300 mg/20 mL	Antihypertensive	1 - 3 mg/kg IV repeated at intervals of 5 - 15 minutes (max.: 150 mg in a single injection).
Dibucaine	NUPERCAINAL	Oint: 1%	Local Anesthetic Antihemorrhoidal	Apply to affected areas AM and PM and after each bowel movement.

GENERIC NAME	COMMON TRADE NAMES	THERAPEUTIC CATEGORY	PREPARATIONS	COMMON ADULT DOSAGE
Dichlorphenamide	DARANIDE	Anti-Glaucoma Agent	Tab: 50 mg	Initially, a priming dose of 100 - 200 mg po, followed by 200 mg q 12 h po until the desired response occurs. The maintenance dosage is 25 - 50 mg once daily to tid po.
Diclofenac Potassium (*)	CATAFLAM	Antiinflammatory, Non-Opioid Analgesic	Tab: 50 mg	**Osteoarthritis:** 100 - 150 mg/day po in divided doses (50 mg bid or tid). **Rheumatoid Arthritis:** 150 - 200 mg/day po in divided doses (50 mg tid or qid). **Ankylosing Spondylitis:** 100 - 125 mg/day po as: 25 mg qid with an extra 25 mg hs, prn. **Analgesia and Primary Dysmenorrhea:** 50 mg tid po or 100 mg initially, followed by 50 mg doses po. Except for the first day when the total dose may be 200 mg, do not exceed 150 mg daily.
Diclofenac Sodium (*)	VOLTAREN	Antiinflammatory	Delayed-Rel. Tab: 25, 50, 75 mg	**Osteoarthritis:** 100 - 150 mg/day po in divided doses (50 mg bid or tid, or 75 mg bid). **Rheumatoid Arthritis:** 150 - 200 mg/day po in div. doses (50 mg tid or qid, or 75 mg bid). **Ankylosing Spondylitis:** 100 - 125 mg/day po as: 25 mg qid with an extra 25 mg hs, prn.
		Antiinflammatory (Topical)	Ophth Solution: 0.1%	**Following Cataract Surgery:** 1 drop into the affected eye(s) qid beginning 24 h after cataract surgery and continuing for the first 2 weeks of the postoperative period. **Corneal Refractive Surgery:** 1 or 2 drops into the affected eye within 1 h prior to surgery. Instill 1 - 2 drops within 15 min after surgery and continue qid for up to 3 days.
	VOLTAREN-XR	Antiinflammatory	Extended-Rel. Tab: 100 mg	**Osteoarthritis & Rheumatoid Arthritis:** 100 mg once daily po.
	SOLARAZE	Drug for Actinic Keratoses	Gel: 3%	Apply to lesions twice daily for 60 - 90 days.

84

Drug	Class	Forms	Dosage
Dicloxacillin Sodium (*)	Antibacterial	**Powd for Susp:** 62.5 mg/5 mL **Cpsl:** 250, 500 mg	**Mild to Moderate Infections:** 125 mg q 6 h po. **More Severe Infections:** 250 mg q 6 h po.
Dicyclomine Hydrochloride (*)	Anticholinergic	**Syrup:** 10 mg/5 mL **Cpsl:** 10 mg **Tab:** 20 mg **Inj:** 10 mg/mL	Initially 80 mg/day po (in 4 equally divided doses). Dosage may be increased during the first week, if necessary, to 160 mg/day po. 80 mg daily IM (in 4 equally divided doses).
Didanosine (*)	Antiviral	**Chewable/Dispersible Tab:** 25, 50, 100, 150, 200 mg	**< 60 kg:** 250 mg once daily po or 125 mg bid q 12 h po. **≥ 60 kg:** 400 mg once daily po or 200 mg bid q 12 h po. Take at least 2 of the appropriate strength tablets at each dose for adequate buffering buffering and to prevent degradation by gastric acid. Chew or crush and disperse the tablets in at least 1 fl. oz. of water prior to consumption. Take on an empty stomach.
		Powd for Solution: 100, 167, 250 mg packets	**< 60 kg:** 167 mg bid q 12 h po. **≥ 60 kg:** 250 mg bid q 12 h po. Dissolve contents of packet in 4 fl. oz. of water and drink on an empty stomach.
VIDEX EC		**Delayed-Rel. Cpsl (with enteric-coated beadlets):** 125, 200, 250, 400 mg	**< 60 kg:** 250 mg once daily po. **≥ 60 kg:** 400 mg once daily po. Take each dose on an empty stomach and swallow the capsule intact.
Dienestrol ORTHO DIENESTROL	Estrogen	**Cream:** 0.01%	1 - 2 applicatorfuls intravaginally daily for 1 - 2 weeks, then gradually reduce to 1/2 initial dosage for a similar period. Maintenance dosage is 1 applicatorful 1 - 3 times a week.
Diethylpropion Hydrochloride (*) (C-IV) TENUATE TENUATE DOSPAN	Anorexiant	**Tab:** 25 mg **Controlled-Rel. Tab:** 75 mg	25 mg tid, 1 h ac po. 75 mg daily po in the midmorning.

GENERIC NAME	COMMON TRADE NAMES	THERAPEUTIC CATEGORY	PREPARATIONS	COMMON ADULT DOSAGE
Diflorasone Diacetate	FLORONE, MAXIFLOR	Corticosteroid (Topical)	Cream & Oint: 0.05%	Apply to the affected area once daily to qid, depending on the severity of the condition.
	FLORONE E		Emollient Cream: 0.05%	Apply to the affected area once daily to tid, depending on the severity of the condition.
Diflunisal (*)	DOLOBID	Non-Opioid Analgesic, Antiinflammatory	Tab: 250, 500 mg	**Analgesic:** Initially 1000 mg po, followed by 500 mg q 12 h; or initially 500 mg po, followed by 250 mg q 8 - 12 h may also be appropriate. **Rheumatoid Arthritis & Osteoarthritis:** 250 to 500 mg bid po.
Digoxin (*)	LANOXIN ELIXIR PEDIATRIC LANOXIN	Heart Failure Drug, Inotropic Agent	Elixir: 50 μg/mL (10% alcohol) Tab: 125, 250 μg Inj: 250 μg/mL	Variable; see Digoxin Dosage Tables, pp. 308 to 311.
	LANOXICAPS		Cpsl: 50, 100, 200 μg	Variable; see Digoxin Dosage Tables, pp. 308 to 311.
Dihydrotachysterol	DHT HYTAKEROL	Vitamin D Analog	Tab: 0.125, 0.2, 0.4 mg Solution: 0.2 mg/mL Cpsl: 0.125 mg	**Initial:** 0.8 - 2.4 mg daily po for several days. **Maintenance:** 0.2 - 1.75 mg daily po. The average dose is 0.6 mg daily po.
Diltiazem Hydrochloride (*)	CARDIZEM	Antianginal	Tab: 30, 60, 90, 120 mg	Initially, 30 mg qid po ac & hs. Dosage should be increased gradually at 1 - 2 day intervals. Usual optimum dosage: 180 - 360 mg/day.
	CARDIZEM SR	Antihypertensive	Sustained-Rel. Cpsl: 60, 90, 120 mg	Initially, 60 - 120 mg bid po; dosage may be adjusted after 14 days. Usual dosage: 240 to 360 mg/day.
	CARDIZEM CD	Antihypertensive, Antianginal	Extended-Rel. Cpsl: 120, 180, 240, 300, 360 mg	**Hypertension:** Initially, 180 - 240 mg once daily po. Dosage may be increased up to 480 mg once daily po (over 14 days). Usual dosage: 240 - 360 mg once daily. **Angina:** Initially, 120 or 180 mg once daily po. Dosage may be increased up to 480 mg once daily po (over 7 - 14 days).

Generic	Brand	Class	Forms	Dosage
	DILACOR XR	Antihypertensive, Antianginal	Extended-Rel. Cpsl: 120, 180, 240 mg	**Hypertension:** 180 - 240 mg once daily po. **Angina:** Initially, 120 mg once daily po. May be titrated to doses of up to 480 mg once daily over a 7 - 14 day period.
	TIAZAC	Antihypertensive	Extended-Rel. Cpsl: 120, 180, 240, 300, 360, 420 mg	**Hypertension:** Initially, 120 - 240 mg once daily po. Usual dosage range: 120 - 540 mg once daily po.
	CARDIZEM	Antiarrhythmic	Inj: 5 mg/mL	**IV Bolus (given over 2 min):** Initially, 0.25 mg/kg; if response is inadequate, in 15 min. give 0.35 mg/kg. Individualize subsequent IV bolus doses. **Continuous IV Infusion (following IV bolus):** Initially, 5 - 10 mg/hr; rate may be increased in 5 mg/hr increments up to 15 mg/hr prn for up to 24 h.
Dimenhydrinate	DRAMAMINE	Antivertigo Agent, Antiemetic	Liquid: 12.5 mg/5 mL; Tab & Chewable Tab: 50 mg; Inj: 50 mg/mL	50 - 100 mg q 4 - 6 h po. 50 - 100 mg q 4 - 6 h po. 50 mg q 4 - 6 h IM or slow IV.
Diphenhydramine Hydrochloride (*)	BENADRYL DYE-FREE	Antihistamine	Liquid: 12.5 mg/5 mL; Softgel Cpsl: 25 mg	25 - 50 mg (10 - 20 mL) q 4 - 6 h po. 25 - 50 mg q 4 - 6 h po.
	BENADRYL ALLERGY	Antihistamine, Antiemetic, Antiparkinsonian	Liquid: 12.5 mg/5 mL; Chewable Tab: 12.5 mg; Cpsl & Tab: 25 mg	25 - 50 mg (10 - 20 mL) q 4 - 6 h po. 25 - 50 mg q 4 - 6 h po. 25 - 50 mg q 4 - 6 h po.
	BENADRYL		Inj (per mL): 50 mg	10 - 50 mg IV or deep IM.
	NYTOL QUICK CAPS, SIMPLY SLEEP	Sedative	Cplt: 25 mg	50 mg po hs, prn.
	UNISOM SLEEPGELS NYTOL SOFTGELS	Sedative	Cpsl: 50 mg; Softgel: 50 mg	50 mg po hs, prn.
	BENADRYL ITCH STOPPING GEL	Antihistamine (Topical)	Gel: 1, 2%	Apply to affected areas not more than tid or qid.

GENERIC NAME	COMMON TRADE NAMES	THERAPEUTIC CATEGORY	PREPARATIONS	COMMON ADULT DOSAGE
Dipyridamole	PERSANTINE	Platelet Aggregation Inhibitor	Tab: 25, 50, 75 mg	75 - 100 mg qid po.
Dirithromycin	DYNABAC	Antibacterial	Enteric-Coated Tab: 250 mg	500 mg once daily po with for 7 - 14 days. Administer with food or within 1 h of eating.
Disopyramide Phosphate (*)	NORPACE NORPACE CR	Antiarrhythmic	Cpsl: 100, 150 mg Extended-Rel. Cpsl: 100, 150 mg	600 mg/day po given in divided doses, e.g., 150 mg q 6 h. For patients under 110 lbs, 400 mg/day po, e.g., 100 mg q 6 h. 600 mg/day po given in divided doses, e.g., 300 mg q 12 h. For patients under 110 lbs, 400 mg/day po, e.g., 200 mg q 12 h.
Disulfiram (*)	ANTABUSE	Antialcoholic	Tab: 250, 500 mg	Initial: A maximum of 500 mg po, given as a single dose for 1 - 2 weeks. Maintenance: 250 mg daily po.
Divalproex Sodium (*)	DEPAKOTE	Antiepileptic, Antimaniacal, Antimigraine Agent	Delayed-Rel. Tab: 125, 250, 500 mg	Epilepsy: Initially, 10 - 15 mg/kg/day po; increase at 1 week intervals by 5 - 10 mg/kg/day (Maximum: 60 mg/kg/day). If the total daily dosage exceeds 250 mg. it should be given in divided doses. Acute Mania: Initially, 750 mg daily po in divided doses. The dose should be increased as rapidly as possible to achieve the lowest therapeutic dose that produces the desired clinical effect or the desired range of plasma concentrations (trough = 50 - 125 μg/mL). Maximum dosage is 60 mg/kg/day. Migraine: 250 mg bid po.
	DEPAKOTE	Antiepileptic	Sprinkle Cpsl: 125 mg	Epilepsy: Initially, 10 - 15 mg/kg/day po; increase at 1 week intervals by 5 - 10 mg/kg/day (Maximum: 60 mg/kg/day). If the total daily dosage exceeds 250 mg. it should be given in divided doses.

Generic	Brand	Category	Formulation	Dosage
	DEPAKOTE ER	Antimigraine Agent	Extended-Rel. Tab: 500 mg	500 mg once daily po for 1 week; then 1000 mg once daily po.
Dobutamine Hydrochloride (*)	DOBUTREX	Sympathomimetic	Powd for Inj: 250 mg	2.5 - 15 μg/kg/min by IV infusion.
Docosanol	ABREVA	Cold Sores/Fever Blisters Drug	Cream: 10%	Apply to affected area at the first sign of cold sores/fever blister (tingling). Use 5 times daily until healed.
Docusate Calcium	SURFAK LIQUIGELS	Stool Softener	Cpsl: 240 mg	240 mg daily po.
Docusate Sodium	COLACE	Stool Softener	Syrup: 20 mg/5 mL, Cpsl: 50, 100 mg	50 - 200 mg daily po.
	EX-LAX STOOL SOFTENER		Cplt: 100 mg	100 mg once daily to tid po.
	PHILLIPS LIQUI-GELS		Liqui-Gel: 100 mg	100 mg once daily to tid po.
Dolasetron Mesylate	ANZEMET	Antiemetic	Tab: 50, 100 mg	**Prevention of Chemotherapy-Induced Nausea and Vomiting:** 100 mg po within 1 h before chemotherapy. **Prevention or Treatment of Postoperative Nausea and Vomiting:** 100 mg po 2 h before surgery.
			Inj: 20 mg/mL	**Prevention of Chemotherapy-Induced Nausea and Vomiting:** 1.8 mg/kg IV as a single dose about 30 min before chemotherapy. Alternatively, 100 mg IV (over 30 sec). **Prevention or Treatment of Postoperative Nausea and Vomiting:** 12.5 mg IV as a single dose about 15 min before the cessation of anesthesia or as soon as nausea or vomiting presents.
Donepezil Hydrochloride	ARICEPT	Drug for Alzheimer's Disease	Tab: 5, 10 mg	5 - 10 mg once daily po.

GENERIC NAME	COMMON TRADE NAMES	THERAPEUTIC CATEGORY	PREPARATIONS	COMMON ADULT DOSAGE
Dopamine Hydrochloride	INTROPIN	Sympathomimetic	Inj (per mL): 40, 80, 160 mg	2 - 10 μg/kg/min by IV infusion.
Dorzolamide Hydrochloride	TRUSOPT	Anti-Glaucoma Agent	Ophth. Solution: 2%	1 drop in the affected eye(s) tid.
Doxacurium Chloride	NUROMAX	Neuromuscular Blocker	Inj: 1 mg/mL	Initially, 0.025 - 0.05 mg/kg IV (depending on duration of effect desired and other drugs given); then, 0.005 - 0.01 mg/kg IV prn.
Doxazosin Mesylate (*)	CARDURA	Antihypertensive, Benign Prostatic Hyperplasia Drug	Tab: 1, 2, 4, 8 mg (as the base)	**Hypertension:** Initially, 1 mg once daily po. After 24 hours, dosage may be increased to 2 mg and thereafter, if needed, to 4, 8, and 16 mg daily. **Benign Prostatic Hyperplasia:** Initially, 1 mg once daily po. Depending on the condition, dosage may then be increased to 2 mg and thereafter 4 and 8 mg once daily (suggested titration interval is 1 - 2 weeks).
Doxepin Hydrochloride (*)	SINEQUAN	Antianxiety Agent, Antidepressant	Cpsl: 10, 25, 50, 75, 100, 150 mg Oral Concentrate: 10 mg/mL	75 mg daily po in single or divided doses. The usual optimum dosage range is 75 - 150 mg daily.
	ZONALON	Antihistamine (Topical)	Cream: 5%	Apply a thin film to affected areas qid, with at least 3 or 4 hours between applications.
Doxorubicin Hydrochloride	ADRIAMYCIN PFS ADRIAMYCIN RDF	Antineoplastic	Inj: 2 mg/mL Powd for Inj: 10, 20, 50 mg	60 - 75 mg/m² as a single IV injection given at 21-day intervals. Alternative: 20 mg/m² IV at weekly intervals.
Doxorubicin Hydrochloride Liposome Injection	DOXIL	Antineoplastic	Inj: 2 mg/mL (encapsulated in liposomes)	20 mg/m² as a single IV injection (over 30 min.) once every 3 weeks.

Doxycycline Calcium (*)	VIBRAMYCIN	Antibacterial, Antimalarial	Syrup: 50 mg/5 mL	**Usual Dosage:** 100 mg q 12 h po for the first day, followed by a maintenance dose of 100 mg/day given as 50 mg q 12 h or 100 mg once daily. **Urinary Tract Infections:** 100 mg q 12 h po. **Malaria Prophylaxis:** 100 mg once daily po.
Doxycycline Hyclate (*)	VIBRAMYCIN VIBRA-TAB	Antibacterial, Antimalarial	Cpsl: 50, 100 mg Tab: 100 mg	Same dosages as for VIBRAMYCIN Syrup.
	DORYX		Cpsl (with coated pellets): 100 mg	Same dosages as for VIBRAMYCIN Syrup.
	VIBRAMYCIN INTRAVENOUS	Antibacterial	Powd for Inj: 100, 200 mg	**Usual Dosage:** 200 mg on the first day given in 1 or 2 IV infusions, then 100 - 200 mg a day, with 200 mg given in 1 or 2 infusions. **Syphilis:** 300 mg daily by IV infusion for at least 10 days.
	PERIOSTAT	Periodontitis Drug	Tab: 20 mg	20 mg bid po, 1 h before or 2 h after meals.
Doxycycline Monohydrate (*)	VIBRAMYCIN	Antibacterial, Antimalarial	Powd for Susp: 25 mg/5 mL	Same dosages as for VIBRAMYCIN Syrup.
Doxylamine Succinate (*)	UNISOM	Sedative	Tab: 25 mg	25 mg po, 30 minutes before retiring.
Dronabinol (C-III)	MARINOL	Antiemetic, Appetite Stimulant	Cpsl: 2.5, 5, 10 mg	**Emesis:** 5 mg/m^2 po, 1 - 3 h prior to chemotherapy, then q 2 - 4 h after chemotherapy for a total of 4 - 6 doses/day. **Anorexia in AIDS patients:** Initially, 2.5 mg bid po, before lunch and supper. For patients who cannot tolerate this dosage, reduce to 2.5 mg once daily with supper or hs. When adverse reactions are absent or minimal or for further therapeutic effect, increase to 2.5 mg before lunch and 5 mg before supper (or 5 mg at lunch and 5 mg after supper). Approx. 50% of patients tolerate 10 mg bid.

GENERIC NAME	COMMON TRADE NAMES	THERAPEUTIC CATEGORY	PREPARATIONS	COMMON ADULT DOSAGE
Dyphylline (*)	LUFYLLIN	Bronchodilator	**Tab**: 200, 400 mg **Elixir**: 100 mg/15 mL (20% alcohol)	Variable: up to 15 mg/kg q 6 h po.
Econazole Nitrate	SPECTAZOLE	Antifungal (Topical)	**Cream**: 1%	**Tinea Infections**: Apply topically to affected areas once daily. **Cutaneous Candidiasis**: Apply to affected areas bid.
Edrophonium Chloride (*)	ENLON, TENSILON	Cholinomimetic	**Inj**: 10 mg/mL	**Diagnosis of Myasthenia**: 2 mg IV; if no reaction occurs after 45 seconds, give 8 mg IV. Test may be repeated in 30 minutes. May also administer 10 mg IM. Subject who shows hyperreactivity (cholinergic reaction), retest after 30 minutes with 2 mg IM. **Evaluation of Treatment Requirements**: 1 - 2 mg IV, 1 hour after oral intake of the drug being used in treatment. **Curare Antagonism**: 10 mg IV, given slowly over 30 - 45 seconds. May be repeated prn, up to a maximum of 40 mg.
Efavirenz	SUSTIVA	Antiviral	**Cpsl**: 50, 100, 200 mg **Tab**: 600 mg	600 mg once daily po in combination with a protease inhibitor or nucleoside analog reverse transcriptase inhibitor.
Eflornithine Hydrochloride	ORNIDYL	Antiprotozoal	**Inj**: 200 mg/mL	100 mg/kg/dose by IV infusion (over a minimum of 45 minutes) q 6 h for 14 days.
Eflornithine Hydrochloride	VANIQA	Facial Hair Retardant	**Cream**: 13.9%	Apply a thin layer to affected areas of face and adjacent areas under the chin bid (at least 8 hours apart). Rub in well. Do not wash the areas for at least 4 hours.
Emedastine Difumarate	EMADINE	Antihistamine (Topical)	**Ophth Solution**: 0.05%	1 drop in the affected eye(s) up to qid.

92

Enalapril Maleate (*)	VASOTEC	Antihypertensive, Heart Failure Drug	**Tab:** 2.5, 5, 10, 20 mg	**Hypertension:** 5 mg once daily po. Usual dosage range is 10 - 40 mg/day as a single dose or in 2 divided doses. **Heart Failure:** As adjunctive therapy with a diuretic or digoxin, use 2.5 mg once daily or bid po. Usual dosage range is 5 - 20 mg/day in 2 divided doses.
Enalaprilat	VASOTEC I.V.	Antihypertensive	**Inj:** 1.25 mg/mL	1.25 mg q 6 h IV (over 5 minutes).
Enoxaparin Sodium	LOVENOX	Anticoagulant	**Inj:** 30 mg/0.3 mL, 40 mg/0.4 mL, 60 mg/0.6 mL, 80 mg/0.8 mL, 100 mg/mL	**Deep Vein Thrombosis (DVT) Prophylaxis:** **Hip or Knee Replacement Surgery:** 30 mg SC (within 12 - 24 h postoperatively provided hemostasis has been established), then 30 mg q 12 h SC for 7 - 14 days. For Hip Replacement Surgery, consider 40 mg once daily SC, given initially 9 - 15 h prior to surgery. Continue for 3 weeks. **Abdominal Surgery:** 40 mg once daily SC with the initial dose given 2 h prior to surgery. The usual duration is 7 - 10 days. **Medical Patients during Acute Illness:** 40 mg once daily SC. The usual duration is 6 - 11 days. **Deep Vein Thrombosis (DVT) Treatment:** **Deep Vein Thrombosis/Pulmonary Embolism:** **Outpatients (e.g., Acute DVT without PE):** 1 mg/kg SC q 12 h. **Inpatients (e.g., Acute DVT with PE):** 1 mg/kg SC q 12 h or 1.5 mg/kg SC once daily (at the same time each day).
Entacapone (*)	COMTAN	Antiparkinsonian	**Tab:** 200 mg	200 mg po given concomitantly with each levodopa/carbidopa dose to a maximum of 8 times daily (1600 mg).
Ephedrine Sulfate (*)		Bronchodilator	**Cpsl:** 25 mg **Inj:** 50 mg/mL	12.5 - 25 mg q 4 h po. 25 - 50 mg SC or IM.

GENERIC NAME	COMMON TRADE NAMES	THERAPEUTIC CATEGORY	PREPARATIONS	COMMON ADULT DOSAGE
Epinephrine	PRIMATENE MIST	Bronchodilator	Aerosol: 0.2 mg/spray	1 inhalation, then wait at least 1 minute. If not relieved, use once more. Do not use again for at least 3 h.
			Inj: 5 mg/mL (1:200)	0.1 - 0.3 mL SC. Do not use more often than q 6 h.
Epinephrine Bitartrate		Bronchodilator	Aerosol: 0.35 mg/spray (equal to 0.16 mg of epinephrine)	1 inhalation, then wait at least 1 minute. If not relieved, use once more. Do not use again for at least 3 h.
Epinephrine Hydrochloride	ADRENALIN CHLORIDE	Sympathomimetic, Bronchodilator	Solution: 1:100 (10 mg/mL) Inj: 1:1000 (1 mg/mL)	Variable, by nebulizer. 0.2 - 1.0 mg SC or IM.
	EPIPEN, EPI E-Z PEN		Auto-injector: 1:1000 soln (0.3 mg delivered per injection of 0.3 mL)	0.3 mg IM.
Eplerenone	INSPRA	Antihypertensive	Tab: 25, 50, 100 mg	Initially, 50 mg once daily po. If necessary, dosage may be increased to 50 mg bid.
Eprosartan Mesylate	TEVETEN	Antihypertensive	Tab: 400, 600 mg	Initially, 600 mg once daily po. Usual range: 400 - 800 mg/day given as a single dose or in 2 divided doses.
Ergotamine Tartrate (*)	ERGOMAR	Antimigraine Agent	Sublingual Tab: 2 mg	2 mg under tongue stat; repeat q 30 minutes, prn, for a maximum of 6 mg per 24 hours.
Ertapenem	INVANZ	Antibacterial	Powd for Inj: 1 g	1 g by IV infusion (over 30 min) for up to 14 days or 1 g by IM injection for up to 7 days.

Erythromycin (*)	A/T/S ERYCETTE T-STAT 2%	Anti-Acne Agent	Solution & Gel: 2% Solution: 2% Solution & Pads: 2%	Apply to affected areas bid.
	ERY-TAB ERYC	Antibacterial	Delayed-Rel. Tab: 250, 333, 500 mg Delayed-Rel. Cpsl: 250 mg	**Usual Dosage:** 250 mg qid po: 333 mg q 8 h po; or 500 mg bid (q 12 h) po. **Streptococcal Infections:** Administer the usual dosage for at least 10 days.
	ERYTHROMYCIN BASE FILMTAB		Tab: 250, 500 mg	**Primary Syphilis:** 20 - 40 g po in divided doses over a period of 10 - 15 days.
	PCE		Dispersable Tab: 333, 500 mg	**Acute Pelvic Inflammatory Disease due to *N. gonorrhoeae*:** After initial treatment with erythromycin lactobionate, give 250 mg q 6 h po for 7 days or 333 mg q 8 h for 7 days. **Urogenital Infections during pregnancy and Uncomplicated Urethral, Endocervical, or Rectal Infections due to *C. trachomatis*:** 500 mg qid po or 666 mg q 8 h po for at least 7 days. **Dysenteric Amebiasis:** 250 mg qid po or 333 mg q 8 h po for 10 - 14 days. **Legionnaires Disease:** 1 - 4 g daily po in divided doses.
Erythromycin Estolate (*)	ILOSONE	Antibacterial	Susp (per 5 mL): 125, 250 mg Cpsl: 250 mg Tab: 500 mg	**Usual Dosage:** 250 mg q 6 h po or 500 mg q 12 h po. **Streptococcal Infections:** Administer the usual dosage for at least 10 days. **Primary Syphilis:** 20 - 40 g po in divided doses over a period of 10 - 15 days. **Urogenital Infections during pregnancy and Uncomplicated Urethral, Endocervical, or Rectal Infections due to *C. trachomatis*:** 500 mg qid po for at least 7 days. **Dysenteric Amebiasis:** 250 mg qid po for 10 to 14 days. **Legionnaires Disease:** 1 - 4 g daily po in divided doses.

GENERIC NAME	COMMON TRADE NAMES	THERAPEUTIC CATEGORY	PREPARATIONS	COMMON ADULT DOSAGE
Erythromycin Ethylsuccinate (*)	E.E.S.	Antibacterial	Gran for Susp (per 5 mL): 200 mg Susp (per 5 mL): 200, 400 mg Tab: 400 mg	**Usual Dosage:** 400 mg q 6 h po or 800 mg q 12 h po. **Streptococcal Infections:** Administer the usual dosage for at least 10 days. **Primary Syphilis:** 48 - 64 g po in divided doses over a period of 10 - 15 days.
	ERYPED		Powd for Susp (per 5 mL): 200, 400 mg Chewable Tab: 200 mg	**Urethritis due to *C. trachomatis* or *U. urealyticum*:** 800 mg tid po for 7 days. **Intestinal Amebiasis:** 400 mg qid po for 10 to 14 days. **Legionnaires Disease:** 1.6 - 4 g daily po in divided doses.
Erythromycin Gluceptate (*)	ILOTYCIN GLUCEPTATE	Antibacterial	Powd for Inj: 1 g	**Usual Dosage:** 5 - 20 mg/kg/day by continuous IV infusion or in divided doses q 6 h IV. **Acute Pelvic Inflammatory Disease due to *N. gonorrhoeae*:** 500 mg q 6 h IV for at least 3 days, followed by 250 mg of oral erythromycin q 6 h for 7 days.
Erythromycin Lactobionate (*)	ERYTHROCIN IV	Antibacterial	Powd for Inj: 500 mg; 1 g	**Severe Infections:** 15-20 mg/kg/day by contin. IV infusion or by intermittent IV infusion in 20 - 60 min periods at intervals of ≤ 6 h.
Erythromycin Stearate (*)	ERYTHROCIN STEARATE	Antibacterial	Tab: 250, 500 mg	**Usual Dosage:** 250 mg q 6 h po or 500 mg q 12 h po on an empty stomach or ac. **Streptococcal Infections:** Administer the usual dosage for at least 10 days. **Acute Pelvic Inflammatory Disease due to *N. gonorrhoeae*:** After initial treatment with erythromycin lactobionate, give 250 mg q 6 h po for 7 days. **Urogenital Infections during pregnancy and Uncomplicated Urethral, Endocervical, or Rectal Infections due to *C. trachomatis*:** 500 mg qid po for at least 7 days. **Intestinal Amebiasis:** 250 mg qid po for 10 to 14 days.

96

Escitalopram Oxalate	LEXAPRO	Antidepressant	**Tab:** 5, 10, 20 mg (as the base)	Initially, 10 mg once daily po.
Esmolol Hydrochloride (*)	BREVIBLOC	Antiarrhythmic	**Inj (per mL):** 10, 250 mg	500 μg/kg/min IV for 1 minute followed by a 4-minute infusion of 50 μg/kg/min. If an adequate effect is not seen within 5 min., repeat loading dose followed by a 4-minute infusion of 100 μg/kg/min. Continue process as above, increasing maintenance infusion by increments of 50 μg/kg/min. As the desired effect is reached, omit loading dose & lower incremental dose in maintenance infusion from 50 μg/kg/min to 25 μg/kg/min or lower.
Esomeprazole Magnesium	NEXIUM	Gastric Acid Pump Inhibitor, Anti-Ulcer Agent	**Delayed-Rel. Cpsl:** 20, 40 mg	**Duodenal Ulcer Associated with *H. pylori*:** 40 mg of esomeprazole once daily po (1 h ac) + 1 g of amoxicillin and 500 mg of clarithromycin bid po for 10 days. **Erosive Esophagitis:** **Treatment of:** 20 - 40 mg once daily po (1 h ac) for 4 - 8 weeks. **Maintenance of Healing Esophagitis:** 20 mg once daily po (1 h ac). **Symptomatic GERD:** 20 mg once daily po (1 h ac) for 4 weeks.
Estazolam (*) (C-IV)	PROSOM	Hypnotic	**Tab:** 1, 2 mg	1 - 2 mg hs po.
Estradiol (*)	ESTRACE	Estrogen	**Tab:** 0.5, 1, 2 mg	**Menopausal Symptoms:** 1 - 2 mg daily po. **Prostatic Cancer:** 1 - 2 mg tid po. **Breast Cancer:** 10 mg tid po for at least 3 mos. **Osteoporosis Prevention:** 0.5 mg daily po cyclically (23 days on, 5 days off) as soon as possible after menopause.

[Continued on the next page]

GENERIC NAME	COMMON TRADE NAMES	THERAPEUTIC CATEGORY	PREPARATIONS	COMMON ADULT DOSAGE
Estradiol [Continued]	ESTRACE		Vaginal Cream: 0.01%	**Initial:** 2 - 4 g intravaginally daily for 1 - 2 weeks, then gradually reduce to 1/2 initial dose for a similar period. **Maintenance:** 1 g intravag. 1 - 3 times a week.
	ESTRING		Vaginal Ring: 2 mg	**Urogenital Symptoms associated with Postmenopausal Vaginal Atrophy:** Insert 1 ring as deeply as possible into the upper third of the vagina. Leave in place for 3 mos, then remove and replace if necessary.
	FEMPATCH		Transdermal: rate = 0.025 mg/24 h	**Vulval or Vaginal Atrophy, Hypoestrogenism, and Vasomotor Symptoms associated with Menopause:** Initially, apply 1 patch to the skin on the buttocks once a week. If symptoms are not relieved after 4 - 6 weeks, 2 patches may be applied weekly.
	ESTRADERM		Transdermal: rate = 0.05, 0.1 mg/24 h	**Vulval or Vaginal Atrophy, Hypoestrogenism, and Vasomotor Symptoms associated with Menopause:** Initially, apply 1 patch (0.05 mg) to the skin on the trunk of the body (including the abdomen and buttocks) once a week (CLIMARA) or twice a week (ALORA, ESTRADERM and VIVELLE). Adjust dosage as necessary (with the lowest dosage needed to control symptoms, especially in women with a intact uterus).
	ALORA		Transdermal: rate = 0.05, 0.075, 0.1 mg/24 h	
	CLIMARA		Transdermal: rate = 0.025, 0.05, 0.075, 0.1 mg/24 h	
	VIVELLE, VIVELLE-DOT		Transdermal: rate = 0.025, 0.0375, 0.05, 0.075, 0.1 mg/24 h	**Prophylactic Therapy to Prevent Postmenopausal Bone Loss:** Initiate with 0.05 mg/day as soon as possible after menopause. Adjust dosage as needed to control symptoms. **Therapeutic Regimen:** May give continuously to patients who do not have an intact uterus. In patients with an intact uterus, may give on a cyclic schedule (3 weeks on the drug, followed by 1 week off the drug).

Generic	Brand	Category	Form	Dosage
Estradiol Cypionate (*)	DEPO-ESTRADIOL	Estrogen	Inj (per mL): 5 mg (in oil)	**Menopausal Symptoms:** 1 - 5 mg IM q 3 - 4 weeks. **Female Hypogonadism:** 1.5 - 2 mg IM monthly.
Estradiol Hemihydrate (*)	VAGIFEM	Estrogen	Vaginal Tab: 25 μg	**Atrophic Vaginitis:** Initial Dose: Insert 1 tab vaginally once daily (at the same time each day) for 2 weeks. **Maintenance:** Insert 1 tab vaginally twice weekly.
Estradiol Valerate (*)	DELESTROGEN	Estrogen	Inj (per mL): 10, 20, 40 mg (in oil)	**Menopausal Symptoms:** 10 - 20 mg IM q 4 weeks. **Female Hypogonadism:** 10 - 20 mg IM q 4 weeks given cyclically.
Estramustine Phosphate	EMCYT	Antineoplastic	Cpsl: 140 mg	14 mg/kg/day (1 cpsl per 22 lb) in 3 or 4 divided doses po.
Estrogens, Conjugated (*)	PREMARIN	Estrogen, Antineoplastic	Tab: 0.3, 0.625, 0.9, 1.25, 2.5 mg	**Female Hypogonadism:** 2.5 - 7.5 mg daily po in divided doses for 20 days, followed by a rest period of 10 days. If bleeding does not occur by the end of this period, the same dosage schedule is repeated. If bleeding occurs before the end of the 10 day period, begin a 20 day regimen with 2.5 - 7.5 mg daily po in divided doses; add an oral progestin during the last 5 days of therapy. If bleeding occur before before this regimen ends, therapy is discontinued and may be resumed on the 5th day of bleeding. **Vasomotor Symptoms of Menopause:** 1.25 mg daily po. Administer on a cyclic schedule (3 weeks on the drug, 1 week off the drug). **Atrophic Vaginitis:** 0.3 - 1.25 mg daily po. Administer cyclically as noted above. **Osteoporosis:** 0.625 mg daily po, cyclically (3 weeks on, 1 week off). **Mammary Carcinoma:** 10 mg tid po for at least 3 months. **Prostatic Carcinoma:** 1.25 - 2.5 mg tid po.

[Continued on the next page]

GENERIC NAME	COMMON TRADE NAMES	THERAPEUTIC CATEGORY	PREPARATIONS	COMMON ADULT DOSAGE
Estrogens, Conjugated [Continued]	PREMARIN	Estrogen	Vaginal Cream: 0.625 mg/g	2 - 4 g (1/2 - 1 applicatorful) intravaginally daily. Administration should be cyclic (3 weeks on, 1 week off).
Estrogens, A Synthetic Conjugated (*)	CENESTIN	Estrogen	Tab: 0.3, 0.625, 0.9, 1.25 mg	**Vasomotor Symptoms associated with Menopause:** Initially, 0.625 mg daily po. Administer on a cyclic schedule (3 weeks on the drug, followed by 1 week off the drug). May titrate dose to 1.25 mg/day.
Estrogens, Esterified (*)	ESTRATAB, MENEST	Estrogen, Antineoplastic, Antiosteoporotic	Tab: 0.3, 0.625, 1.25, 2.5 mg	**Female Hypogonadism:** 2.5 - 7.5 mg daily po, in divided doses for 20 days, followed by a rest period of 10 days. If bleeding does not occur by the end of this period, the same dosage schedule is repeated. If bleeding occurs before the end of the 10 day period, begin a 20 day regimen with 2.5 - 7.5 mg daily po in divided doses; add an oral progestin during the last 5 days of therapy. If bleeding occur before before this regimen ends, therapy is discontinued and may be resumed on the 5th day of bleeding. **Vasomotor Symptoms:** 1.25 mg daily po. Administration should be cyclic (3 weeks on the drug, followed by 1 week off). **Atrophic Vaginitis and Kraurosis Vulvae:** 0.3 to 1.25 mg daily po. Administer cyclically. **Osteoporosis Prevention:** 0.3 mg daily po and increase to a maximum of 1.25 mg daily po, if necessary. **Prostatic Cancer:** 1.25 - 2.5 mg tid po. **Breast Cancer in Men and Postmenopausal Women:** 10 mg tid po for at least 3 months.

Drug	Brand	Category	Form/Strength	Dosage
Estropipate (*)	OGEN	Estrogen, Antiosteoporotic	**Tab:** 0.75, 1.5, 3 mg (equivalent to sodium estrone sulfate: 0.625, 1.25, 2.5 mg respectively)	**Female Hypogonadism:** 1.5 - 9 mg daily po for the first 3 weeks of a theoretical cycle, followed by a rest period of 8 - 10 days. If bleeding does not occur by the end of this period, the same dosage schedule is repeated. If bleeding does not occur, an oral progestin may be added during the third week of the cycle. **Vasomotor Symptoms and Vulval and Vaginal Atrophy:** 0.75 - 6 mg daily po. Administration should be cyclic (3 weeks on the drug, followed by 1 week off). **Prevention of Osteoporosis:** 0.75 mg daily po for 25 days of a 31 day cycle per month.
	ORTHO-EST		**Tab:** 0.75, 1.5 mg (equivalent to sodium estrone sulfate: 0.625, 1.25 mg respectively)	
	OGEN	Estrogen	**Vaginal Cream:** 1.5 mg/g	2 - 4 g intravaginally daily. Administration should be cyclic (3 weeks on, 1 week off).
Etanercept	ENBREL	Antirheumatic	**Powd for Inj:** 25 mg	25 mg twice weekly by SC injection, 72 to 96 h apart.
Ethacrynate Sodium	SODIUM EDECRIN	Diuretic	**Powd for Inj:** 50 mg	0.5 - 1.0 mg/kg IV (maximum: 100 mg).
Ethacrynic Acid	EDECRIN	Diuretic	**Tab:** 25, 50 mg	50 - 100 mg daily po.
Ethambutol Hydrochloride	MYAMBUTOL	Tuberculostatic	**Tab:** 100, 400 mg	**Initial:** 15 mg/kg po as a single dose q 24 h. **Retreatment:** 25 mg/kg po as a single dose q 24 h. After 60 days, decrease dose to 15 mg/kg po as a single dose q 24 h.
Ethinyl Estradiol (*)	ESTINYL	Estrogen, Antineoplastic	**Tab:** 0.02, 0.05, 0.5 mg	**Vasomotor Symptoms associated with Menopause:** 0.02 - 0.05 mg daily po. Administration should be cyclic (3 weeks on, 1 week off). **Prostatic Cancer:** 0.15 - 2.0 mg daily po. **Breast Cancer:** 1.0 mg tid po.
Ethionamide (*)	TRECATOR-SC	Tuberculostatic	**Tab:** 250 mg	15 - 20 mg/kg daily po taken once daily (up to a maximum of 1 g/day).

GENERIC NAME	COMMON TRADE NAMES	THERAPEUTIC CATEGORY	PREPARATIONS	COMMON ADULT DOSAGE
Ethotoin (*)	PEGANONE	Antiepileptic	Tab: 250, 500 mg	**Initial:** 1 g or less daily po in 4 - 6 divided doses, with gradual increases over a period of several days. Take after meals. **Maintenance:** Usually 2 - 3 g daily po in 4 - 6 divided doses after food.
Etidronate Disodium	DIDRONEL IV	Bone Stabilizer	Inj: 300 mg/6 mL	7.5 mg/kg daily by IV infusion (over at least 2 h) for 3 days. Daily dose must be diluted in at least 250 mL of sterile normal saline.
Etodolac	LODINE	Non-Opioid Analgesic, Antiinflammatory	Cpsl: 200, 300 mg Tab: 400, 500 mg	**Analgesia:** 200 - 400 mg q 6 - 8 h po. **Osteoarthritis & Rheumatoid Arthritis:** Initially, 300 mg bid or tid po, 400 mg bid po, or 500 mg bid po. Adjust dosage within 600 to 1200 mg/day po prn for maintenance.
	LODINE XL	Antiinflammatory	Extended-Rel. Tab: 400, 500, 600 mg	**Osteoarthritis & Rheumatoid Arthritis:** 400 to 1000 mg once daily po.
Etoposide (*)	VEPESID	Antineoplastic	Inj: 100 mg/5 mL	**Testicular Cancer:** Ranges from 50 - 100 mg/m^2/day IV for days 1 - 5 to 100 mg/m^2/day IV for day 1, 3 and 5. Repeat at 3 - 4 week intervals. **Small Cell Lung Cancer:** Ranges from 35 mg/m^2/day IV for 4 days to 50 mg/m^2/day IV for 5 days. Repeat at 3 - 4 week intervals.
			Cpsl: 50 mg	**Small Cell Lung Cancer:** Twice the IV dose po, rounded to the nearest 50 mg.
Ezetimibe	ZETIA	Antihyperlipidemic	Tab: 10 mg	10 mg once daily po.
Famciclovir (*)	FAMVIR	Antiviral	Tab: 125, 250, 500 mg	**Herpes zoster:** 500 mg q 8 h po for 7 days. **Genital Herpes (Recurrent):** 125 mg bid po for 5 days.

102

Famotidine (*)	PEPCID	Histamine H$_2$-Blocker, Anti-Ulcer Agent	Powd for Susp: 40 mg/5 mL Tab: 20, 40 mg	**Duodenal Ulcer:** **Acute:** 40 mg hs po; or 20 mg bid po. **Maintenance:** 20 mg hs po. **Active Benign Gastric Ulcer:** 40 mg hs po. **Pathol. Hypersecr. Conditions:** 20 mg q 6 h po. **Gastroesophageal Reflux Disease:** 20 mg bid po for up to 6 weeks.
	PEPCID INJECTION PEPCID INJECTION PREMIXED		Inj: 10 mg/mL Inj: 20 mg/50 mL	20 mg q 12 h IV. 20 mg q 12 h by IV infusion (over 15 - 30 minutes).
	PEPCID AC MYLANTA AR ACID REDUCER	Histamine H$_2$-Blocker	Tab & Gelcap: 10 mg Chewable Tab: 10 mg Tab: 10 mg	**Heartburn, Acid Indigestion & Sour Stomach:** **Treatment:** 10 mg po with water up to bid. **Prevention:** 10 mg po 1 h prior to eating symptom-causing foods or drinks. Repeat up to bid.
Felbamate (*)	FELBATOL	Antiepileptic	Tab: 400, 600 mg Susp: 600 mg/5 mL	**Monotherapy:** Begin at 1200 mg/day po, in 3 to 4 divided doses. Titrate under close supervision, increasing the dosage in 600 mg increments q 2 weeks to 2400 mg/day, and thereafter to 3600 mg/day if indicated. **Adjunctive Therapy:** Add 1200 mg/day po (in 3 to 4 divided doses) while lowering the dose of present antiepileptic drug by 20%. Further reductions in these drug may be necessary to minimize adverse effects due to drug interactions. Raise the dosage of felbamate by 1200 mg/day increments at weekly intervals to 3600 mg/day if necessary.
Felodipine	PLENDIL	Antihypertensive	Extended-Rel. Tab: 2.5, 5, 10 mg	Initially, 5 mg once daily po. Dosage may be decreased to 2.5 mg or increased to 10 mg once daily po after 2 weeks.

GENERIC NAME	COMMON TRADE NAMES	THERAPEUTIC CATEGORY	PREPARATIONS	COMMON ADULT DOSAGE
Fenofibrate	TRICOR	Antihyperlipidemic	Tab: 54, 160 mg	**Primary Hypercholesterolemia and Mixed Hyperlipidemia:** Initially, 160 mg daily po. **Hypertriglyceridemia:** Initially 54 - 160 mg daily po with meals. The maximum dose is 160 mg daily.
Fenoprofen Calcium (*)	NALFON	Non-Opioid Analgesic, Antiinflammatory	**Cpsl:** 200, 300 mg **Tab:** 600 mg	**Analgesia:** 200 mg q 4 - 6 h po, prn. **Rheumatoid Arthritis and Osteoarthritis:** 300 to 600 mg tid to qid po.
Fentanyl (*) (C-II)	DURAGESIC	Opioid Analgesic	**Transdermal:** rate = 25, 50, 75, 100 μg/hr	Individualize dosage. Each system may be worn for up to 72 h.
Fentanyl Citrate (*) (C-II)	SUBLIMAZE	Opioid Analgesic	**Inj:** 50 μg/mL (as the base)	2 - 50 μg/kg IM or IV.
	FENTANYL ORALET	Opioid Analgesic	**Lozenge:** 100, 200, 300, 400 μg	Administer only in a hospital setting. Individualize dosage. Fentanyl transmucosal doses of 5 μg/kg (400 μg) provide effects similar to usual doses of fentanyl citrate given IM, i.e., 0.75 - 1.25 μg/kg. Oral administration should begin 20 - 40 minutes prior to anticipated need of desired effect.
	ACTIQ		**Lozenge on a Stick:** 200, 400, 600, 800, 1200, 1600 μg	Initial dose to treat episodes of breakthrough cancer pain should be 200 μg consumed over a 15-min. period. Prescribe an initial titration supply of six 200 μg units. Advise patients to use all units before increasing to a higher dose. Redosing should not occur more often than q 30 min. Dose increases may be occur after evaluation over several episodes of breakthrough cancer pain.
Ferrous Gluconate (*) (11.6% iron)	FERGON	Hematinic	**Tab:** 320 mg	320 mg daily po.

Drug	Brand	Class	Form/Strength	Dosage
Ferrous Sulfate (*) (20% iron)	FEOSOL	Hematinic	Elixir: 220 mg/5 mL (5% alcohol)	5 - 10 mL tid po, preferably between meals.
	FER-IN-SOL		Syrup: 90 mg/5 mL (5% alc.)	5 mL daily po.
	FERO-GRADUMET		Controlled-Rel. Tab: 525 mg	525 mg once daily or bid po.
Ferrous Sulfate, Exsiccated (30% iron)	FEOSOL	Hematinic	Tab: 200 mg Cpsl: 159 mg	200 mg tid - qid po pc & hs. 159 - 318 mg daily po.
	FER-IN-SOL		Cpsl: 190 mg	1 capsule daily po.
	SLOW FE		Slow Release Tab: 160 mg	160 - 320 mg daily po.
Fexofenadine Hydrochloride (*)	ALLEGRA	Antihistamine	Tab: 30, 60, 180 mg Cpsl: 60 mg	**Chronic Idiopathic Urticaria:** 60 mg bid po. **Seasonal Allergic Rhinitis:** 180 mg once daily po or 60 mg bid po.
Finasteride	PROSCAR	Benign Prostatic Hyperplasia Drug	Tab: 5 mg	5 mg once daily po.
	PROPECIA	Hair Growth Stimulator	Tab: 1 mg	1 mg once daily po.
Flavoxate Hydrochloride	URISPAS	Urinary Tract Antispasmodic	Tab: 100 mg	100 - 200 mg tid or qid po.
Flecainide Acetate (*)	TAMBOCOR	Antiarrhythmic	Tab: 50, 100, 150 mg	Initially, 100 mg q 12 h po. May increase in increments of 50 mg bid q 4 days.
Floxuridine	STERILE FUDR	Antineoplastic	Powd for Inj: 500 mg	0.1 - 0.6 mg/kg/day by intra-arterial infusion.

GENERIC NAME	COMMON TRADE NAMES	THERAPEUTIC CATEGORY	PREPARATIONS	COMMON ADULT DOSAGE
Fluconazole (*)	DIFLUCAN	Antifungal	Tab: 50, 100, 150, 200 mg Powd for Susp: 10, 40 mg/mL Inj: 200 mg/100 mL, 400 mg/200 mL	**Oropharyngeal Candidiasis:** 200 mg on the first day, followed by 100 mg once daily po or IV. Continue treatment for at least 2 weeks. **Esophageal Candidiasis:** 200 mg on the first day, followed by 100 mg once daily po or IV. Doses up to 400 mg may be used based on the patient response. Continue treatment for a minimum of 3 weeks and at least 2 weeks following resolution of symptoms. **Systemic Candidiasis and Cryptococcal Meningitis:** 400 mg on the first day, followed by 200 mg once daily po or IV. **Vaginal Candidiasis:** 150 mg po as a single dose.
Flucytosine (*)	ANCOBON	Antifungal	Cpsl: 250, 500 mg	50 - 150 mg/kg/day po in divided doses at 6-hour intervals.
Fludrocortisone Acetate	FLORINEF ACETATE	Mineralocorticoid	Tab: 0.1 mg	0.1 mg daily po. If transient hypertension develops, reduce dosage to 0.05 mg daily.
Flumazenil (*)	ROMAZICON	Benzodiazepine Antagonist	Inj: 0.1 mg/mL	**Reversal of Conscious Sedation or in General Anesthesia:** Initially 0.2 mg IV (over 15 seconds). After 45 seconds, a further dose of 0.2 mg can be injected and repeated at 60-second intervals where necessary (up to a maximum of 4 additional times) to a maximum total dose of 1 mg. **Management of Suspected Benzodiazepine Overdose:** Initially 0.2 mg IV (over 30 seconds). After 30 seconds, a further dose of 0.3 mg can be injected (over 30 seconds). Further doses of 0.5 mg can be given (over 30 seconds) at 60-second intervals up to a cumulative dose of 3 mg.

Flunisolide		Corticosteroid (Topical)	Aerosol: 250 μg/spray	2 inhalations bid AM and PM.
	NASALIDE, NASAREL		Spray: 25 μg/spray	2 sprays in each nostril bid.
Fluocinolone Acetonide	SYNALAR	Corticosteroid (Topical)	Cream: 0.01, 0.025% Oint: 0.025% Solution: 0.01%	Apply as a thin film bid - qid.
	SYNALAR-HP		Cream: 0.2%	Apply as a thin film bid - qid.
Fluocinonide	LIDEX	Corticosteroid (Topical)	Cream, Oint & Solution: 0.05%	Apply as a thin film bid - qid.
Fluorometholone	FML	Corticosteroid (Topical)	Ophth Susp: 0.1%	1 drop into affected eye(s) bid - qid. During the initial 24 - 48 hours, the frequency of dosing may be increased if necessary.
	FML FORTE		Ophth Susp: 0.25%	1 drop into affected eye(s) bid - qid.
	FML		Ophth Oint: 0.1%	Apply 1/2 inch ribbon to eye(s) q 4 h for the 1st 24 - 48 h. When a favorable response is observed, reduce dosage to 1 - 3 times daily.
Fluorometholone Acetate	FLAREX	Corticosteroid (Topical)	Ophth Susp: 0.1%	1 - 2 drops into affected eye(s) qid. May initiate with 2 drops q 2 h during the initial 24 - 48 hours; then, the frequency of dosing may be decreased.
Fluorouracil (*)	FLUOROURACIL INJECTION	Antineoplastic	Inj: 500 mg/10 mL	12 mg/kg daily IV for 4 days. If no toxicity is observed, 6 mg/kg are given on days 6, 8, 10 and 12. May repeat course in 30 days.
	EFUDEX	Antineoplastic (Topical)	Cream: 5% Solution: 2, 5%	**Actinic or Solar Keratosis:** Cover lesions bid; continue therapy for at least 2 - 4 weeks. **Superficial Basal Cell Carcinomas:** Use only 5% cream or solution. Cover lesions bid; continue therapy for at least 3 - 6 weeks.

[Continued on the next page]

GENERIC NAME	COMMON TRADE NAMES	THERAPEUTIC CATEGORY	PREPARATIONS	COMMON ADULT DOSAGE
Fluorouracil [Continued]	FLUOROPLEX	Antineoplastic (Topical)	**Cream & Solution:** 1%	Cover all lesions bid. Continue therapy for 2 to 6 weeks.
	CARAC	Drug for Actinic Keratoses	**Cream:** 0.5% (0.35% in microspheres)	**Actinic or Solar Keratosis:** Apply a thin film to skin where lesions appear once daily for up to 4 weeks.
Fluoxetine Hydrochloride (*)	PROZAC	Antidepressant, Drug for Obsessive-Compulsive Disorder	**Cpsl:** 10, 20, 40 mg (as the base) **Tab:** 10 mg (as the base) **Liquid:** 20 mg/5 mL (as the base) (0.23% alcohol)	20 mg daily po in the AM. May increase dose after several weeks to 20 mg bid po. Do not exceed maximum dose of 80 mg/day.
	PROZAC WEEKLY	Antidepressant	**Delayed-Rel. Cpsl:** 90 mg (as the base)	90 mg once weekly po. Initiate 7 days after the last 20 mg daily dose.
	SARAFEM	Drug for Premenstrual Dysphoric Disorder	**Cpsl:** 10, 20 mg (as the base)	20 mg once daily po.
Fluoxymesterone (C-III)	HALOTESTIN	Androgen	**Tab:** 2, 5, 10 mg	**Male Hypogonadism:** 5 - 20 mg daily po as a single dose or in 3 - 4 divided doses. **Breast Cancer:** 10 - 40 mg daily po in 3 - 4 divided doses.
Fluphenazine Decanoate (*)	PROLIXIN DECANOATE	Antipsychotic	**Inj:** 25 mg/mL	12.5 - 25 mg IM or SC.
Fluphenazine Hydrochloride (*)	PROLIXIN	Antipsychotic	**Tab:** 1, 2.5, 5, 10 mg **Elixir:** 2.5 mg/5 mL (14% alcohol) **Inj:** 2.5 mg/mL	2.5 - 10 mg daily po in divided doses at 6- to 8-hour intervals. 1.25 - 10 mg daily IM in divided doses at 6- to 8-hour intervals.
Flurandrenolide	CORDRAN	Corticosteroid (Topical)	**Cream & Oint:** 0.025, 0.05% **Lotion:** 0.05% **Tape:** 4 mcg/cm²	Apply as a thin film to affected areas bid - tid and rub in gently. Apply to affected areas; replace q 12 h.

Generic	Brand	Class	Form/Strength	Dosage
Flurazepam Hydrochloride (*) (C-IV)	DALMANE	Hypnotic	Cpsl: 15, 30 mg	15 - 30 mg hs po.
Flurbiprofen (*)	ANSAID	Antiinflammatory	Tab: 50, 100 mg	200 - 300 mg daily, given bid, tid or qid po.
Flurbiprofen Sodium	OCUFEN	Antiinflammatory (Topical)	Ophth Solution: 0.03%	1 drop in eye q 30 minutes, beginning 2 h before surgery (total of 4 drops).
Flutamide	EULEXIN	Antineoplastic	Cpsl: 125 mg	250 mg tid po at 8-hour intervals.
Fluticasone Propionate	CUTIVATE	Corticosteroid (Topical)	Oint: 0.005% Cream: 0.05%	Apply a thin film to affected skin areas bid. Rub in gently.
	FLONASE		Nasal Spray: 50 μg/spray	Initially, 2 sprays in each nostril once daily or 1 spray in each nostril twice daily (morning and evening). May decrease to 1 spray in each nostril once daily based on response. **For Adolescents over 12 yrs:** Initially, 1 spray in each nostril once daily; may increase to 2 sprays in each nostril once daily, then may decrease to 1 spray in each nostril once daily based on response.
	FLOVENT 44 mcg FLOVENT 110 mcg FLOVENT 220 mcg		Aerosol: 44 μg/spray Aerosol: 110 μg/spray Aerosol: 220 μg/spray	**Patients Previously Using Bronchodilators Only:** 88 μg bid. **Patients Previously Using Inhaled Corticosteroids:** 88 - 220 μg bid. **Patient Previously Using Oral Corticosteroids:** 880 μg bid.
	FLOVENT DISKUS		Powd for Inhalation: 50, 100, 250 μg/actuation	**Patients Previously Using Bronchodilators Only:** 100 μg bid. **Patients Previously Using Inhaled Corticosteroids:** 100 - 250 μg bid. **Patient Previously Using Oral Corticosteroids:** 500 - 1000 μg bid.

GENERIC NAME	COMMON TRADE NAMES	THERAPEUTIC CATEGORY	PREPARATIONS	COMMON ADULT DOSAGE
Fluvastatin Sodium	LESCOL	Antihyperlipidemic	Cpsl: 20, 40 mg	For an LDL cholesterol reduction of at least 25%, start with 40 mg po in the evening or 40 mg bid. For less LDL cholesterol reduction, a starting dose of 20 mg is recommended. Adjust dosage after about 4 weeks.
	LESCOL XL		Extended-Rel. Tab: 80 mg	For an LDL cholesterol reduction of at least 25%, 80 mg once daily po in the evening.
Fluvoxamine Maleate (*)	LUVOX	Drug for Obsessive-Compulsive Disorder	Tab: 25, 50, 100 mg	Initially, 50 mg hs po. Increase dose in 50 mg increments q 4 - 7 days, as tolerated, until maximum therapeutic benefit occurs. Daily dosages over 100 mg should be given in divided doses (bid). Maximum: 300 mg/day.
Folic Acid		Vitamin	Tab: 0.4, 0.8, 1 mg	Usual Therapeutic Dose: up to 1 mg daily po.
Formoterol Fumarate	FORADIL AEROLIZER	Bronchodilator	Inhalation Powd in Cpsl:	Maintenance of Asthma and COPD Therapy: 12 µg using the Aerolizer Inhaler. Treatment of Exercise-Induced Bronchospasm: 12 µg by inhalation at least 15 min before exercise, administered prn.
Foscarnet Sodium	FOSCAVIR	Antiviral	Inj: 24 mg/mL	CMV Retinitis: Initial: 60 mg/kg IV (at a constant rate over a minimum of 1 h) q 8 h for 2 - 3 weeks. Maintenance: 90 mg/kg/day by IV infusion (over 2 h). Herpes Simplex Infection: Initial: 40 mg/kg by IV infusion (over at least 1 h) q 8 or 12 h for 2 - 3 weeks or until healed. Maintenance: 90 mg/kg/day by IV infusion (over 2 h).

Fosfomycin Tromethamine	MONUROL	Urinary Ant-Infective	**Granules:** 3 g	**Women > 18 yrs:** Pour the contents of 1 packet into 3 - 4 fl. oz. of water; stir to dissolve. Drink immediately.
Fosinopril Sodium	MONOPRIL	Antihypertensive, Heart Failure Drug	**Tab:** 10, 20, 40 mg	**Hypertension:** Initially, 10 mg once daily po. May increase dosage to usual range: 20 to 40 mg daily. **Heart Failure:** Initially, 10 mg once daily po. Increase dosage over several weeks to a maximal and tolerated dose not to exceed 40 mg once daily.
Fosphenytoin Sodium (*)	CEREBYX	Antiepileptic	**Powd for Inj:** 150 mg (100 mg of phenytoin sodium), 750 mg (500 mg of phenytoin sodium)	Dosages given as phenytoin sodium equivalent units (PE). **Status Epilepticus:** Loading Dose of 15 - 20 mg PE/kg IV given at 100 - 150 mg PE/min. **Nonemergent and Maintenance Dosing:** **Loading Dose:** 10 - 20 mg PE/kg IM or IV (at a rate ≤ 150 mg PE/min). **Maintenance Dose:** 4 - 6 PE/kg/day.
Frovatriptan Succinate	FROVA	Antimigraine Agent	**Tab:** 2.5 mg	2.5 mg po with fluids. May repeat after 2 h. Maximum: 7.5 mg in 24 h.
Furazolidone	FUROXONE	Antibacterial	**Liquid:** 50 mg/15 mL **Tab:** 100 mg	100 mg qid po.
Furosemide (*)	LASIX	Diuretic, Antihypertensive	**Solution:** 10 mg/mL (11.5% alcohol) **Tab:** 20, 40, 80 mg	**Diuresis:** 20 - 80 mg daily po. May repeat in 6 to 8 h if needed. **Hypertension:** 40 mg bid po.
		Diuretic	**Inj:** 10 mg/mL	**Diuresis:** 20 - 40 mg IM or IV (over 1 - 2 min). **Acute Pulmonary Edema:** 40 mg IV (over 1 - 2 min). If response is not adequate after 1 h, dose may be doubled.
Gabapentin (*)	NEURONTIN	Antiepileptic, Drug for Postherpetic Neuralgia	**Oral Solution:** 250 mg/5 mL **Cpsl:** 100, 300, 400 mg **Tab:** 600, 800 mg	Titrate with 300 mg po on day 1, 300 mg bid po on day 2, and 300 mg tid po on day 3. If necessary, the dosage may be increased by using 300 - 400 mg tid up to 1800 mg/day.

GENERIC NAME	COMMON TRADE NAMES	THERAPEUTIC CATEGORY	PREPARATIONS	COMMON ADULT DOSAGE
Galantamine Hydrobromide	REMINYL	Drug for Alzheimer's Disease	Tab: 4, 8, 12 mg Oral Solution: 4 mg/mL	Initially, 4 mg bid po. After a minimum of 4 weeks, if well tolerated, increase to 8 mg bid po. Attempt to further increase to 12 mg bid after only a minimum of 4 weeks at the previous dose.
Ganciclovir	CYTOVENE	Antiviral	Cpsl: 250, 500 mg	**CMV Retinitis (Maintenance):** Following the IV induction treatment with CYTOVENE-IV (see below), 1000 mg tid po with food. Alternatively, 500 mg 6 times daily po (q 3 h during waking hours) with food. **Prevention of CMV in Patients with Advanced HIV Infection:** 1000 mg tid po with food.
Ganciclovir Sodium	CYTOVENE-IV	Antiviral	Powd for Inj: 500 mg	**CMV Retinitis:** **Induction:** 5 mg/kg IV (at a constant rate over 1 hour), q 12 h for 14 - 21 days. **Maintenance:** 5 mg/kg IV (at a constant rate over 1 hour), once daily 7 days each week, or 6 mg/kg IV once daily on 5 days each week. **Prevention of CMV in Transplant Recipients:** Initially, 5 mg/kg IV (at a constant rate over 1 hour), q 12 h for 7 - 14 days; then, 5 mg/kg IV once daily 7 days each week, or 6 mg/kg IV once daily on 5 days each week.
Gatifloxacin Sesquihydrate	TEQUIN	Antibacterial	Tab: 200, 400 mg Inj: 10, 20 mg/mL	**Urinary Tract Infections (Complicated) & Acute Pyelonephritis:** 400 mg once daily po or by slow IV infusion for 7 - 10 days. **Urinary Tract Infections (Uncomplicated):** 200 mg once daily po or by slow IV infusion for 3 days, or 400 mg po or by slow IV infusion as a single dose. **Community-Acquired Pneumonia:** 400 mg once daily po or by slow IV infusion for 7 - 14 days.

				Acute Bacterial Exacerbation of Chronic Brochitis: 400 mg once daily po or by slow IV infusion for 5 days. **Acute Sinusitis:** 400 mg once daily po or by slow IV infusion for 10 days. **Gonorrhea:** 400 mg po or by slow IV infusion as a single dose.
Gemfibrozil	LOPID	Antihyperlipidemic	**Tab:** 600 mg	600 mg bid po 30 minutes before the morning and evening meal.
Gentamicin Sulfate (*)	GARAMYCIN	Antibacterial (Topical)	**Cream & Oint:** 0.1%	Apply to affected areas tid to qid.
			Ophth Solution: 3 mg/mL	1 - 2 drops into affected eye(s) q 4 h. In severe infections, dosage may be increased to as much as 2 drops once every hour.
			Ophth Oint: 3 mg/g	Apply to affected eye(s) bid or tid.
		Antibacterial	**Inj:** 40 mg/mL	**Usual Dosage:** 3 mg/kg/day IM or IV divided in 3 doses at 8-hour intervals. **Life-Threatening Infections:** Up to 5 mg/kg/day may be administered in 3 or 4 equal doses.
Glatiramer Acetate	COPAXONE	Multiple Sclerosis Drug	**Powd for Inj:** 20 mg	20 mg daily SC.
Glimepiride	AMARYL	Hypoglycemic Agent	**Tab:** 1, 2, 4 mg	**Initial:** 1 - 2 mg once daily po, given with breakfast or the first main meal. **Maintenance:** 1 - 4 mg once daily po. After a dose of 2 mg is reached, increase the dose at increments of ≤ 2 mg at 1 - 2 week intervals based on patient's blood glucose.
Glipizide	GLUCOTROL	Hypoglycemic Agent	**Tab:** 5, 10 mg	**Initial:** 5 mg daily po before breakfast. **Titration:** As determined by blood glucose response, increase dosage in increments of 2.5 - 5 mg. At least several days should elapse between titration steps. **Maintenance:** Total daily doses above 15 mg should ordinarily be divided, e.g., bid.

[Continued on the next page]

GENERIC NAME	COMMON TRADE NAMES	THERAPEUTIC CATEGORY	PREPARATIONS	COMMON ADULT DOSAGE
Glipizide [Continued]	GLUCOTROL XL		Extended-Rel. Tab: 2.5, 5, 10 mg	Initially, 5 mg daily po with breakfast. Usual dosage range: 5 - 10 mg daily po.
Glyburide (*)	DIAβETA, MICRONASE	Hypoglycemic Agent	Tab: 1.25, 2.5, 5 mg	Initial: 1.25 - 5 mg daily po with breakfast. Maintenance: 1.25 - 20 mg daily po as a single dose or in divided doses.
Glyburide Micronized	GLYNASE PRESTAB	Hypoglycemic Agent	Tab: 1.5, 3, 6 mg	Initial: 0.75 - 3 mg daily po with breakfast. Maintenance: 0.75 - 12 mg daily po as a single dose or in divided doses.
Glycopyrrolate	ROBINUL	Anticholinergic	Tab: 1 mg	Initial: 1 mg tid po (in the morning, early afternoon, and hs. Maintenance: 1 mg bid po is often adequate.
	ROBINUL FORTE		Tab: 2 mg	2 mg bid or tid po at equally spaced intervals.
Gold Sodium Thiomalate		Antirheumatic	Inj (per mL): 50 mg	Weekly IM injections as follows: 1st— 10 mg; 2nd— 25 mg; 3rd and subsequent— 25 - 50 mg until toxicity or major improvement. Maintenance doses: 25 - 50 mg every other week for 2 - 20 weeks. If condition remains stable, give 25 - 50 mg every 3rd week.
Goserelin Acetate	ZOLADEX	Antineoplastic	Powd for Inj: 3.6 mg	3.6 mg q 28 days by SC injection into the upper abdominal wall.
Granisetron Hydrochloride	KYTRIL	Antiemetic	Tab: 1.12 mg (1 mg as the base)	1 mg bid po. The 1st dose is given up to 1 h before chemotherapy and the 2nd dose 12 h after the 1st, only on the days chemotherapy is given.
			Inj: 1.12 mg/mL (1 mg/mL as the base)	10 μg/kg, infused IV over 5 minutes, beginning within 30 minutes before initiation of chemotherapy, and only on the days that chemotherapy is given.

Griseofulvin Microsize	FULVICIN U/F	Antifungal	**Tab:** 250, 500 mg	500 mg daily po as a single dose or in divided doses.
	GRIFULVIN V		**Susp:** 125 mg/5 mL **Tab:** 250, 500 mg	500 mg daily po.
Griseofulvin Ultramicrosize	FULVICIN P/G	Antifungal	**Tab:** 125, 165, 250, 330 mg	330 - 375 mg daily po as a single dose or in divided doses.
	GRIS-PEG		**Tab:** 125, 250 mg	375 mg daily po (single dose or in div. doses).
Guaifenesin (*)	ROBITUSSIN	Expectorant	**Syrup:** 100 mg/5 mL	10 - 20 mL (100 - 400 mg) q 4 h po.
	ORGANIDIN NR		**Liquid:** 100 mg/5 mL **Tab:** 200 mg	200 - 400 mg q 4 h po. 200 - 400 mg q 4 h po.
	HUMIBID L.A.		**Sustained-Rel. Tab:** 600 mg	
	DURATUSS G		**Long-Acting Tab:** 1200 mg	1200 mg q 12 h po.
Guanabenz Acetate	WYTENSIN	Antihypertensive	**Tab:** 4, 8 mg	Initially, 4 mg bid po. May increase dosage in increments of 4 - 8 mg/day q 1 - 2 weeks.
Guanadrel Sulfate	HYLOREL	Antihypertensive	**Tab:** 10, 25 mg	Initially, 5 mg bid po. Adjust dosage weekly; most require 20 - 75 mg/day (given bid).
Guanethidine Monosulfate (*)	ISMELIN	Antihypertensive	**Tab:** 10, 25 mg	**Ambulatory Patients:** Initially, 10 mg daily po. Dosage should be increased gradually, no more often than every 5 - 7 days. Average daily dose is 25 - 50 mg po. **Hospitalized Patients:** Initially, 25 - 50 mg po. May increase by 25 or 50 mg daily or every other day.
Guanfacine Hydrochloride	TENEX	Antihypertensive	**Tab:** 1, 2 mg	1 mg daily po hs. Dose may be increased after 3 - 4 weeks to 2 mg if necessary.
Halcinonide	HALOG	Corticosteroid (Topical)	**Cream, Oint & Solution:** 0.1%	Apply to affected areas bid to tid.

GENERIC NAME	COMMON TRADE NAMES	THERAPEUTIC CATEGORY	PREPARATIONS	COMMON ADULT DOSAGE
Halobetasol Propionate	ULTRAVATE	Corticosteroid (Topical)	Cream & Oint: 0.05%	Apply a thin layer to affected skin once or twice daily. Rub in gently and completely.
Halofantrine Hydrochloride	HALFAN	Antimalarial	Tab: 250 mg	**Non-Immune Patients:** 500 mg q 6 h po for 3 doses, with a repeat course of therapy given 7 days after the first. **Semi-Immune Patients:** 500 mg q 6 h po for 3 doses. A second course of therapy given 7 days after the first is optional. Give on an empty stomach at least 1 h ac or 2 h pc.
Haloperidol (*)	HALDOL	Antipsychotic	Tab: 0.5, 1, 2, 5, 10, 20 mg	0.5 - 5 mg bid to tid po.
Haloperidol Decanoate	HALDOL DECANOATE 50 HALDOL DECANOATE 100	Antipsychotic	Inj: 70.5 mg/mL (50 mg/mL as the base) Inj: 141.0 mg/mL (100 mg/mL as the base)	Administer once q 4 wks by deep IM injection. For patients previously maintained on antipsychotics, the recommended initial dose is 10 - 15 times the previous daily dose in oral haloperidol equivalents. The initial dose should not exceed 100 mg.
Haloperidol Lactate	HALDOL	Antipsychotic	Liquid Conc: 2 mg/mL Inj: 5 mg/mL	0.5 - 5 mg bid to tid po. 2 - 5 mg q 4 - 8 h IM.
Heparin Sodium (*)		Anticoagulant	Inj: 1,000 - 40,000 units/mL	**Deep SC:** 5000 units IV, followed by 10,000 to 20,000 units SC. Then 8,000 - 10,000 units q 8 h or 15,000 - 20,000 units q 12 h. **Intermittent IV:** 10,000 units undiluted or in 50 - 100 mL of 0.9% sodium chloride injection. Then 5,000 - 10,000 units undiluted or in sodium chloride injection q 4 - 6 h. **IV Infusion:** 5,000 units IV; then 20,000 to 40,000 units/24 h in 1,000 mL of 0.9% NaCl injection by continuous IV infusion.

Generic	Brand	Class	Forms	Dosage
Homatropine Hydrobromide	ISOPTO HOMATROPINE	Mydriatic - Cycloplegic	Ophth Solution: 2, 5%	**Refraction:** Instill 1 - 2 drops in the eye(s). May be repeated in 5 - 10 min, if necessary. **Uveitis:** Instill 1 - 2 drops in the eye(s) q 3 - 4 h.
Hydralazine Hydrochloride (*)	APRESOLINE	Antihypertensive	Tab: 10, 25, 50, 100 mg	Initiate therapy in gradually increasing doses: 10 mg qid for 2 - 4 days, increase to 25 mg qid for the rest of the week. For the 2nd and subsequent weeks, raise to 50 mg qid. 20 - 40 mg IM or IV, repeated as necessary.
			Inj: 20 mg/mL	
Hydrochlorothiazide (*)	MICROZIDE	Antihypertensive	Cpsl: 12.5 mg	12.5 mg once daily po.
	ESIDRIX, HYDRODIURIL	Diuretic, Antihypertensive	Tab: 25, 50, 100 mg	**Diuresis:** 25 - 100 mg daily or bid po. **Hypertension:** 50 - 100 mg daily po in the AM.
Hydrocortisone	HYDROCORTONE	Corticosteroid	Tab: 10 mg	Initial dosage varies from 20 - 240 mg daily po depending on the disease being treated and the patient's response.
	CORTEF	Corticosteroid	Tab: 5, 10, 20 mg	
	CORTENEMA	Corticosteroid (Topical)	**Retention Enema:** 100 mg/60 mL	Use 1 enema rectally nightly for 21 days or until patient comes into remission.
	ANUSOL-HC 2.5%, PROCTOCREAM-HC 2.5%	Corticosteroid (Topical)	Cream: 2.5%	Apply as a thin film to affected areas bid - qid.
	CORT-DOME	Corticosteroid (Topical)	Cream: 0.5, 1%	Apply as a thin film to affected areas bid - qid.
	HYTONE	Corticosteroid (Topical)	Cream, Oint & Lotion: 2.5%	Apply as a thin film to affected areas bid - qid.
Hydrocortisone Acetate	HYDROCORTONE ACETATE	Corticosteroid	Inj (per mL): 25, 50 mg [low solubility; provides a prolonged effect]	**Only for Intra-articular, Intralesional and Soft Tissue Injection:** Dose and frequency of injection are variable and must be individualized on the basis of the disease and the response of the patient. The initial dosage varies from 5 - 75 mg a day.

[Continued on the next page]

117

GENERIC NAME	COMMON TRADE NAMES	THERAPEUTIC CATEGORY	PREPARATIONS	COMMON ADULT DOSAGE
Hydrocortisone Acetate [Continued]	ANUSOL HC-1 ANUSOL-HC	Corticosteroid (Topical)	Oint: 1% Rectal Suppos: 25 mg	Apply as a thin film to affected areas bid - qid. Insert 1 rectally AM and PM for 2 weeks. In more severe cases, 1 rectally tid or 2 bid.
	CORTICAINE		Cream: 0.5, 1%	Apply as a thin film to affected areas up to qid.
	CORTIFOAM		Aerosol: 10% (with rectal applicator)	1 applicatorful rectally once or twice daily for 2 - 3 weeks, and every 2nd day thereafter.
Hydrocortisone Buteprate	PANDEL	Corticosteroid (Topical)	Cream: 1%	Apply a thin film to affected areas once or twice daily.
Hydrocortisone Butyrate	LOCOID	Corticosteroid (Topical)	Cream, Oint & Solution: 0.1%	Apply to affected area as a thin film bid to tid.
Hydrocortisone Sodium Phosphate	HYDROCORTONE PHOSPHATE	Corticosteroid	Inj: 50 mg/mL [water soluble; rapid onset, short duration]	For IV, IM & SC Injection: Dose requirements vary and must be individualized on the basis of the disease and the response of the patient. Initial daily dose: from 15 - 240 mg.
Hydrocortisone Sodium Succinate	SOLU-CORTEF	Corticosteroid	Powd for Inj: 100, 250, 500, 1000 mg	100 - 500 mg IM, IV, or by IV infusion. Repeat at intervals of 2, 4, or 6 h.
Hydrocortisone Valerate	WESTCORT	Corticosteroid (Topical)	Cream & Oint: 0.2%	Apply to affected areas as a thin film bid to tid.
Hydroflumethiazide	DIUCARDIN, SALURON	Diuretic, Antihypertensive	Tab: 50 mg	Diuresis: 50 mg once or twice daily po. Hypertension: 50 mg bid po.
Hydromorphone Hydrochloride (*) (C-II)	DILAUDID	Opioid Analgesic	Tab: 2, 3, 4, 8 mg Oral Liquid: 5 mg/5 mL Inj: 1, 2, 4 mg/mL Rectal Suppos: 3 mg	2 mg q 4 - 6 h po, prn. More severe pain may require 4 mg or more q 4 - 6 h po. 2.5 - 10 mg (2.5 - 10 mL) q 3 - 6 h po. 1 - 2 mg q 4 - 6 h SC or IM, prn. For IV use, give dose slowly over at least 2 - 3 minutes. Insert 1 suppository rectally q 6 - 8 h.
	DILAUDID-HP	Opioid Analgesic	Inj: 10 mg/mL Powd for Inj: 250 mg	1 - 2 mg q 4 - 6 h SC or IM.

118

Generic	Brand	Class	Formulation	Dosing
Hydroxyurea	HYDREA	Antineoplastic	Cpsl: 500 mg	**Solid Tumors:** **Intermittent Therapy:** 80 mg/kg po as a single dose every 3rd day. **Continuous Therapy:** 20 - 30 mg/kg po as a single dose daily. **Resistant Chronic Myelocytic Leukemia:** 20 to 30 mg/kg po as a single dose daily.
Hydroxyzine Hydrochloride (*)	ATARAX	Sedative, Antipruritic, Antianxiety Agent	Syrup: 10 mg/5 mL. (0.5% alcohol) Tab: 10, 25, 50, 100 mg	**Sedation:** 50 - 100 mg po. **Pruritis:** 25 mg tid or qid po. **Anxiety:** 50 - 100 mg qid po.
	VISTARIL	Antiemetic, Antipruritic, Antianxiety Agent, Sedative	Inj (per mL): 25, 50 mg	**Nausea & Vomiting:** 25 - 100 mg IM. **Pruritis:** 25 mg tid or qid IM. **Anxiety:** 50 - 100 mg qid IM. **Sedation:** 50 - 100 mg IM.
Hydroxyzine Pamoate	VISTARIL	Sedative, Antipruritic, Antianxiety Agent	Susp: 25 mg/5 mL Cpsl: 25, 50, 100 mg	**Sedation:** 50 - 100 mg po. **Pruritis:** 25 mg tid or qid po. **Anxiety:** 50 - 100 mg qid po.
Hyoscyamine Sulfate	LEVSIN	Anticholinergic, Antispasmodic	Solution: 0.125 mg/mL (5% alcohol) Elixir: 0.125 mg/5 mL (20% alcohol) Tab & Subling Tab: 0.125 mg Inj: 0.5 mg/mL	0.125 - 0.25 mg q 4 h po. 0.125 - 0.25 mg q 4 h po. 0.125 - 0.25 mg q 4 h po or sublingually. 0.25 - 0.5 mg SC, IM, or IV up to qid at 4-hour intervals.
	NULEV	Anticholinergic, Antispasmodic	Oral Disintegrating Tab: 0.125 mg	Dissolve on tongue; swallow with or without water. 0.125 - 0.25 mg q 4 h po prn.
	LEVSINEX TIMECAPS	Anticholinergic, Antispasmodic	Timed-Rel. Cpsl: 0.375 mg	0.375 - 0.750 mg q 12 h po.
	LEVBID	Anticholinergic, Antispasmodic	Extended-Rel. Tab: 0.375 mg	0.375 - 0.750 mg q 12 h po.

GENERIC NAME	COMMON TRADE NAMES	THERAPEUTIC CATEGORY	PREPARATIONS	COMMON ADULT DOSAGE
Ibuprofen (*)	ADVIL, MOTRIN IB, NUPRIN	Non-Opioid Analgesic, Antipyretic	Tab: 200 mg	200 - 400 mg q 4 - 6 h po.
	MOTRIN MIGRAINE PAIN	Non-Opioid Analgesic	Cplt: 200 mg	200 - 400 mg q 4 - 6 h po.
	MOTRIN	Non-Opioid Analgesic, Antiinflammatory	Susp: 100 mg/5 mL. Tab: 400, 600, 800 mg	**Analgesia:** 400 mg q 4 - 6 h po prn pain. **Dysmenorrhea:** 400 mg q 4 h po prn pain. **Rheumatoid Arthritis and Osteoarthritis:** 1200 to 3200 mg daily po in divided doses (300 mg qid or 400, 600, or 800 mg tid or qid).
Ibutilide Fumarate	CORVERT	Antiarrhythmic	Inj: 0.1 mg/mL	**≥ 60 kg:** Infuse 1 mg (1 vial) IV over 10 mins. If the arrhythmia does not terminate within 10 minutes after the initial infusion, a second infusion of equal strength may be given 10 minutes after completion of the first infusion. **< 60 kg:** Infuse 0.1 mL/kg (0.01 mg/kg) IV over 10 minutes. If the arrhythmia does not terminate within 10 minutes after the initial infusion, a second infusion of equal strength may be given 10 minutes after completion of the first infusion.
Idarubicin Hydrochloride	IDAMYCIN	Antineoplastic	Powd for Inj: 5, 10, 20 mg	12 mg/m² daily for 3 days by slow IV (10 - 15 minutes) in combination with cytarabine.
Imipramine Hydrochloride (*)	TOFRANIL	Antidepressant	Tab: 10, 25, 50 mg	**Outpatients:** Initially, 75 mg/day po in divided doses, increased to 150 mg/day. **Hospitalized Patients:** Initially, 100 mg/day po in divided doses, gradually increased to 200 mg/day po as required.
Imipramine Pamoate	TOFRANIL-PM	Antidepressant	Cpsl: 75, 100, 125, 150 mg	**Outpatients:** Initially, 75 mg/day po; may raise dosage to 150 mg/day (dosage at which the optimum response usually occurs). The usual maintenance dosage is 75 - 150 mg daily as a single dose hs or in divided doses.

Inamrinone Lactate (*)	Inotropic Agent	Inj: 5 mg/mL	**Hospitalized Patients:** Initially, 100 - 150 mg daily po; may increase to 200 mg/day. If no response in 2 wks, give 250 - 300 mg/day. 0.75 mg/kg IV bolus (over 2 - 3 minutes), then 5 - 10 μg/kg/min by IV infusion.
Indapamide	Diuretic, Antihypertensive	Tab: 1.25, 2.5 mg	**Edema of CHF:** 2.5 mg daily po as a single dose in the AM. If response is not satisfactory, may double dose in 1 week. **Hypertension:** 1.25 mg daily po as a single dose in the AM. If response is not satisfactory, may double dose in 4 weeks.
Indinavir Sulfate	Antiviral	Cpsl: 100, 200, 333, 400 mg	800 mg (two 400 mg cpsls) q 8 h po, 1 h before or 2 h after a meal.
Indomethacin (*)	Antiinflammatory	Susp: 25 mg/5 mL Cpsl: 25, 50 mg Rectal Suppos: 50 mg	**Rheumatoid Arthritis:** 25 mg bid or tid po pc; if well tolerated, increase the daily dosage by 25 or 50 mg. In persistent night pain or AM stiffness, giving a large portion of the daily dose (up to 100 mg) hs po or by suppository may be helpful. **Acute Painful Shoulder:** 75 - 150 mg daily po pc in 3 - 4 divided doses for 7 - 14 days. **Acute Gout:** 50 mg tid po pc until pain is tolerable.
		Sustained-Rel. Cpsl: 75 mg	75 mg daily po.
INDOCIN SR			

121

GENERIC NAME	COMMON TRADE NAMES	THERAPEUTIC CATEGORY	PREPARATIONS	COMMON ADULT DOSAGE
Infliximab	REMICADE	Drug for Crohn's Disease, Antiarthritic	Powd for Inj: 100 mg	**Crohn's Disease (Moderate to Severe):** 5 mg/kg given as a single IV infusion at 0, 2, and 6 weeks followed by a maintenance regimen of 5 mg/kg q 6 weeks thereafter. **Crohn's Disease (Fistulizing):** 5 mg/kg by IV infusion followed by additional 5 mg/kg infusion followed by additional 5 mg/kg doses at 2 and 6 weeks after the first dose. **Rheumatoid Arthritis:** 3 mg/kg given as an IV infusion followed by additional doses at 2 and 6 weeks after the first infusion, then every 8 weeks thereafter. Give in combination with methotrexate.
Insulin (*)	ILETIN, HUMULIN, etc.	Hypoglycemic Agent	Inj: 100 units/mL	Variable: inject SC. See the Insulin Table, pp. 316 to 319 for preparations.
Insulin Aspart	NOVOLOG	Hypoglycemic Agent	Inj: 100 units/mL	Variable: inject SC. See p. 316.
Insulin Glargine (*)	LANTUS	Hypoglycemic Agent	Inj: 100 units/mL	Variable: inject once daily SC hs.
Insulin Lispro (*)	HUMALOG	Hypoglycemic Agent	Inj: 100 units/mL	Variable: inject SC. See pp. 316.
Interferon alfa-2a (*)	ROFERON-A	Antineoplastic	Inj (per mL): 3, 6, 9, 36 million IUnits Powd for Inj: 6 million IUnits	**Hairy Cell Leukemia:** For Induction- 3 million IU daily for 16 - 24 weeks SC or IM. For Maintenance- 3 million IU 3 times a week SC or IM. **Kaposi's Sarcoma:** For Induction- 36 million IU daily for 10 - 12 weeks SC or IM. For Maintenance- 36 million IU 3 times a week SC or IM. **Chronic Myelogenous Leukemia:** 9 milion IU daily SC or IM.

Interferon alfa-2b	INTRON A	Antineoplastic, Antiviral	**Powd for Inj:** 3, 5, 10, 18, 25, 50 million IUnits/vial; **Solution for Inj:** 3, 5, 10, 18, 25 million IUnits/vial	**Hairy Cell Leukemia:** 2 million IU/m² IM or SC 3 times a week for up to 6 months. **Kaposi's Sarcoma:** 30 million IU/m² IM or SC 3 times a week. **Chronic Hepatitis B:** 30 - 35 million IU per week SC or IM, either as 5 million IU daily or 10 million IU 3 times a week for 16 weeks. **Chronic Hepatitis C:** 3 million IU 3 times per week SC or IM. At 16 weeks of therapy, extend treatment to 18 - 24 months at 3 million IU 3 times a week. **Follicular Lymphoma:** 5 million IU 3 times a week SC or IM for up to 18 months in conjunction with an anthracycline-containing chemotherapy regimen. **Condylomata Acuminata (10 million IU vial):** 1 million IU into the base of each wart SC 3 times a week on alternate days, for 3 weeks. To reduce side effects, administer in the evening if possible with acetaminophen. **Malignant Melanoma:** Initially, 20 million IU/m² IV on 5 consecutive days per week for 4 weeks. Maintenance dose is 10 million IU/m² SC 3 times weekly for 48 weeks.
Interferon alfa-n3	ALFERON N	Antineoplastic	**Inj:** 5 million IUnits/vial of 1 mL	**Condylomata Acuminata:** 250,000 IU per wart. Maximum dose per treatment session is 2.5 million IU SC at the base of each wart. Use twice weekly for up to 8 weeks.
Interferon alfacon-1	INFERGEN	Antiviral	**Inj:** 9, 15 µg	**Chronic Hepatitis C Infection:** 9 µg SC as a single dose 3 times weekly for 24 weeks. At least 48 h should elapse between doses.

123

GENERIC NAME	COMMON TRADE NAMES	THERAPEUTIC CATEGORY	PREPARATIONS	COMMON ADULT DOSAGE
Interferon beta-1a	AVONEX	Multiple Sclerosis Drug	Powd for Inj: 6.6 million IUnits (33 µg)	6 million IU (30 µg) IM once a week.
	REBIF		Powd for Inj: 22, 44 µg	Initially, 8.8 µg SC 3 times a week. Administer at the same time (preferably in the late afternoon or evening) on the same 3 days (e.g., Monday, Wednesday, Friday) at least 48 h apart each week). Gradually increase over a 4 week period to 44 µg SC 3 times a week.
Interferon beta-1b	BETASERON	Multiple Sclerosis Drug	Powd for Inj: 9.6 million IUnits (0.3 mg)	8 million IU (0.25 mg) SC every other day.
Iodoquinol	YODOXIN	Amebicide	Tab: 210, 650 mg	630 - 650 mg tid po after meals for 20 days.
Ipratropium Bromide	ATROVENT	Bronchodilator	Aerosol: 18 µg/spray Solution: 500 µg/2.5 mL	2 inhalations (36 µg) qid. 500 µg by nebulization tid - qid (q 6 - 8 h).
			Nasal Spray: 0.03, 0.06% (21, 42 µg/spray, respectively)	0.03%: 2 sprays (42 µg) per nostril bid - tid. 0.06%: 2 sprays (84 µg) per nostril tid - qid.
Irbesartan	AVAPRO	Antihypertensive, Drug for Nephropathy in Type II Diabetes	Tab: 75, 150, 300 mg	Hypertension: Initially 150 mg once daily po. May increase to 300 mg once daily po. Nephropathy: The recommended target maintenance dose is 300 mg once daily po.
Isocarboxazid	MARPLAN	Antidepressant	Tab: 10 mg	10 mg bid po. If tolerated, increase dosage by 10 mg q 2 - 4 days to achieve a dosage of 40 mg by the end of the 1st week. Increase dosage by increments of up to 20 mg/week, if needed and tolerated, to a maximum dosage of 60 mg per day. Daily dosage should be divided into 2 - 4 doses.

124

Drug	Class	Dosage Form	Dosage
Isoetharine	Bronchodilator	Solution for Inhalation: 1%	**Hand Nebulizer:** 4 inhalations, up to q 4 h. **Oxygen Aerosolization:** 0.5 mL, diluted 1:3 with saline or other diluent, administered with O_2 flow adjusted to 4 - 6 L/min, over 15 - 20 minutes. **IPPB:** 0.5 mL, diluted 1:3 with saline or other diluent (with an inspiratory flow rate of 15 L/min at a cycling pressure of 15 cm H_2O).
Isoniazid (*) INH NYDRAZID	Tuberculostatic	Tab: 300 mg Inj: 100 mg/mL	300 mg daily po. **Treatment:** 5 mg/kg (up to 300 mg daily) IM in a single dose, or 15 mg/kg (up to 900 mg) daily 2 - 3 times weekly. **Preventive Therapy:** 300 mg daily IM in a single dose.
Isoproterenol Hydrochloride (*) ISUPREL	Bronchodilator	Solution: 1:200 (0.5%), 1:100 (1.0%)	**Acute Bronchial Asthma (Hand-Bulb Nebulizer):** 5 - 15 inhalations (of 1:200) or 3 - 7 inhalations (of 1:100) up to 5 times daily. **Bronchospasm in COPD:** **Hand-Bulb Nebulizer:** Same dosage as for Acute Bronchial Asthma above. **Nebulization by Compressed Air or Oxygen:** 0.5 mL (of 1:200) diluted to 2 - 2.5 mL with water or isotonic saline. Flow rate is regulated to deliver over 10 - 20 minutes. Breath in mist up to 5 times daily. **IPPB:** 0.5 mL (of 1:200) diluted to 2 - 2.5 mL with water or isotonic saline. The IPPB treatments are usually given for 15 - 20 minutes, up to 5 times daily.
Isosorbide ISMOTIC	Osmotic Diuretic	Solution: 100 g/220 mL (45%)	Initially 1.5 g/kg po, followed by 1 - 3 g/kg bid - qid po as indicated.

GENERIC NAME	COMMON TRADE NAMES	THERAPEUTIC CATEGORY	PREPARATIONS	COMMON ADULT DOSAGE
Isosorbide Dinitrate (*)	ISORDIL	Antianginal	**Sublingual Tab:** 2.5, 5, 10 mg **Oral Tab:** 5, 10, 20, 30, 40 mg **Controlled-Rel. Cpsl & Tab:** 40 mg	2.5 - 10 mg q 2 - 3 h sublingually. Initially, 5 - 20 mg po. For maintenance, 10 - 40 mg q 6 h po. Initially, 40 mg po. For maintenance, 40 - 80 mg q 8 - 12 h po.
	SORBITRATE		**Sublingual Tab:** 2.5, 5 mg **Chewable Tab:** 5, 10 mg **Oral Tab:** 5, 10, 20, 30, 40 mg	2.5 - 5 mg q 2 - 3 h sublingually. 5 - 10 mg q 2 - 3 h po. Initially, 5 - 20 mg po. For maintenance, 10 - 40 mg q 6 h po.
	DILATRATE-SR		**Sustained-Rel. Cpsl:** 40 mg	Initially, 40 mg po. For maintenance, 40 - 80 mg q 8 - 12 h po.
Isosorbide Mononitrate	ISMO	Antianginal	**Tab:** 20 mg	20 mg bid po, with the doses given 7 h apart.
	MONOKET		**Tab:** 10, 20 mg	20 mg bid po, with the doses given 7 h apart.
	IMDUR		**Extended-Rel. Tab:** 30, 60, 120 mg	Initially, 30 - 60 mg once daily po. May increase to 120 mg once daily po.
Isotretinoin	ACCUTANE	Anti-Cystic Acne Agent	**Cpsl:** 10, 20, 40 mg	0.5 - 2 mg/kg/day divided in 2 doses po for 15 - 20 weeks.
Isradipine	DYNACIRC	Antihypertensive	**Cpsl:** 2.5, 5 mg	Initially, 2.5 mg bid po. May increase in increments of 5 mg/day at 2 - 4 week intervals to a maximum of 20 mg/day.
	DYNACIRC CR		**Controlled-Rel. Tab:** 5, 10 mg	Initially, 5 mg once daily po. May increase in increments of 5 mg at 2 - 4 week intervals to a maximum of 20 mg/day.

126

| Itraconazole | SPORANOX | Antifungal | Cpsl: 100 mg | **Blastomycosis and Chronic Pulmonary Histoplasmosis:** 200 mg once daily po with food. May increase the dosage in 100 mg increments to a maximum of 400 mg daily. Doses over 200 mg/day should be given in 2 divided doses. |

Aspergillosis:
Pulmonary: 200 mg daily po for 3 - 4 mos.
Invasive Pulmonary: 200 mg bid po for 3 - 4 months.
Sporotrichosis: 100 mg daily po for 3 months.
Paracoccidioidomycosis: 100 mg daily po for 6 months.

Onychomycosis:
Toenails with or without Fingernail Involvement: 200 mg once daily po for 12 consecutive weeks.
Fingernails Only: 200 mg bid po for 1 week. After 3 weeks without the drug, repeat the dosage.
Oral Candidiasis: 100 mg daily po for 2 weeks.
Oral/Esophageal Candidiasis: 100 mg daily po for 4 weeks.
Tinea corporis/T. cruris: 100 mg once daily po for 14 consecutive days or 200 mg once daily po for 7 consecutive days.
Tinea pedis: 100 mg once daily po for 28 consecutive days or 200 mg bid po for 7 consecutive days.
Pityriasis versicolor: 200 mg once daily po for 7 consecutive days.

Oral Solution: 10 mg/mL

Vigorously swish solution in the mouth (10 mL at a time) for several seconds and swallow.
Oropharyngeal Candidiasis: 200 mg daily po in single or divided doses for 1 - 2 weeks.
Esophageal Candidiasis: 100 mg daily po for a minimum of 3 weeks. Continue for 2 weeks following resolution of symptoms.

[Continued on the next page]

GENERIC NAME	COMMON TRADE NAMES	THERAPEUTIC CATEGORY	PREPARATIONS	COMMON ADULT DOSAGE
Itraconazole [Continued]			Injection: 10 mg/mL	**Blastomycosis, Histoplasmosis, & Aspergillosis:** 200 mg (by IV infusion over 1 h) bid for 4 doses, followed by 200 mg per day by IV infusion. Continue injection for a maximum of 14 days; then continue with capsules for a minimum of 3 months until the infection has subsided.
Ivermectin (*)	STROMECTOL	Anthelmintic	Tab: 3, 6 mg	See Table below. Take tablets with water.

Dosage for Strongyloidiasis		Dosage for Onchocerciasis	
Body Weight (kg)	Oral Dosage	Body Weight (kg)	Oral Dosage
15 to 24	3 mg	15 to 25	3 mg
25 to 35	6 mg	26 to 44	6 mg
36 to 50	9 mg	45 to 64	9 mg
51 to 65	12 mg	65 to 84	12 mg
66 to 79	15 mg	≥ 85	[150 µg/kg]
≥ 80	[200 µg/kg]		

GENERIC NAME	COMMON TRADE NAMES	THERAPEUTIC CATEGORY	PREPARATIONS	COMMON ADULT DOSAGE
Ketoconazole (*)	NIZORAL	Antifungal	Tab: 200 mg	200 mg once daily po. In very severe infections, 400 mg once daily po.
			Cream: 2% Shampoo: 2%	Apply topically once daily. Shampoo twice a week for 4 weeks with at least 3 days between shampooing; then shampoo intermittently prn.
	NIZORAL A-D	Antidandruff Shampoo	Shampoo: 1%	Shampoo twice a week for up to 8 weeks with at least 3 days between shampooing; then shampoo intermittently prn.

Ketoprofen (*)	ORUDIS KT	Non-Opioid Analgesic, Antiinflammatory	**Tab:** 12.5 mg	12.5 - 25 mg q 4 - 6 h po prn.
	ORUDIS		**Cpsl:** 25, 50, 75 mg	**Analgesia & Dysmenorrhea:** 25 - 50 mg q 6 - 8 h po. **Rheumatoid Arthritis & Osteoarthritis:** 75 mg tid po or 50 mg qid po.
	ORUVAIL	Antiinflammatory	**Extended-Rel. Cpsl:** 100, 150, 200 mg	**Rheumatoid Arthritis & Osteoarthritis:** 200 mg once daily po.
Ketorolac Tromethamine (*)	ACULAR	Antiinflammatory (Topical)	**Ophth Solution:** 0.5%	1 drop into affected eye(s) qid.
	TORADOL [IV/IM]	Non-Opioid Analgesic	**Inj (per mL):** 15, 30 mg	**Single-Dose Treatment (IM or IV*):** < 65 yrs: 1 dose of 60 mg IM or 30 mg IV. ≥ 65 yrs, renally impaired, or under 50 kg (110 lbs): 1 dose - 30 mg IM or 15 mg IV. **Multiple-Dose Treatment (IM or IV*):** < 65 yrs: 30 mg q 6 h IM or IV, not to exceed 120 mg per day. ≥ 65 yrs, renally impaired, or under 50 kg (110 lbs): 15 mg q 6 h IM or IV, not to exceed 60 mg per day. * The IV bolus dose must be given over no less than 15 seconds.
	TORADOL [ORAL]		**Tab:** 10 mg	Indicated only as continuation therapy to TORADOL [IV/IM]. The maximum combined duration of use (parenteral and oral) is 5 days. < 65 yrs: 20 mg po as a first dose for those who received 60 mg IM (single dose), 30 mg IV (single dose), or 30 mg (multiple dose) of TORADOL [IV/IM], followed by 10 mg q 4 - 6 h po, not to exceed 40 mg/day. ≥ 65 yrs, renally impaired, or under 50 kg (110 lbs): 10 mg po as a first dose for those who received 30 mg IM or 15 mg IV (single dose), or 15 mg (multiple dose) of TORADOL [IV/IM], followed by 10 mg q 4 - 6 h po, not to exceed 40 mg/day.

GENERIC NAME	COMMON TRADE NAMES	THERAPEUTIC CATEGORY	PREPARATIONS	COMMON ADULT DOSAGE
Ketotifen Fumarate	ZADITOR	Antihistamine (Topical)	Ophth Solution: 0.025%	1 drop into the affected eye(s) q 8 - 12 h.
Labetalol Hydrochloride (*)	NORMODYNE, TRANDATE	Antihypertensive	Tab: 100, 200, 300 mg	**Initial:** 100 mg bid po. Titrate dosage upward in increments of 100 mg bid q 2 - 3 days. **Maintenance:** Usually, 200 - 400 mg bid po.
			Inj: 5 mg/mL	**Repeated IV:** 20 mg IV (over 2 minutes). May give additional injections of 40 - 80 mg at 10-minute intervals (maximum: 300 mg). **IV Infusion:** 200 mL of a diluted solution (1 mg/mL) given at a rate of 2 mL/min.
Lactulose	DUPHALAC	Laxative	Syrup: 10 g/15 mL	15 - 30 mL (10 - 20 g) daily po. Dose may be increased to 60 mL daily if necessary.
Lamivudine	EPIVIR	Antiviral	Oral Solution: 10 mg/mL Tab: 150, 300 mg	**HIV Infection:** 150 mg bid po or 300 mg once daily po in combination with other antiretroviral agents.
	EPIVIR-HBV		Oral Solution: 5 mg/mL Tab: 100 mg	**Chronic Hepatitis B:** 100 mg once daily po.
Lamotrigine (*)	LAMICTAL	Antiepileptic	Tab: 25, 100, 150, 200 mg	**Monotherapy:** 500 mg/day po in 2 divided doses. **Patients on Enzyme-Inducing Antiepileptic Drugs, but not Valproate:** Initially, 50 mg once daily po for 2 weeks, followed by 100 mg/day po in 2 divided doses for 2 weeks. Thereafter, 300 - 500 mg/day po in 2 divided doses. **Patients on Enzyme-Inducing Antiepileptic Drugs and Valproate:** Initially, 25 mg every other day po for 2 weeks, followed by 25 mg once daily po for 2 weeks. Thereafter, 100 - 400 mg/day po in 1 or 2 divided doses. The usual maintenance dosage when adding lamotrigine to valproate alone is 100 to 200 mg/day.

Lansoprazole	PREVACID	Gastric Acid Pump Inhibitor, Anti-Ulcer Agent	**Delayed-Rel. Cpsl:** 15, 30 mg **Granules for Delayed-Rel. Oral Susp:** 15, 30 mg per packet	**Duodenal Ulcer:** **Treatment of:** 15 mg once daily po for 4 weeks. **Maintenance of Healed Ulcer:** 15 mg once daily po. **Associated with *H. pylori*:** 30 mg of lansoprazole + 500 mg of clarithromycin + 1 g of amoxicillin bid po for 10 or 14 days, or 30 mg of lansoprazole + 1 g of amoxicillin tid for 14 days for those intolerant to or resistant to clarithromycin. **Gastric Ulcer:** **Treatment of:** 30 mg once daily po for up to 8 weeks. **Maintenance of Healed Ulcer Associated with NSAIDs:** 30 mg once daily po for up to 8 weeks. **Risk Reduction from NSAIDs:** 15 mg once daily po for up to 12 weeks. **Erosive Esophagitis:** **Treatment of:** 30 mg once daily po for up to 8 weeks. **Maintenance of Healing Esophagitis:** 15 mg once daily po. **Pathological Hypersecretory Conditions including Zollinger-Ellison Syndrome:** The recommended starting dose is 60 mg once a day po. Adjust to individual patient needs and continue for as long as indicated.
Latanoprost	XALATAN	Anti-Glaucoma Agent	**Ophth Solution:** 0.005% (50 μg/mL)	1 drop into affected eye(s) once daily in the evening.
Leflunomide	ARAVA	Antirheumatic	**Tab:** 10, 20, 100 mg	Initiate with a loading dose of one 100 mg tab po per day for 3 days. Then, 20 mg once daily po.
Letrozole	FEMARA	Antineoplastic	**Tab:** 2.5 mg	2.5 mg once daily po.

GENERIC NAME	COMMON TRADE NAMES	THERAPEUTIC CATEGORY	PREPARATIONS	COMMON ADULT DOSAGE
Levalbuterol Hydrochloride	XOPENEX	Bronchodilator	**Solution for Inhalation:** (0.73 mg/3 mL, equal to 0.63 mg/3 mL of base) **Solution for Inhalation:** (1.44 mg/3 mL, equal to 1.25 mL/3 mL of base)	0.63 mg (base) tid (q 6 - 8 h) by nebulization. For those patients with more severe asthma or for those who do not respond adequately to a lower dose, 1.26 mg (base) tid may be used with close monitoring for adverse effects.
Levetiracetam	KEPPRA	Antiepileptic	**Tab:** 250, 500, 750 mg	Initially 1000 mg/day, given as 500 mg bid po. Doses may be increased by 1000 mg/day q 2 weeks to a maximum of 3000 mg per day.
Levobetaxolol Hydrochloride	BETAXON	Anti-Glaucoma Agent	**Ophth Suspension:** 0.5%	1 drop into the affected eye(s) bid.
Levobunolol Hydrochloride	BETAGAN LIQUIFILM	Anti-Glaucoma Agent	**Ophth Solution:** 0.25, 0.5%	**0.25%:** 1 - 2 drops into the affected eye(s) bid daily. **0.5%:** 1 - 2 drops into the affected eye(s) once daily.
Levocabastine Hydrochloride	LIVOSTIN	Antiallergic, Ophthalmic	**Ophth Solution:** 0.05%	1 drop into affected eye(s) qid for up to 2 weeks.
Levodopa	LARODOPA	Antiparkinsonian	**Tab:** 100, 250, 500 mg	Initially, 500 mg to 1 g daily po divided in 2 or more doses with food. May increase dosage gradually in increments not more than 750 mg q 3 - 7 days. Maximum 8 g daily.
Levofloxacin (*)	QUIXIN	Antibacterial (Topical)	**Ophth Solution:** 0.5%	Instill 1 - 2 drops in the affected eye(s) q 2 h while awake, up to 8 times a day on days 1 and 2. Instill 1 - 2 drops in the affected eye(s) q 4 h while, up to 4 times daily on days 3 - 7.

132

Drug	Class	Forms	Dosing
LEVAQUIN	Antibacterial	**Tab:** 250, 500, 750 mg **Inj:** 5, 25 mg/mL	**Bronchitis:** 500 mg once daily po or by IV infusion (over 60 min) for 7 days. **Pneumonia:** 500 mg once daily po or by IV infusion (over 60 min) for 7 - 14 days. **Sinusitis:** 500 mg once daily po or by IV infusion (over 60 min) for 10 - 14 days. **Skin & Skin Structure Infections (Uncomplicated):** 500 mg once daily po or by IV infusion (over 60 min) for 7 - 10 days. **Skin & Skin Structure Infections (Complicated):** 750 mg once daily po or by IV infusion (over 90 min) for 7 - 10 days. **Urinary Tract Infections (Complicated) and Pyelonephritis:** 250 mg once daily po or by IV infusion (over 60 min) for 10 days. **Urinary Tract Infections (Uncomplicated):** 250 mg once daily po for 3 days.
Levonorgestrel (*)			
NORPLANT SYSTEM	Implant Contraceptive	**Kit:** 6 cpsls (each with 36 mg levonorgestrel) plus trocar, scalpel, forceps, syringe, 2 syringe needles, package of skin closures, gauze sponges, stretch bandages, surgical drapes	Total implanted dose is 216 mg. Perform implantation of all 6 capsules during the first 7 days of the onset of menses. Insertion is subdermal in the mid-portion of the upper arm; distribute capsules in a fan-like pattern, about 15 degrees apart, for a total of 75 degrees.
MIRENA	Intrauterine Contraceptive	**Intrauterine System:** unit containing a reservoir of 52 mg levonorgestrel	Insert a single unit into the uterine cavity within 7 days of the onset of menstruation or immediately after the first trimester abortion. Replace within 5 years.
PLAN B	Emergency Contraceptive	**Tab:** 0.75 mg	0.75 mg po within 72 h after unprotected intercourse; follow with 0.75 mg 12 h later.
Levorphanol Tartrate (*) (C-II)			
LEVO-DROMORAN	Opioid Analgesic	**Tab:** 2 mg **Inj:** 2 mg/mL	2 mg po q 6 - 8 h prn. May be increased to 3 mg q 6 - 8 h if needed. 1 - 2 mg IM or SC q 6 - 8 prn.

GENERIC NAME	COMMON TRADE NAMES	THERAPEUTIC CATEGORY	PREPARATIONS	COMMON ADULT DOSAGE
Levothyroxine Sodium (*)	LEVOTHROID, SYNTHROID	Thyroid Hormone	**Tab:** 25, 50, 75, 88, 100, 112, 125, 137, 150, 175, 200, 300 μg	**Usual Dosage:** 50 μg daily po with increases of 25 - 50 μg at 2 - 4 week intervals until the patient is euthyroid or symptoms preclude further dose increases. The usual maintenance dosage is 100 - 200 μg daily po. **Myxedema Coma or Hypothyroid Patients with Angina:** Starting dose should be 25 μg daily po with increases of 25 - 50 μg at 2 - 4 week intervals as determined by response.
	SYNTHROID		**Powd for Inj:** 200, 500 μg	**Myxedema Coma:** Initially, 200 - 500 μg (100 μg/mL) IV. Then, 100 - 200 μg daily IV. After evaluation of thyroid state, 50 - 100 μg daily IV is usually sufficient.
Lidocaine	XYLOCAINE	Local Anesthetic	**Oint:** 2.5% **Oint:** 5%	Apply topically prn. Apply topically. Maximum single application- 5 g (≈ 6 inches of ointment). Maximum daily application- 1/2 tube (≈ 17 - 20 g).
	LIDODERM		**Adhesive Patch:** 5%	Apply to intact skin, covering the most painful area. To adjust dose, cut patches before removing release liner. May apply up to 3 patches at once for up to 12 hours of a 24-hour period.
	XYLOCAINE		**Oral Spray:** 10%	2 metered doses per quadrant are advised as the upper limit.
Lidocaine Hydrochloride (*)	XYLOCAINE	Antiarrhythmic	**Inj (per mL):** 5 mg (0.5%), 10 mg (1%), 15 mg (1.5%), 20 mg (2%),	**IV Injection:** 50 - 100 mg IV bolus (at a rate of 25 - 50 mg/min). May repeat dose in 5 min. **IV Infusion:** Following bolus administration, give at a rate of 1 - 4 mg/min.
	4% XYLOCAINE-MPF	Local Anesthetic	**Inj:** 40 mg/mL (4%)	**Retrobulbar Inj.:** 3 - 5 mL/70 kg (1.7-3 mg/kg. **Transtracheal Injection:** 2 - 3 mL injected rapidly through a large needle. **Topical:** Spray pharynx with 1 - 5 mL.

134

	XYLOCAINE 2% VISCOUS	Local Anesthetic	Solution: 2%	**Mouth:** 15 mL swished around mouth and spit out. Readminister q 3 - 8 h prn. **Pharynx:** 15 mL gargled & may be swallowed. Readminister q 3 - 8 h prn.
Lindane (*)		Antiparasitic, Scabicide	Lotion: 1%	**Scabies:** Apply to dry skin as a thin layer and rub in thoroughly. Leave on for 8 - 12 h, then remove by thorough washing.
			Shampoo: 1%	**Head & Crab Lice:** Apply 30 - 60 mL to dry hair. Work thoroughly into hair and allow to remain in place for 4 minutes. Add small amounts of water to form a good lather. Rinse thoroughly and towel dry.
Linezolid	ZYVOX	Antibacterial	Inj: 2 mg/mL Tab: 400, 600 mg Powd for Solution: 100 mg/5 mL	**Vancomycin-resistant *Enterococcus faecium* Infections:** 600 mg IV (over 30 - 120 min) or po q 12 h for 14 - 28 days. **Nosocomial Pneumonia, Complicated Skin and Skin Structure Infections, and Community-acquired Pneumonia:** 600 mg IV (over 30 to 120 min) or po q 12 h for 10 - 14 days. **Uncomplicated Skin and Skin Structure Infections:** 400 mg IV (over 30 - 120 min) or po q 12 h for 10 - 14 days.
Liothyronine Sodium (*)	CYTOMEL	Thyroid Hormone	Tab: 5, 25, 50 µg	**Usual Dosage:** 25 µg daily po. Daily dosage may be increased by 12.5 - 25 µg q 1 - 2 weeks. Usual maintenance dose is 25 - 75 µg daily po. **Myxedema:** Starting dose is 5 µg daily po. May increase by 5 - 10 µg daily q 1 - 2 weeks. When 25 µg daily is reached, dosage may be increased by 12.5 - 25 µg q 1 - 2 weeks. Usual maintenance dose is 50 - 100 µg daily.
	TRIOSTAT		Inj: 10 µg/mL	**Myxedema Coma:** Initially, 25 - 50 µg IV. The dosage may be repeated at least 4 h and no more than 12 h apart.

GENERIC NAME	COMMON TRADE NAMES	THERAPEUTIC CATEGORY	PREPARATIONS	COMMON ADULT DOSAGE
Lisinopril (*)	PRINIVIL, ZESTRIL	Antihypertensive, Heart Failure Drug, Post-MI Drug	Tab: 2.5, 5, 10, 20, 30, 40 mg	**Hypertension:** Initially, 10 mg once daily po. Usual dosage range is 20 - 40 mg as a single daily dose. **Heart Failure:** Initially, 5 mg once daily po with diuretics and digitalis. Usual dosage range is 5 - 20 mg once daily. **Acute Myocardial Infarction:** 5 mg po within 24 h of the onset of acute MI symptoms, followed by 5 mg po after 24 h, 10 mg po after 48 h, and then 10 mg once daily po. Continue dosing for 6 weeks.
Lithium Carbonate (*)	ESKALITH	Antimaniacal	Cpsl: 300 mg	**Usual Dosage:** 300 mg tid or qid po. **Acute Mania:** 900 mg bid po or 600 mg tid po. **Long-Term Control:** 900 - 1200 mg daily po in 2 or 3 divided doses.
	ESKALITH CR		Controlled-Rel. Tab: 450 mg	**Usual Dosage:** 450 mg bid po.
	LITHOBID		Slow-Rel. Tab: 300 mg	**Acute Mania:** 900 mg bid po or 600 mg tid po. **Long-Term Control:** 900 - 1200 mg daily po in 2 or 3 divided doses.
	LITHONATE		Cpsl: 300 mg	**Acute Mania:** 600 mg tid po. **Long-Term Control:** 300 mg tid or qid po.
	LITHOTAB		Tab: 300 mg	Same dosages as for LITHONATE above.
Lithium Citrate (*)		Antimaniacal	Syrup: 8 mEq (= 300 mg of lithium carbonate)/5 mL	**Acute Mania:** 10 mL (16 mEq) tid po. **Long-Term Control:** 5 mL (8 mEq) tid or qid po.
Lodoxamide Tromethamine	ALOMIDE	Antiallergic, Ophthalmic	Ophth Solution: 0.1 %	1 - 2 drops in each affected eye qid for up to 3 months.

Lomefloxacin Hydrochloride (*)	MAXAQUIN	Antibacterial	Tab: 400 mg	**Lower Respiratory Tract and Urinary Tract Infections (Uncomplicated)**: 400 mg once daily po for 10 days. **Urinary Tract Infections, Complicated**: 400 mg once daily po for 14 days.
Lomustine	CeeNU	Antineoplastic	Cpsl: 10, 40, 100 mg	130 mg/m^2 po as a single dose q 6 weeks. Dosage adjustments are made in 6 weeks based on platelet and leukocyte counts.
Loperamide Hydrochloride	IMODIUM	Antidiarrheal	Cpsl: 2 mg	4 mg po followed by 2 mg after each unformed stool. Maximum daily dosage- 16 mg.
	IMODIUM A-D, PEPTO DIARRHEA CONTROL		Liquid: 1 mg/5 mL (5.25% alcohol) Cplt: 2 mg	4 mg po followed by 2 mg after each unformed stool. Maximum daily dosage- 8 mg.
Loracarbef (*)	LORABID	Antibacterial	Powd for Susp (per 5 mL): 100, 200 mg Cpsl: 200, 400 mg	**Lower Resp. Tract Infect. (Except Pneumonia)**: 200 - 400 mg q 12 h po for 7 days. **Pneumonia**: 400 mg q 12 h po for 14 days. **Upper Respiratory Tract Infections**: 200 - 400 mg q 12 h po for 10 days. **Skin and Skin Structure Infections**: 200 mg q 12 h po for 7 days. **Urinary Tract Infections (Uncomplicated Cystitis)**: 200 mg q 24 h po for 7 days. **Urinary Tract Infections (Uncomplicated Pyelonephritis)**: 400 mg q 12 h po for 14 days.
Loratadine (*)	CLARITIN	Antihistamine	Syrup: 1 mg/mL Tab: 10 mg	10 mL (10 mg) once daily po. 10 mg once daily po.
Lorazepam (*) (C-IV)	ATIVAN	Antianxiety Agent	Tab: 0.5, 1, 2 mg Inj (per mL): 2, 4 mg	**Anxiety**: 2 - 3 mg daily po given bid or tid. **Insomnia due to Anxiety**: 2 - 4 mg hs po. **Premedicant**: 0.05 mg/kg (maximum 4 mg) IM. **Anxiety**: 0.044 mg/kg (maximum 2 mg) IV.

GENERIC NAME	COMMON TRADE NAMES	THERAPEUTIC CATEGORY	PREPARATIONS	COMMON ADULT DOSAGE
Losartan Potassium	COZAAR	Antihypertensive	Tab: 25, 50, 100 mg	Usual starting dose is 50 mg once daily po. For patients treated with a diuretic, start with 25 mg once daily po. The drug can be given once or twice daily with the total daily dose range of 25 - 100 mg.
Loteprednol Etabonate	ALREX	Corticosteroid (Topical)	Ophth Suspension: 0.2%	1 drop into the affected eye(s) qid.
	LOTEMAX		Ophth Suspension: 0.5%	**Steroid Responsive Disease**: 1 - 2 drops into the affected eye(s) qid. During the initial treatment within the first week, the dosing may be increased up to 1 drop every hour. **Postoperative Inflammation**: 1 - 2 drops into operated eye(s) qid, beginning 24 h after surgery & continuing for 2 weeks.
Lovastatin	MEVACOR	Antihyperlipidemic	Tab: 10, 20, 40 mg	Initially 20 mg once daily po with the evening meal. Dosage adjustments may be made at 4 week intervals. Usual dosage range is 10 to 80 mg/day po in a single or 2 divided doses.
	ALTOCOR		Extended-Rel. Tab: 10, 20, 40, 60 mg	Initially 20, 40, or 60 mg once daily po hs. Dosage adjustments may be made at 4 week intervals. The usual dosage range is 10 - 60 mg/day po in a single dose.
Loxapine Hydrochloride (*)	LOXITANE C	Antipsychotic	Conc Liquid: 25 mg/mL (as the base)	Initially, 10 mg bid po. Dosage should be increased rapidly over 7 - 10 days; usual maintenance range is 60 - 100 mg daily, but many patients do well at 20 - 60 mg daily.
Loxapine Succinate	LOXITANE	Antipsychotic	Cpsl: 5, 10, 25, 50 mg (as the base)	Same dosage as for LOXITANE C above.
Mafenide Acetate	SULFAMYLON	Burn Preparation	Cream: 85 mg/g	Apply to the clean and debrided wound with a sterile gloved hand, once or twice daily, to a thickness of about 1/16 in.

Magnesium Hydroxide	MILK OF MAGNESIA	Antacid, Saline Laxative	Susp: 400 mg/5 mL	**Antacid:** 5 - 15 mL with water, up to qid po. **Laxative:** 30-60 mL followed by 8 oz. of fluid.
	MILK OF MAGNESIA CONCENTRATED	Saline Laxative	Susp: 800 mg/5 mL	**Laxative:** 15 - 30 mL followed by 8 oz. of fluid.
Magnesium Salicylate	MOMENTUM	Non-Opioid Analgesic	Cplt: 467 mg	934 mg (2 cplt) q 6 h po.
Magnesium Sulfate		Anticonvulsant	Inj: 12.5, 50%	**IM:** 4 - 5 g of a 50% solution q 4 h prn. **IV:** 4 g of a 10 - 20% solution (not exceeding 1.5 mL/min of a 10% solution). **IV Infusion:** 4 - 5 g in 250 mL of 5% Dextrose or Sodium Chloride Solution (not exceeding 3 mL/min).
Maprotiline Hydrochloride (*)		Antidepressant	Tab: 25, 50, 75 mg	**Outpatients:** Initially, 75 mg daily po as a single dose or in divided doses. May increase dosage gradually after 2 weeks in increments of 25 mg. Usual maintenance dosage is 75 to 150 mg daily po. **Hospitalized Patients:** Initially, 100 - 150 mg daily po as a single dose or in divided doses. May increase dosage gradually, if needed, up to a maximum dose of 225 mg daily.
Mebendazole (*)	VERMOX	Anthelmintic	Chewable Tab: 100 mg	**Pinworm:** 100 mg daily po (1 dose). **Common Roundworm, Whipworm, Hookworm:** 100 mg bid AM & PM for 3 days po.
Mechlorethamine Hydrochloride	MUSTARGEN	Antineoplastic	Powd for Inj: 10 mg	0.4 mg/kg IV either as a single dose or in divided doses of 0.1 - 0.2 mg/kg/day.
Meclizine Hydrochloride (*)	ANTIVERT ANTIVERT/25 ANTIVERT/50	Antivertigo Agent	Tab: 12.5 mg Tab: 25 mg Tab: 50 mg	**Vertigo:** 25 - 100 mg po in divided doses. **Motion Sickness:** 25 - 50 mg po, 1 hour prior to embarkation; repeat dose q 24 h prn.
	BONINE DRAMAMINE LESS DROWSY FORMULA		Chewable Tab: 25 mg Tab: 25 mg	**Motion Sickness:** 25 - 50 mg po, 1 hour before travel starts, for up to 24 h protection.

GENERIC NAME	COMMON TRADE NAMES	THERAPEUTIC CATEGORY	PREPARATIONS	COMMON ADULT DOSAGE
Meclocycline Sulfosalicylate	MECLAN	Anti-Acne Agent	Cream: 1%	Apply to affected area bid, AM and PM.
Meclofenamate Sodium		Non-Opioid Analgesic, Antiinflammatory	Cpsl: 50, 100 mg	**Analgesia:** 50 - 100 mg q 4 - 6 h po. **Dysmenorrhea:** 100 mg tid po, for up to 6 days, starting at the onset of menses. **Rheumatoid Arthritis & Osteoarthritis:** 200 to 400 mg daily po in 3 or 4 equal doses.
Medroxyprogesterone Acetate (*)	PROVERA, CYCRIN	Progestin	Tab: 2.5, 5, 10 mg	5 - 10 mg daily po for 5 - 10 days.
	DEPO-PROVERA	Antineoplastic	Inj (per mL): 400 mg	Initially, 400 - 1000 mg weekly IM. If improvement is noted within a few weeks, patient may be maintained with as little as 400 mg per month.
		Injectable Contraceptive	Inj: 150 mg/mL	150 mg q 3 months by deep IM injection in the gluteal or deltoid muscle.
Medrysone	HMS	Corticosteroid	Ophth Susp: 1%	1 drop into affected eye(s) up to q 4 h.
Mefenamic Acid (*)	PONSTEL	Non-Opioid Analgesic	Cpsl: 250 mg	500 mg po, then 250 mg q 6 h po with food.
Mefloquine Hydrochloride	LARIAM	Antimalarial	Tab: 250 mg	**Treatment:** 1250 mg po as a single dose with food and with at least 8 oz. of water. **Prophylaxis:** 250 mg once weekly po for 4 weeks, then 250 mg every other week. Take with food and at least 8 oz of water. Start 1 week prior to departure to endemic area.
Megestrol Acetate	MEGACE	Progestin	Susp: 40 mg/mL	**Appetite Stimulant in Patients with AIDS:** 800 mg/day (20 mL/day) po.
		Antineoplastic	Tab: 20, 40 mg Susp: 40 mg/mL	**Breast Cancer:** 40 mg qid po. **Endometrial Cancer:** 40 - 320 mg daily po in divided doses for at least 2 months.

Meloxicam	MOBIC	Antiinflammatory	Tab: 7.5, 15 mg	7.5 mg once daily po.
Melphalan	ALKERAN	Antineoplastic	Tab: 2 mg	**Multiple Myeloma:** 6 mg daily po as a single dose. After 2 - 3 weeks, discontinue drug for up to 4 weeks; when WBC and platelet counts begin rising, maintenance dose of 2 mg daily po may be initiated. **Epithelial Ovarian Cancer:** 0.2 mg/kg daily for 5 days. Repeat q 4 - 5 weeks.
			Powd for Inj: 50 mg	Usual dose is 16 mg/m^2 given as a single IV infusion over 15 - 20 min. Administer at 2 week intervals for 4 doses, then, after recovery from toxicity, at 4 week intervals.
Meperidine Hydrochloride (*) (C-II)	DEMEROL	Opioid Analgesic	Tab: 50, 100 mg Syrup: 50 mg/5 mL Inj (per mL): 25, 50, 75, 100 mg	**Analgesia:** 50 - 150 mg q 3 - 4 h po. IM or SC. **Preoperatively:** 50 - 100 mg IM or SC. 30 - 90 minutes prior to anesthesia. **Obstetrical Analgesia:** 50 - 100 mg IM or SC when pain becomes regular; may repeat at 1 - 3 hour intervals.
Mephenytoin	MESANTOIN	Antiepileptic	Tab: 100 mg	Initially 50 - 100 mg daily po, increasing the daily dose by 50 - 100 mg at weekly intervals to a maintenance dose of 200 to 600 mg daily.
Mephobarbital (*) (C-IV)	MEBARAL	Antiepileptic, Sedative	Tab: 32, 50, 100 mg	**Epilepsy:** 400 - 600 mg daily po. **Sedation:** 32 - 100 mg tid or qid po. Optimum dosage is 50 mg tid or qid po.
Meprobamate (*) (C-IV)	MILTOWN	Antianxiety Agent	Tab: 200, 400 mg	1200 - 1600 mg/day po in 3 - 4 divided doses.
Mercaptopurine	PURINETHOL	Antineoplastic	Tab: 50 mg	**Induction:** 2.5 mg/kg daily po. May increase after 4 weeks to 5 mg/kg daily po. **Maintenance:** 1.5 - 2.5 mg/kg po as a single dose.

GENERIC NAME	COMMON TRADE NAMES	THERAPEUTIC CATEGORY	PREPARATIONS	COMMON ADULT DOSAGE
Meropenem (*)	MERREM IV	Antibacterial	Powd for Inj: 0.5, 1 g	1 g q 8 h by IV infusion (over 15 - 30 min) or as an IV bolus (5 - 20 mL) over 3 - 5 min.
Mesalamine	ASACOL	Bowel Antiinflammatory Agent	Delayed-Rel. Tab: 400 mg	800 mg tid po for 6 weeks.
	PENTASA		Controlled-Rel. Cpsi: 250 mg	1000 mg po for up to 8 weeks.
	ROWASA		Rectal Susp: 4 g/60 mL	One rectal instillation (4 g) once a day, preferably hs, and retained for approx. 8 h.
	CANASA		Rectal Suppos: 500 mg	Insert 1 rectally bid, and retained for 1 - 3 h.
Mesoridazine Besylate (*)	SERENTIL	Antipsychotic	Tab: 10, 25, 50, 100 mg Conc Liquid: 25 mg/mL (0.61% alcohol)	**Schizophrenia:** 50 mg tid po. **Behavioral Problems in Mental Deficiency and Chronic Brain Syndrome:** 25 mg tid po. **Alcoholism:** 25 mg bid po. **Psychoneurotic Manifestations:** 10 mg tid po.
			Inj: 25 mg/mL	25 mg IM. May repeat in 30 - 60 minutes.
Metaproterenol Sulfate	ALUPENT	Bronchodilator	Aerosol: 650 µg/spray	2 - 3 inhalations q 3 - 4 h.
Metaxolone	SKELAXIN	Skeletal Muscle Relaxant	Tab: 400 mg	800 mg tid to qid po.
Metformin Hydrochloride (*)	GLUCOPHAGE	Antihyperglycemic Agent	Tab: 500, 850, 1000 mg	**500 mg:** Usual staring dose is 500 mg bid po. given with the morning and evening meals. Make dosage increases in increments of 500 mg every week, given in divided doses, up to a maximum of 2500 mg/day. Can be given bid up to 2000 mg/day; if 2500 mg per day is required, it may be better tolerated if given tid with meals.

142

Methadone Hydrochloride (*) (C-II)	DOLOPHINE HYDROCHLORIDE	Opioid Analgesic	**Tab:** 5, 10 mg **Inj:** 10 mg/mL

850 mg: Usual staring dose is 850 mg daily po, given with the morning meal. Make dosage increases in increments of 850 mg every other week, given in divided doses, up to a maximum of 2550 mg/day. The usual maintenance dose is 850 mg bid with the morning & evening meals. When necessary, may give 850 mg tid with meals.

2.5 - 10 mg q 3 - 4 h po, IM or SC prn pain.

Methamphetamine Hydrochloride (*) (C-II)	DESOXYN	CNS Stimulant, Anorexiant	**Tab:** 5 mg

Attention Deficit Hyperactivity Disease:
Initially 5 mg once daily or bid po. Dosage may be raised in increments of 5 mg at weekly intervals until optimum response is achieved. Usual dosage 20 - 25 mg daily.
Exogenous Obesity: 5 mg po, 30 min ac.

Methenamine Hippurate	HIPREX, UREX	Urinary Tract Anti-Infective	**Tab:** 1 g

1 g bid (morning and night) po.

Methenamine Mandelate	MANDELAMINE	Urinary Tract Anti-Infective	**Tab:** 0.5, 1 g **Susp:** 0.5 g/5 mL

1 g qid po, pc and hs.
1 g qid po, pc and hs.

Methimazole (*)	TAPAZOLE	Antithyroid Drug	**Tab:** 5, 10 mg

Initial: 15 mg daily po (mild disease), 30 - 40 mg daily po (moderately severe), and 60 mg daily po (severe), divided into 3 doses q 8 h.
Maintenance: 5 - 15 mg daily po.

Methocarbamol (*)	ROBAXIN	Skeletal Muscle Relaxant	**Tab:** 500 mg

Initial: 1500 mg qid po.
Maintenance: 1000 mg qid po.

	ROBAXIN-750		**Tab:** 750 mg

Initial: 1500 mg qid po.
Maintenance: 750 mg q 4 h po or 1500 mg tid po.

GENERIC NAME	COMMON TRADE NAMES	THERAPEUTIC CATEGORY	PREPARATIONS	COMMON ADULT DOSAGE
Methotrexate Sodium (*)		Anti-Psoriasis Agent	**Tab:** 2.5 mg **Powd for Injection:** 20 mg **Inj:** 25 mg/mL	Individualize dosage. A test dose may be given prior to therapy to detect extreme sensitivity. 10 - 25 mg once a week po, IM, or IV until response is achieved. For po use, may given 2.5 mg q 12 h for 3 doses, once a week. Do not exceed 30 mg per week.
Methsuximide (*)	CELONTIN	Antiepileptic	**Cpsl:** 150, 300 mg	300 mg daily po for the 1st week. May raise dosage at weekly intervals by 300 mg/day for 3 weeks to a daily dosage of 1200 mg.
Methyclothiazide	ENDURON	Diuretic, Antihypertensive	**Tab:** 2.5, 5 mg	**Diuresis:** 2.5 - 10 mg once daily po. **Hypertension:** 2.5 - 5 mg once daily po.
Methylcellulose	CITRUCEL CITRUCEL (Sugar-Free)	Bulk Laxative	**Powder:** 2 g/heaping tablespoonful (19 g) **Powder:** 2 g/heaping tablespoonful (10.2 g)	1 heaping tablespoonful stirred into 8 fl. oz. of cold water 1 - 3 times daily po at the first sign of constipation.
Methyldopa (*)	ALDOMET	Antihypertensive	**Susp:** 250 mg/5 mL (1% alcohol) **Tab:** 125, 250, 500 mg	**Initial:** 250 mg bid or tid po for the first 48 h. Adjust dosage at intervals of not less than 2 days. **Maintenance:** 500 mg - 2 g daily po in 2 - 4 divided doses.
Methyldopate Hydrochloride (*)	ALDOMET	Antihypertensive	**Inj:** 50 mg/mL	250 - 500 mg q 6 h IV.
Methylergonovine (*)	METHERGINE	Oxytocic	**Tab:** 0.2 mg **Inj:** 0.2 mg/mL	0.2 mg tid or qid po for a maximum of 1 week. 0.2 mg q 2 - 4 h IM.
Methylphenidate Hydrochloride (*) (C-II)	RITALIN, METHYLIN	CNS Stimulant	**Tab:** 5, 10, 20 mg	10 - 30 mg daily po in divided doses 2 or 3 times daily, preferably 30 - 45 minutes ac.
	RITALIN LA		**Extended-Rel. Cpsl:** 20, 30, 40 mg	Initially 20 mg once daily po in the AM. The dosage may be adjusted in weekly 10 mg increments to a maximum of 60 mg daily once daily po in the AM.

	RITALIN SR METHYLIN ER		**Sustained-Rel. Tab**: 20 mg **Extended-Rel. Tab**: 10, 20 mg	20 mg q 8 h po, preferably 30 - 45 minutes ac. 10 - 20 mg q 8 h po, preferably 30 - 45 minutes ac.
	CONCERTA		**Extended-Rel. Tab**: 18, 27, 36, 54 mg	18 mg once daily po. May increase dosage by 18 mg once daily po at intervals of 1 week. Maximum dose is 54 mg daily. Swallow the tablets whole; do not crush, chew, or divide.
Methylprednisolone	MEDROL	Corticosteroid	**Tab**: 2, 4, 8, 16, 24, 32 mg	Initial dosage varies from 4 - 48 mg daily po, depending on the disease being treated. This dosage should be maintained or adjusted until the patient's response is satisfactory.
Methylprednisolone Acetate	DEPO-MEDROL	Corticosteroid	**Inj (per mL)**: 40, 80 mg	Initial dosage varies from 20 - 80 mg weekly to monthly, depending on the disease being treated; the dosage may be given intra-articularly or IM. The dosage should be maintained or adjusted until the patient's response is satisfactory.
Methylprednisolone Sodium Succinate	SOLU-MEDROL	Corticosteroid	**Powd for Inj**: 40, 125, 500 mg: 1, 2 g	30 mg/kg IV (administered over at least 30 minutes) q 4 - 6 h for 48 hours.
Methyltestosterone (C-III)	ANDROID, TESTRED	Androgen, Antineoplastic	**Cpsl**: 10 mg	**Replacement Therapy in Males**: 10 - 50 mg daily po. **Breast Carcinoma in Females**: 50 - 200 mg daily po.
Methysergide Maleate	SANSERT	Antimigraine Agent	**Tab**: 2 mg	4 - 8 mg daily with meals po.
Metipranolol Hydrochloride	OPTIPRANOLOL	Anti-Glaucoma Agent	**Ophth Solution**: 0.3%	1 drop into affected eye(s) bid.

145

GENERIC NAME	COMMON TRADE NAMES	THERAPEUTIC CATEGORY	PREPARATIONS	COMMON ADULT DOSAGE
Metoclopramide Hydrochloride	REGLAN	GI Stimulant, Antiemetic	Inj: 5 mg/mL	**Diabetic Gastroparesis (severe symptoms):** 10 mg slow IV (over 1 - 2 minutes) for up to 10 days; then switch to oral therapy. **Nausea and Vomiting associated with Cancer Chemotherapy:** 1 - 2 mg/kg slow IV (over 15 minutes), 30 min before beginning cancer therapy; repeat q 2 h for 2 doses, then q 3 h for 3 doses. **Postoperative Nausea and Vomiting:** 10 mg IM. **Facilitate Small Bowel Intubation:** 10 mg slow IV (over 1 - 2 minutes).
			Syrup: 5 mg/5 mL **Tab:** 5, 10 mg	**Gastroesophageal Reflux:** 10 - 15 mg po up to qid 30 minutes ac & hs. If symptoms are intermittent, single doses of up to 20 mg may be used prior to the provoking stimulus. **Diabetic Gastroparesis (early symptoms):** 10 mg po 30 minutes ac & hs for 2 - 8 weeks.
Metolazone	MYKROX	Antihypertensive	**Tab:** 0.5 mg	0.5 mg once daily po in the AM. If necessary, the dose may be increased to 1 mg daily po.
	ZAROXOLYN	Diuretic, Antihypertensive	**Tab:** 2.5, 5, 10 mg	**Diuresis:** 5 - 20 mg once daily po. **Hypertension:** 2.5 - 5 mg once daily po.
Metoprolol Succinate	TOPROL XL	Antihypertensive, Antianginal	**Extended-Rel. Tab:** 23.75, 47.5, 95, 190 mg (equivalent to 25, 50, 100, 200 mg of metoprolol tartrate, respectively)	**Hypertension:** Initially, 50 - 100 mg daily po in a single dose. May increase dosage at weekly (or longer) intervals up to a maximum of 400 mg daily. **Angina:** Initially 100 mg daily po in a single dose. May increase dosage at weekly intervals up to a maximum of 400 mg daily.
Metoprolol Tartrate (*)	LOPRESSOR	Post-MI Drug	Inj: 1 mg/mL	**Post-Myocardial Infarction:** Start with 3 bolus IV injections of 5 mg each, at approximately 2-minute intervals. Then, switch to oral dosing as described below.

146

Metronidazole (*)

Antihypertensive, Antianginal, Post-MI Drug

Tab: 50, 100 mg

Hypertension and Angina: Initially, 100 mg daily po in a single or divided doses. May increase at weekly intervals. The effective dosage range is 100 - 400 mg/day.

Post-Myocardial Infarction:

Early Treatment: In patients who tolerate the full IV dose (15 mg; see below), 50 mg po q 6 h, initiated 15 minutes after the last IV dose and continue for 48 h. Then give a maintenance dose of 100 mg bid po. In patients who do not tolerate the full IV dose, 25 - 50 mg po q 6 h, initiated 15 minutes after the last IV dose or as soon as their condition allows.

Late Treatment: Patients who appear not to tolerate full Early Treatment or those with contraindications to treatment, 100 mg po bid, as soon as their condition allows.

FLAGYL
FLAGYL 375

Antitrichomonal, Amebicide, Antibacterial

Tab: 250, 500 mg
Cpsl: 375 mg

Trichomoniasis: 250 mg tid po for 7 days; 375 mg bid po for 7 days; or 2 g as a single dose po.

Acute Intestinal Amebiasis: 750 mg tid po for 5 - 10 days.

Amebic Liver Abscess: 500 - 750 mg tid po for 5 - 10 days.

Anaerobic Bacterial Infections: Following IV dosing (as described below), 7.5 mg/kg po q 6 h for 7 - 10 days.

FLAGYL ER

Antitrichomonal, Antibacterial

Tab: 750 mg

Bacterial Vaginosis: 750 mg once daily po for 7 days. Take at least 1 h ac or 2 h pc.

METROGEL
METROCREAM

Anti-Acne Agent

Gel: 0.75%
Cream: 0.75%

Apply and rub in a thin film to affected areas bid, morning and evening.

METROGEL VAGINAL

Antibacterial (Topical)

Vaginal Gel: 0.75%

Insert 1 applicatorful intravaginally once daily hs or bid, morning and evening, for 5 days.

GENERIC NAME	COMMON TRADE NAMES	THERAPEUTIC CATEGORY	PREPARATIONS	COMMON ADULT DOSAGE
Metronidazole Hydrochloride	FLAGYL I.V. FLAGYL I.V. RTU	Antibacterial	Powd for Inj: 500 mg Inj: 500 mg/100 mL	**Treatment of Anaerobic Infections:** 15 mg/kg infused IV (over 1 h) as a loading dose; then, 7.5 mg/kg infused IV (over 1 h) q 6 h. **Surgical Prophylaxis:** 15 mg/kg infused IV (over 30 - 60 minutes) and completed 1 hour before surgery; then 7.5 mg/kg infused IV (over 30 - 60 minutes) at 6 and 12 h after the initial dose.
Metyrosine	DEMSER	Antihypertensive	Cpsl: 250 mg	250 mg qid po. This may be increased by 250 to 500 mg every day to a maximum of 4.0 g per day in divided doses.
Mexiletine Hydrochloride (*)	MEXITIL	Antiarrhythmic	Cpsl: 150, 200, 250 mg	Initially, 200 mg q 8 h po with food or antacid. After 2 - 3 days, dosage may be adjusted in 50 or 100 mg increments. For rapid control of arrhythmias, 400 mg po may be used as an initial loading dose.
Miconazole Nitrate	DESENEX, MICATIN	Antifungal (Topical)	Liquid Spray, Powder & Spray Powder: 2%	Apply to affected areas bid, AM and PM.
	MONISTAT-DERM, MICATIN		Cream: 2%	Apply to affected areas bid, AM and PM.
	MONISTAT 3		Vaginal Suppos: 200 mg	200 mg intravaginally once daily hs for 3 days.
	MONISTAT 7		Vaginal Cream: 2%	Insert 1 applicatorful intravaginally once daily hs for 7 days.
			Vaginal Suppos: 100 mg	100 mg intravaginally once daily hs for 7 days.
Midazolam Hydrochloride (*) (C-IV)	VERSED	Sedative - Hypnotic	Inj (per mL): 1, 5 mg	**Preoperative Sedation:** 0.07 - 0.08 mg/kg deep IM (approx. 5 mg) 1 h before surgery. **Conscious Sedation:** Titrate IV dose slowly to the desired effect. Give no more than 2.5 mg (over at least 2 minutes). Wait another 2 minutes to fully evaluate effect. If further titration is needed, use small increments.

148

Midodrine Hydrochloride	PRO-AMATINE	Drug for Orthostatic Hypotension	**Tab:** 2.5, 5 mg	10 mg tid po (during the daytime, e.g., at 4 hour intervals).
Miglitol	GLYSET	Hypoglycemic Agent	**Tab:** 25, 50, 100 mg	**Initial:** 25 mg tid po with the first bite of each main meal. **Maintenance:** After 4 - 8 weeks at the 25 mg dose, give 50 mg tid po with the first bite of each main meal.
Milrinone Lactate	PRIMACOR	Inotropic Agent	**Inj:** 1 mg/mL **Inj (Premixed):** 200 μg/mL in 5% Dextrose Injection	**Loading Dose:** 50 μg/kg IV (over 10 minutes). **Maintenance:** 0.375 - 0.75 μg/kg/min by IV infusion. Total daily dosage: 0.59 - 1.13 mg/kg per 24 hours.
Mineral Oil	FLEET MINERAL OIL ENEMA	Emollient Laxative	**Rectal Liquid:** (pure)	Administer 1 bottle (118 mL) rectally as a single dose.
Minocycline Hydrochloride	MINOCIN IV	Antibacterial	**Powd for Inj:** 100 mg	200 mg initially IV, followed by 100 mg q 12 h IV.
	DYNACIN		**Cpsl:** 50, 75, 100 mg	200 mg initially po, followed by 100 mg q 12 h po; or, 100 - 200 mg initially po, followed by 50 mg qid po.
Minoxidil (*)	LONITEN	Antihypertensive	**Tab:** 2.5, 10 mg	Initially, 5 mg once daily po. May increase to 10, 20 and then to 40 mg daily po as a single dose or in divided doses. Intervals between dosage adjustments should be at least 3 days.
	ROGAINE	Hair Growth Stimulator	**Solution:** 20 mg/mL (2%)	Apply 1 mL to the total affected areas of the scalp bid.
	ROGAINE EXTRA STRENGTH		**Solution:** 50 mg/mL (5%)	Apply 1 mL to the total affected areas of the scalp bid.
Mirtazapine (*)	REMERON REMERON SOFTAB	Antidepressant	**Tab & Oral Disintegrating Tab:** 15, 30, 45 mg	15 mg/day po, preferably in the evening prior to sleep.
Misoprostol	CYTOTEC	Anti-Ulcer Agent	**Tab:** 100, 200 μg	200 μg qid with food po.

GENERIC NAME	COMMON TRADE NAMES	THERAPEUTIC CATEGORY	PREPARATIONS	COMMON ADULT DOSAGE
Mivacurium Chloride	MIVACRON	Neuromuscular Blocker	Inj (per mL): 0.5, 2 mg	**Initial:** 0.15 mg/kg IV (over 5-15 sec), or 0.20 mg/kg IV (over 30 sec), or 0.25 mg/kg IV (0.15 mg/kg followed in 30 sec by 0.10 mg/kg) for tracheal intubation. **Maintenance:** 0.1 mg/kg IV.
Modafinil (*)	PROVIGIL	CNS Stimulant	Tab: 100, 200 mg	Narcolepsy: 200 mg once daily po in the AM.
Moexipril Hydrochloride	UNIVASC	Antihypertensive	Tab: 7.5, 15 mg	**Initial:** 7.5 mg once daily po, 1 h ac. **Maintenance:** 7.5 - 30 mg daily po in 1 or 2 divided doses, 1 h ac.
Molindone Hydrochloride (*)	MOBAN	Antipsychotic	Conc Liquid: 20 mg/mL (alcohol) Tab: 5, 10, 25, 50, 100 mg	**Initial:** 50 - 75 mg/day po; increase to 100 mg/day in 3 - 4 days. **Maintenance:** 5 - 15 mg tid or qid po (mild); 10 - 25 mg tid or qid po (moderate); 225 mg/day may be needed (severe psychosis).
Mometasone Furoate	ELOCON NASONEX	Corticosteroid (Topical)	Cream, Oint & Lotion: 0.1% Nasal Spray: 50 µg/spray	Apply a thin film to affected areas once daily. **Allergic Rhinitis:** 2 sprays in each nostril once daily. For prophylaxis, begin 2 - 4 weeks prior to anticipated start of pollen season.
Montelukast Sodium (*)	SINGULAIR	Drug for Asthma	Tab: 5, 10 mg (as the base)	10 mg daily po, taken in the evening.
Moricizine Hydrochloride (*)	ETHMOZINE	Antiarrhythmic	Tab: 200, 250, 300 mg	600 - 900 mg/day po, given q 8 h in 3 equally divided doses. Within this range, the dosage can be adjusted in increments of 150 mg/day at 3-day intervals.

Morphine Sulfate (*) (C-II)	ASTRAMORPH/PF, DURAMORPH	Opioid Analgesic	Inj (per mL): 0.5, 1 mg	IV: 2 - 10 mg/70 kg. **Epidural:** Initially, 5 mg in the lumbar region; after 1 hour, incremental doses of 1 - 2 mg at interval sufficient to assess effectiveness may be given carefully. **Max:** 10 mg/24 h. **Intrathecal:** 0.2 - 1 mg in the lumbar area.
	INFUMORPH		Inj (per mL): 10, 25 mg	**Intrathecal Infusion:** Initially, 0.2 - 1 mg/day (patients with no opioid tolerance) and 1 - 10 mg/day (opioid tolerance) in the lumbar area. **Epidural Infusion:** 3.5 - 7.5 mg/day (patients with no opioid tolerance) and 4.5 - 10 mg/day (opioid tolerance).
	KADIAN		Sustained-Rel. Cpsl: 20, 50, 100 mg	Variable po dosages based on patient tolerance to opioids and type of conversion, e.g., from oral morphine, parenteral morphine, or other opioid analgesics. Commonly used q 24 h.
	MS CONTIN		**Controlled-Rel. Tab:** 15, 30, 60, 100, 200 mg	Variable po dosages based on patient tolerance to opioids and type of conversion, e.g., from oral morphine, parenteral morphine, or other opioid analgesics. Commonly used q 12 h.
	ORAMORPH SR		**Sustained-Rel. Tab:** 15, 30, 60, 100 mg	
	MSIR		Solution (per 5 mL): 10, 20 mg **Conc Solution:** 20 mg/mL **Cpsl & Tab:** 15, 30 mg	5 - 30 mg q 4 h po prn pain.
	RMS		Rectal Suppos: 5, 10, 20, 30 mg	10 - 20 mg q 4 h rectally.
	ROXANOL		Oral Solution: 20 mg/mL	10 - 30 mg q 4 h po prn pain.
	ROXANOL 100		Oral Solution: 100 mg/5 mL	10 - 30 mg q 4 h po prn pain.

151

GENERIC NAME	COMMON TRADE NAMES	THERAPEUTIC CATEGORY	PREPARATIONS	COMMON ADULT DOSAGE
Moxifloxacin Hydrochloride	AVELOX AVELOX I.V.	Antibacterial	**Tab:** 400 mg **Inj:** 400 mg/250 mL	**Acute Bacterial Exacerbation of Chronic Bronchitis:** 400 mg once daily po or by IV infusion (over 60 min) for 5 days. **Acute Bacterial Sinusitis:** 400 mg once daily po or by IV infusion (over 60 min) for 10 days. **Community-Acquired Pneumonia:** 400 mg once daily po or by IV infusion (over 60 min) for 7 - 14 days. **Skin & Skin Structure Infections (Uncomplic.):** 400 mg once daily po or by IV infusion (over 60 min) for 7 days.
Mupirocin	BACTROBAN	Antibacterial (Topical)	**Oint:** 2%	Apply a small amount to affected area tid.
Mupirocin Calcium	BACTROBAN NASAL	Antibacterial (Topical)	**Oint:** 2%	Apply approximately 1/2 of the ointment from the single-use tube into each nostril bid (morning & evening) for 5 days.
	BACTROBAN		**Cream:** 2%	Apply a small amount to affected area tid for 10 days.
Mycophenolate Mofetil	CELLCEPT	Immunosuppressant	**Cpsl:** 250 mg **Tab:** 500 mg **Powd for Oral Susp:** 200 mg/mL (when reconst.) **Powd for Inj:** 500 mg (as the HCl)	**Renal Transplantation:** 1 g po or IV (over ≥ 2 h) bid. **Cardiac Transplantation:** 1.5 g po of IV (over ≥ 2 h) bid. **Hepatic Transplantation:** 1 g bid IV (over ≥ 2 h) or 1.5 g bid po. Give the initial oral dose as soon as possible following transplantation. Give on an empty stomach. IV administration is recommended for patients unable to take cpls or tabs. Use within 24 h of transplantation and for ≤ 14 days. Switch to the oral medication ASAP.

Nabumetone (*)	RELAFEN	Antiinflammatory	Tab: 500, 750 mg	Initially 1000 mg po as a single dose with or without food. Dosage may be increased to 1500 - 2000 mg/day as a single dose or in 2 divided doses.
Nadolol (*)	CORGARD	Antihypertensive, Antianginal	Tab: 20, 40, 80, 120, 160 mg	**Hypertension:** Initially, 40 mg once daily po. May increase dosage in increments of 40 to 80 mg until optimal response occurs. Usual maintenance dose is 40 - 80 mg once daily. **Angina:** Initially, 40 mg once daily po. May increase dosage in increments of 40 - 80 mg at 3 - 7 day intervals until optimal response occurs. Usual maintenance dosage is 40 to 80 mg once daily.
Nafcillin Sodium (*)		Antibacterial	Cpsl: 250 mg	**Mild to Moderate Infections:** 250 - 500 mg q 4 to 6 h po. **Severe Infections:** 1000 mg q 4 - 6 h po.
Naftifine Hydrochloride	NAFTIN	Antifungal (Topical)	Cream: 1% Gel: 1%	Gently massage into affected areas once daily. Gently massage into affected areas bid, morning and evening.
Nalbuphine Hydrochloride (*)	NUBAIN	Opioid Analgesic	Inj (per mL): 10, 20 mg	10 mg/70 kg SC, IM, or IV; dose may be repeated q 3 - 6 h prn.
Nalidixic Acid (*)	NEG-GRAM	Urinary Tract Anti-Infective	Susp: 250 mg/5 mL Cplt: 250, 500 mg; 1 g	Initially, 1 g qid po for 1 - 2 weeks. For prolonged therapy, may reduce dosage to 500 mg qid after the initial treatment period.

GENERIC NAME	COMMON TRADE NAMES	THERAPEUTIC CATEGORY	PREPARATIONS	COMMON ADULT DOSAGE
Nalmefene Hydrochloride	REVEX	Opioid Antagonist	Inj (per mL): 100 μg, 1.0 mg.	**Opioid Overdose (Known or Suspected):** Use the 1.0 mg/mL strength. **Non-Opioid Dependent Patients:** 0.5 mg/70 kg IM, SC, or IV. If needed, this may be followed by a 2nd dose of 1.0 mg/70 kg, 2 - 5 minutes later. **Suspected Opioid-Dependent Patients:** An initial challenge dose of 0.1 mg/70 kg should be used. If no evidence of withdrawal occurs, use the above dosage. **Postoperative Opioid Respiratory Depression:** Use the 100 μg/mL strength. Initially 0.25 μg/kg IM, SC or IV, followed by 0.25 μg/kg incremental doses at 2 - 5 minute intervals, stopping as soon as the desired degree of opioid reversal occurs.
Naloxone Hydrochloride (*)	NARCAN	Opioid Antagonist	Inj (per mL): 0.4, 1 mg	**Opioid Overdose (Known or Suspected):** Initially, 0.4 - 2 mg IV. Dose may be repeated at 2 - 3 min intervals. Max: 10 mg. **Postoperative Opioid Respiratory Depression:** 0.1 - 0.2 mg IV at 2 - 3 minute intervals. Doses may be repeated in 1 - 2 hours.
Naltrexone Hydrochloride (*)	REVIA	Opioid Antagonist	Tab: 50 mg	50 mg once daily po for most patients.
Nandrolone Decanoate (C-III)	DECA-DURABOLIN	Anabolic Steroid	Inj (per mL): 50, 100, 200 mg (in oil)	**Women:** 50 - 100 mg per week by deep IM. **Men:** 100 - 200 mg per week by deep IM.
Naphazoline Hydrochloride	PRIVINE	Nasal Decongestant	Nasal Solution & Spray: 0.05%	1 - 2 drops or sprays in each nostril no more than q 6 h.
	NAPHCON NAPHCON FORTE	Ocular Decongestant	Ophth Solution: 0.012% Ophth Solution: 0.1%	1 - 2 drops into the affected eye(s) up to qid. 1 - 2 drops into the affected eye(s) q 3 - 4 h.

Naproxen (*)	NAPROSYN	Non-Opioid Analgesic, Antiinflammatory	**Susp:** 125 mg/5 mL **Tab:** 250, 375, 500 mg	**Analgesia, Dysmenorrhea, Acute Tendonitis and Bursitis:** 500 mg po, followed by 250 mg po q 6 - 8 h prn. **Acute Gout:** 750 mg po, followed by 250 mg po q 8 h until the attack has subsided. **Rheumatoid Arthritis, Osteoarthritis and Ankylosing Spondylitis:** 250 - 500 mg bid po, morning and evening. **Juvenile Arthritis:** 5 mg/kg bid po.
	EC-NAPROSYN	Antiinflammatory	**Delayed-Rel. Tab:** 375, 500 mg	**Rheumatoid Arthritis, Osteoarthritis and Ankylosing Spondylitis:** 375 - 500 mg bid po, morning and evening.
Naproxen Sodium	ALEVE	Non-Opioid Analgesic, Antipyretic	**Cplt, Tab & Gelcap:** 220 mg	**Analgesia & Fever:** 220 mg q 8 - 12 h po with a full glass of liquid, while symptoms persist or 440 mg initially, followed by 220 mg 12 h later.
	ANAPROX ANAPROX DS	Non-Opioid Analgesic, Antiinflammatory	**Tab:** 275 mg **Tab:** 550 mg	**Analgesia, Dysmenorrhea, Acute Tendonitis and Bursitis:** 550 mg po, followed by 275 mg po q 6 - 8 h prn. **Acute Gout:** 825 mg po, followed by 275 mg po q 8 h until the attack has subsided. **Rheumatoid Arthritis, Osteoarthritis and Ankylosing Spondylitis:** 275 or 550 mg bid po, morning and evening.

[Continued on the next page]

155

GENERIC NAME	COMMON TRADE NAMES	THERAPEUTIC CATEGORY	PREPARATIONS	COMMON ADULT DOSAGE
Naproxen Sodium [Continued]	NAPRELAN	Non-Opioid Analgesic, Antiinflammatory	Controlled-Rel. Tab: 412.5, 550 mg (equivalent to 375 and 500 mg of naproxen, respectively)	**Analgesia, Dysmenorrhea, Acute Tendonitis and Bursitis:** 1000 mg once daily po. **Acute Gout:** 1000 - 1500 mg once daily po on the first day, followed by 1000 mg once daily until the attack has subsided. **Rheumatoid Arthritis, Osteoarthritis and Ankylosing Spondylitis:** 750 - 1000 mg once daily po.
Naratriptan Hydrochloride	AMERGE	Antimigraine Agent	Tab: 1, 2.5 mg	1 - 2.5 mg po taken with fluid. If the headache returns or if the patient has only a partial response, the dose may be repeated after 4 h. Do not exceed 5 mg within 24 h.
Natamycin	NATACYN	Antifungal (Topical)	Ophth Susp: 5%	**Fungal Keratitis:** 1 drop into the affected eye(s) at 1 or 2 hour intervals. The frequency of application can usually be reduced to 1 drop 6 - 8 times daily after the first 3 or 4 days. **Fungal Blepharitis & Conjunctivitis:** 4 to 6 daily applications may be sufficient.
Nateglinide	STARLIX	Hypoglycemic	Tab: 60, 120 mg	120 mg tid po. 1 - 30 min ac.
Nedocromil Sodium	TILADE	Drug for Asthma	Aerosol: 1.75 mg/spray	2 inhalations qid at regular intervals.
	ALOCRIL	Antiallergic, Ophthalmic	Ophth Solution: 2%	1 - 2 drops in each eye bid at regular intervals.
Nefazodone Hydrochloride (*)	SERZONE	Antidepressant	Tab: 50, 100, 150, 200, 250 mg	Initially, 100 mg bid po. Effective dose range is 300 - 600 mg/day; therefore, increase dose in increments of 100 - 200 mg/day (given on a bid basis) at interval of no less than 1 week.
Nelfinavir Mesylate	VIRACEPT	Antiviral	Tab: 250 mg	750 mg (3 tablets) tid or 1250 mg (6 tablets), po, with meals or a light snack, in combination with nucleoside analogues.

156

Neostigmine Methylsulfate	PROSTIGMIN	Cholinomimetic	Inj (per mL): 0.5, 1 mg	**Myasthenia Gravis:** 0.5 mg SC or IM. Adjust subsequent doses based on response. **Postoperative Distension & Urinary Retention: Prevention:** 0.25 mg SC or IM as soon as possible after operation; repeat q 4 - 6 h for 2 - 3 days. **Treatment:** 0.5 mg SC or IM. **Reversal of Neuromuscular Blockade:** 0.5 - 2 mg by slow IV, repeated as required. Also administer IV atropine sulfate, 0.6 - 1.2 mg.
Netilmicin Sulfate (*)	NETROMYCIN	Antibacterial	Inj: 100 mg/mL	**Urinary Tract Infections (Complicated):** 1.5 - 2.0 mg/kg q 12 h IM or IV. **Serious Systemic Infections:** 1.3 - 2.2 mg/kg q 8 h IM or IV; or, 2.0 - 3.25 mg/kg q 12 h IM or IV.
Nevirapine	VIRAMUNE	Antiviral	Tab: 200 mg Suspension: 50 mg/5 mL	**Initial:** 200 mg once daily po for 14 days. **Maintenance:** 200 mg bid po in combination with a nucleoside analog antiretroviral drug.
Niacin	NIACOR	Antihyperlipidemic	Tab: 500 mg	Start with 250 mg once daily po following the evening meal. Frequency of dosing and total daily dose can be increased q 4 - 7 days until the desired response is attained or the first-level therapeutic dose of 1.5 - 2 g daily is reached. If response is not adequate after 2 months, the dosage can be increased at 2 to 4 week intervals to 3 grams/day (1 g tid po). The usual dose is 1 - 2 g bid to tid po.
	NIASPAN		Extended-Rel. Tab: 500, 750, 1000 mg	Take hs with a low-fat meal or snack. 500 mg once daily hs po for 1 - 4 weeks; then 1000 mg once daily hs po during weeks 5 - 8. After week 8, titrate to the patient's response. Maximum: 2000 mg/day.

GENERIC NAME	COMMON TRADE NAMES	THERAPEUTIC CATEGORY	PREPARATIONS	COMMON ADULT DOSAGE

Nicardipine Hydrochloride (*)

CARDENE — Antianginal, Antihypertensive — Cpsl: 20, 30 mg

Angina: Initially, 20 mg tid po; may increase dosage after 3 days. Doses in the range of 20 - 40 mg tid are effective.
Hypertension: Initially, 20 mg tid po. Doses in the range of 20 - 40 mg tid are effective.

CARDENE SR — Antihypertensive — Sustained-Rel. Cpsl: 30, 45, 60 mg

Initially, 30 mg bid po. Effective doses range from 30 - 60 mg bid po.

CARDENE I.V. — Antihypertensive — Inj: 2.5 mg/mL

Initiation in a Drug-free Patient: Administer by contin. IV infusion at a conc. of 0.1 mg/mL.
Titration: For gradual reduction in blood pressure, start at 5 mg/h (50 mL/h); may increase rate by 2.5 mg/h (25 mL/h) q 15 min up to a max. of 15 mg/h (150 mL/h). For rapid reduction in blood pressure, begin at 5 mg/h (50 mL/h); may increase rate by 2.5 mg/h (25 mL/h) q 5 min up to a maximum of 15 mg/h (150 mL/h). In either case, after desired effect is achieved reduce infusion rate to 30 mL/h.
Maintenance: Adjust infusion rate as needed.
Substitution for Oral Nicardipine: Use the infusion rate as indicated in the table below:

Oral Dose	Equivalent IV Infusion Rate
20 mg q 8 h	0.5 mg/h
30 mg q 8 h	1.2 mg/h
40 mg q 8 h	2.2 mg/h

158

Nicotine (*)	Smoking Deterrent		
HABITROL, NICODERM CQ		Transdermal: rate = 7, 14, 21 mg/24 hr	Apply to clean, dry, non-hairy site on upper body or upper outer arm. Initially, one 21 mg/24 h patch daily for 6 weeks; then, one 14 mg/24 h patch daily for 2 - 4 weeks; then, one 7 mg/24 h patch daily for 2 - 4 weeks.
NICOTROL		Transdermal: rate = 15 mg/16 hr	Apply to clean, dry, non-hairy site on upper body or upper outer arm. Apply one patch daily for 6 weeks.
NICOTROL STEP 1		Transdermal: rate = 15 mg/16 hr	Apply to clean, dry, non-hairy site on upper body or upper outer arm. Apply one patch daily for 6 weeks (Weeks 1 through 6).
NICOTROL STEP 2		Transdermal: rate = 10 mg/16 hr	Apply to clean, dry, non-hairy site on upper body or upper outer arm. Apply one patch daily for 2 weeks (Weeks 7 and 8).
NICOTROL STEP 3		Transdermal: rate = 5 mg/16 hr	Apply to clean, dry, non-hairy site on upper body or upper outer arm. Apply one patch daily for 2 weeks (Weeks 9 and 10).
NICOTROL INHALER		Inhaler: 10 mg/cartridge (4 mg delivered)	Individualize dosage. The most successful patients used between 6 and 16 cartridges per day. The recommended duration of therapy is 3 months, after which patients may be weaned from the inhaler by gradual reduction of the daily dose over the following 6 to 12 weeks.
NICOTROL NS		Nasal Spray: 0.5 mg/spray	1 spray in each nostril. Start with 1 - 2 doses per hour, which may be increased up to a maximum of 5 doses per hour (40 doses per day).

GENERIC NAME	COMMON TRADE NAMES	THERAPEUTIC CATEGORY	PREPARATIONS	COMMON ADULT DOSAGE
Nicotine Polacrilex (*)	NICORETTE	Smoking Deterrent	Chewing Gum: 2 mg/piece	**Less Dependent Smokers:** Chew 1 piece slowly and intermittently for 30 minutes. Most patients require 9 - 12 pieces of gum per day. Maximum: 30 pieces per day.
	NICORETTE DS		Chewing Gum: 4 mg/piece	**Highly Dependent Smokers:** Chew 1 piece slowly and intermittently for 30 minutes. Most patients require 9 - 12 pieces of gum per day. Maximum: 20 pieces per day.
Nifedipine (*)	ADALAT, PROCARDIA	Antianginal	Cpsl: 10, 20 mg	Initially, 10 mg tid po; may increase dosage over a 7 - 14 day period. Usual effective dosage range is 10 - 20 mg tid po.
	ADALAT CC, PROCARDIA XL	Antianginal, Antihypertensive	Extended-Rel. Tab: 30, 60, 90 mg	Initially, 30 or 60 mg once daily po: adjust the dosage over a 7 - 14 day period.
Nilutamide	NILANDRON	Antineoplastic	Tab: 50, 150 mg	300 mg once daily po for 30 days, followed by 150 mg once daily.
Nisoldipine (*)	SULAR	Antihypertensive	Extended-Rel. Tab: 10, 20, 30, 40 mg	Initially 20 mg once daily po, then increase the dose by 10 mg per week, or longer intervals, to adequate control of blood pressure. The usual maintenance dosage is 20 - 40 mg once daily po.
Nitrofurantoin	FURADANTIN	Urinary Tract Anti-infective, Antibacterial	Oral Susp: 25 mg/5 mL	50 - 100 mg qid po with food. For long-term suppressive therapy, reduce dosage to 50 - 100 mg po hs.
Nitrofurantoin Macrocrystals	MACRODANTIN	Urinary Tract Anti-infective, Antibacterial	Cpsl: 25, 50, 100 mg	**Usual Dosage:** 50 - 100 mg qid po with food. **Urinary Tract Infections (Uncomplicated):** 50 mg qid po with food.
Nitrofurantoin Monohydrate	MACROBID	Urinary Tract Anti-infective	Cpsl: 100 mg	100 mg q 12 h po with food for 7 days.
Nitrofurazone	FURACIN	Burn Preparation	Cream & Soluble Dressing: 0.2%	Apply directly to the lesion or place on gauze. Reapply daily or every few days.

Nitroglycerin (*)		Antianginal		
	DEPONIT		**Transdermal: rate = 0.2, 0.4 mg/h**	Apply a 0.2 mg/h or 0.4 mg/h patch for 12 to 14 h daily as a starting dose.
	MINITRAN		**Transdermal: rate = 0.1, 0.2, 0.4, 0.6 mg/h**	Same dosage as for DEPONIT above.
	NITRODISC		**Transdermal: rate = 0.2, 0.3, 0.4 mg/h**	Same dosage as for DEPONIT above.
	NITRO-DUR		**Transdermal: rate = 0.1, 0.2, 0.3, 0.4, 0.6, 0.8 mg/h**	Same dosage as for DEPONIT above.
	TRANSDERM-NITRO		**Transdermal: rate = 0.1, 0.2, 0.4, 0.6 mg, 0.8 mg/h**	Same dosage as for DEPONIT above.
	NITRO-BID		**Oint: 2%**	Apply 0.5 inch of ointment to a 1 x 3-inch area of skin q 8 h. Titrate upward (1 inch on a 2 x 3-in area q 8 h) until angina is controlled.
	NITROSTAT		**Subling. Tab: 0.3, 0.4, 0.6 mg**	Place 1 tablet under tongue or in the buccal pouch at the first sign of an acute anginal attack. Repeat approx. q 5 min. until relief is obtained. Take no more than 3 tabs within 15 minutes.
	NITROGARD		**Extended-Rel. Buccal Tab: 1, 2, 3 mg**	Place tablet under the upper lip or in the buccal pouch; allow tablet to dissolve slowly over a 3 - 5 hour period. Initial dose is 1 mg, with subsequent increases guided by symptoms and side effects.
	NITROLINGUAL PUMP SPRAY		**Spray: 0.4 µg/spray**	1 - 2 sprays onto or under tongue at onset of attack. No more than 3 sprays within a 15 minute period.
	NITRO-BID IV		**Inj (per mL): 5 mg**	Initially, 5 µg/min by IV infusion. Titrate dosage based upon clinical situation; increases of 5 µg/min can be made at 3 - 5 min intervals. If no response occurs at 20 µg/min, increments of 10 and later 20 µg/min can be used.

GENERIC NAME	COMMON TRADE NAMES	THERAPEUTIC CATEGORY	PREPARATIONS	COMMON ADULT DOSAGE
Nizatidine (*)	AXID	Histamine H$_2$-Blocker, Anti-Ulcer Agent	Cpsl: 150, 300 mg	**Active Duodenal Ulcer or Benign Gastric Ulcer:** 300 mg once daily po hs or 150 mg bid po. **Maintenance of Healed Duodenal Ulcer:** 150 mg once daily po hs. **Gastroesophageal Reflux Disease:** 150 mg bid po.
	AXID AR	Histamine H$_2$-Blocker	Tab: 75 mg	**Prevention of Heartburn, Acid Indigestion, and Sour Stomach:** 75 mg po with water 30 - 60 min. before consuming food and beverages that may cause symptoms. May be used up to bid.
Norethindrone (*)	ORTHO MICRONOR, NOR-Q.D.	Oral Contraceptive (Progestin-Only)	Tab: 0.35 mg	1 tablet daily po, every day of the year starting on the first day of menstruation.
Norethindrone Acetate (*)	AYGESTIN	Progestin	Tab: 5 mg	**Amenorrhea:** 2.5 - 10 mg once daily po, for 5 to 10 days during the second half of the menstrual cycle. **Endometriosis:** 5 mg once daily po for 2 weeks, with increments of 2.5 mg/day q 2 weeks until 15 mg/day is reached.
Norfloxacin (*)	NOROXIN	Urinary Tract Anti-Infective	Tab: 400 mg	**Urinary Tract Infections:** **Uncomplicated, due to _E. coli, K. pneumonia, or P. mirabilis:_** 400 mg q 12 h po for 3 days. **Uncomplicated, due to Other Organisms:** 400 mg q 12 h po for 7 - 10 days. **Complicated:** 400 mg q 12 h po for 10 - 21 days. **Gonorrhea (Uncomplicated):** 800 mg po (as a single dose). **Prostatitis:** 400 mg q 12 h po for 28 days.
Norgestrel	OVRETTE	Oral Contraceptive (Progestin-Only)	Tab: 0.075 mg	1 tablet daily po, every day of the year starting on the first day of menstruation.

Nortriptyline Hydrochloride (*)	PAMELOR	Antidepressant	**Solution:** 10 mg/5 mL (3.4% alcohol) **Cpsl:** 10, 25, 50, 75 mg	25 mg tid or qid po; or total daily dosage may be given once daily hs po.
Nystatin	MYCOSTATIN	Antifungal	**Susp:** 100,000 Units/mL **Tab:** 500,000 Units **Pastilles:** 200,000 Units **Vaginal Tab:** 100,000 Units **Cream & Oint:** 100,000 Units/g **Powder:** 100,000 Units/g	400,000 - 600,000 Units qid po (1/2 dose in each side of the mouth). 500,000 - 1,000,000 Units tid po. 200,000 - 400,000 Units 4 or 5 times daily po. Allow to dissolve slowly in the mouth. 1 tablet daily intravaginally for 2 weeks. Apply liberally to affected areas bid. Apply to candidal lesions bid or tid.
Ofloxacin (*)	FLOXIN FLOXIN I.V.	Antibacterial	**Tab:** 200, 300, 400 mg **Inj (per mL):** 10, 20 mg	**Lower Respiratory Tract, Skin & Skin Structure Infections:** 400 mg q 12 h po or by IV infusion (over 60 min.) for 10 days. **Gonorrhea (Uncomplicated):** 400 mg po or by IV infusion (over 60 min.) as a single dose. **Cervicitis or Urethritis due to _N. gonorrhoeae_ and/or _C. trachomatis_:** 300 mg q 12 h po or by IV infusion (over 60 min.) for 7 days. **Acute Pelvic Inflammatory Disease:** 400 mg q 12 h po or by IV infusion (over 60 min.) for 10 - 14 days. **Cystitis due to _E. coli_ or _K. pneumoniae_:** 200 mg q 12 h po or by IV infusion (over 60 min.) for 3 days. **Cystitis due to other Organisms:** 200 mg q 12 h po or by IV infusion (over 60 min.) for 7 days. **Urinary Tract Infections (Complicated):** 200 mg q 12 h po or by IV infusion (over 60 min.) for 10 days. **Prostatitis:** 300 mg q 12 h po for 6 weeks or by IV infusion (over 60 min.) for up to 10 days, then switch to oral therapy.

163

[Continued on the next page]

GENERIC NAME	COMMON TRADE NAMES	THERAPEUTIC CATEGORY	PREPARATIONS	COMMON ADULT DOSAGE
Ofloxacin [Continued]	OCUFLOX	Antibacterial (Topical)	**Ophth Solution:** 0.3%	**Bacterial Conjunctivitis:** 1 - 2 drops in affected eye(s) q 2 - 4 h for 2 days, then 1 - 2 drops qid for up to 5 more days. **Bacterial Corneal Ulcer:** On Days 1 and 2 instill 1 - 2 drops in affected eye(s) q 30 min. while awake; awaken at approximately 4 and 6 h after retiring and instill 1 or 2 drops. On Days 3 through 7 - 9 instill 1 or 2 drops hourly while awake. On Days 7 - 9 to end of therapy instill 1 or 2 drops qid.
	FLOXIN OTIC	Antibacterial (Topical)	**Otic Solution:** 0.3%	**Otitis Externa:** 10 drops (0.5 mL) instilled into the affected ear bid for 10 days. **Chronic Suppurative Otitis Media w/Perforated Tympanic Membranes:** 10 drops (0.5 mL) instilled into the affected ear bid for 14 days.
Olanzapine (*)	ZYPREXA ZYPREXA ZYDIS	Antipsychotic, Antimaniacal	**Tab:** 2.5, 5, 7.5, 10, 15, 20 mg **Oral Disintegrating Tab:** 5, 10, 15, 20 mg	**Schizophrenia:** Initially 5 - 10 mg once daily po, with a target dose of 10 mg/day within several days of initiation. Adjust dosage at 5 mg increments at intervals of not less than 1 week. Continue at the lowest dose needed to maintain remission. **Bipolar Mania:** Initially 10 - 15 mg once daily po. Adjust dosage at 5 mg increments at intervals of not less than 24 hours.
Olmesartan Medoxomil	BENICAR	Antihypertensive	**Tab:** 5, 20, 40 mg	**Monotherapy (Not Volume Depleted):** Initially 20 mg once daily po. May increase to a max. of 40 mg once daily after 2 weeks. **With a Diuretic (Volume Depleted):** Consider a lower initial dose.
Olopatadine Hydrochloride	PATANOL	Antihistamine	**Ophth Solution:** 0.1%	1 - 2 drops in each affected eye bid at an interval of 6 - 8 h.
Olsalazine Sodium	DIPENTUM	Bowel Antinflam. Agent	**Cpsl:** 250 mg	1000 mg daily po in 2 divided doses.

Omeprazole (*)	PRILOSEC	Gastric Acid Pump Inhibitor, Anti-Ulcer Agent	Delayed-Rel. Cpsl: 10, 20, 40 mg	**Acute Duodenal Ulcer, Severe Erosive Esophagitis or Poorly Responsive Gastro-esophageal Reflux Disease (GERD):** 20 mg once daily po for up to 4 - 8 weeks. **Maintenance of Healing Erosive Esophagitis:** 20 mg daily po. **Active Duodenal Ulcer Associated with** *Helicobacter pylori* **Infection:** 40 mg po each AM plus clarithromycin 500 mg tid po for days 1 - 14; then 20 mg po each AM for days 15 - 28. **Pathological Hypersecretory Conditions:** 60 mg once daily po, initially; adjust dosage as indicated. Daily dosages over 80 mg po should be given in divided doses.
Ondansetron Hydrochloride (*)	ZOFRAN	Antiemetic	Tab: 4, 8, 24 mg Oral Solution: 4 mg/5 mL Inj: 2 mg/mL Inj (premixed): 32 mg/50 mL	**Highly Emetogenic Chemotherapy:** 24 mg po as a single dose 30 minutes before the start of single-day chemotherapy. **Moderately Emetogenic Chemotherapy:** 8 mg po q 8 h for 2 doses 30 minutes before chemotherapy, then 8 mg q 12 h for 1 - 2 days after chemotherapy is completed. **Prevention of Postoperative Nausea and Vomiting:** 16 mg po as a single dose 1 hour before induction of anesthesia. **Nausea & Vomiting Associated With Cancer Chemotherapy:** Three 0.15 mg/kg doses IV: The first dose is infused over 15 minutes beginning 30 minutes before the start of emetogenic chemotherapy. Alternatively, 32 mg IV (infused over 15 min) beginning 30 minutes before the start of emetogenic chemotherapy. Subsequent doses are given 4 and 8 h after the first dose. **Prevention of Postoperative Nausea and Vomiting:** Immediately before induction of anesthesia or postoperatively, 4 mg IV (over 2 to 5 min).

GENERIC NAME	COMMON TRADE NAMES	THERAPEUTIC CATEGORY	PREPARATIONS	COMMON ADULT DOSAGE
Orlistat (*)	XENICAL	Lipase Inhibitor	Cpsl: 120 mg	120 mg tid po with each main meal containing fat (during or up to 1 hour pc).
Orphenadrine Citrate (*)	NORFLEX	Skeletal Muscle Relaxant	Extended-Rel. Tab: 100 mg Inj: 60 mg/2 mL	100 mg bid po, AM and PM. 60 mg q 12 h IM or IV.
Oseltamivir Phosphate	TAMIFLU	Antiviral	Cpsl: 75 mg Powd for Susp: 12 mg/mL	**Treatment of Influenza:** 75 mg bid po for 5 days. Begin treatment within 2 days of symptom onset. **Prophylaxis of Influenza:** 75 mg once daily po for at least 7 days. Begin therapy within 2 days of exposure.
Oxacillin Sodium (*)	BACTOCILL	Antibacterial	Cpsl: 250, 500 mg Powd for Inj: 250, 500 mg; 1, 2, 4 g	**Mild to Moderate Infections of the Skin, Soft Tissue or Upper Respiratory Tract:** 500 mg q 4 - 6 h po for a minimum of 5 days. **Serious or Life-Threatening Infections:** After initial parenteral treatment, 1 g q 4 - 6 h po. **Mild to Moderate Upper Respiratory and Local Skin and Soft Tissue Infections:** 250 - 500 mg q 4 - 6 h IM or IV. **Severe Lower Respiratory or Disseminated Infections:** 1 g q 4 - 6 h IM or IV.
Oxandrolone (C-III)	OXANDRIN	Anabolic Steroid	Tab: 2.5 mg	2.5 mg bid - qid po. Usually a course of therapy of 2 - 4 weeks is adequate.
Oxaprozin	DAYPRO	Antiinflammatory	Tab: 600 mg	1200 mg once daily po. For patients of low body weight or mild disease, an initial dose of 600 mg once a day may be appropriate.
Oxazepam (*) (C-IV)	SERAX	Antianxiety Agent	Cpsl: 10, 15, 30 mg Tab: 15 mg	10 - 30 mg tid or qid po. 15 - 30 mg tid or qid po.

Oxcarbazepine	TRILEPTAL	Antiepileptic	**Tab:** 150, 300, 600 mg **Susp:** 300 mg/5 mL	**Adjunctive Therapy:** Initially 300 mg bid po. If clinically indicated, the dose may be increased by a maximum of 600 mg/day at approximately weekly intervals; the recommended daily dose is 1200 mg/day. **Conversion to Monotherapy:** Initially 300 mg bid po while simultaneously initiating the reduction of the dose of the concomitant antiepileptic drugs (AEDs). The concomitant AEDs should be completely withdrawn over 3 - 6 weeks, while the maximum dose of oxcarbazepine should be reached in 2 - 4 weeks. Increase as clinically indicated by a maximum increment of 600 mg/day at approximately weekly intervals to achieve a recommended daily dose of 2400 mg/day. **Initiation of Monotherapy:** Initially 300 mg bid po. The dose should be increased by 300 mg/day every third day to a dose of 1200 mg/day.
Oxiconazole Nitrate	OXISTAT	Antifungal (Topical)	**Cream & Lotion:** 1%	**Tinea pedis:** Apply to affected areas once daily or bid for 1 month. **Tinea corporis, and T. cruris:** Apply to affected areas once daily or bid for 2 weeks. **Tinea versicolor:** Apply to affected areas once daily for 2 weeks.
Oxtriphylline		Bronchodilator	**Tab:** 100, 200 mg	7.8 mg/kg po, followed by 4.7 mg/kg q 8 h po (in nonsmokers) and 4.7 mg/kg q 6 h po (in smokers).
	CHOLEDYL SA		**Sustained-Action Tab:** 400, 600 mg	Therapy should be initiated and daily dosage requirements established using a non-sustained-action form of oxtriphylline. If the total daily dosage of the nonsustained prep. is 1200 mg, then 600 mg of CHOLEDYL SA may be used q 12 h. Similarly, if the total daily dosage is 800 mg, then 400 mg of CHOLEDYL SA may be used q 12 h.

GENERIC NAME	COMMON TRADE NAMES	THERAPEUTIC CATEGORY	PREPARATIONS	COMMON ADULT DOSAGE
Oxybutynin Chloride	DITROPAN	Urinary Tract Antispasmodic	Syrup: 5 mg/5 mL Tab: 5 mg	5 mg bid - tid po.
	DITROPAN XL		Extended-Rel. Tab: 5, 10, 15 mg	Initially, 5 mg once daily po. May increase weekly in 5 mg increments. Maximum: 30 mg daily po.
Oxycodone Hydrochloride (*) (C-II)	ROXICODONE	Opioid Analgesic	Solution: 5 mg/5 mL Conc Solution: 20 mg/mL Tab: 5 mg	5 mg q 6 h po prn pain.
	OXYCONTIN		Controlled-Rel. Tab: 10, 20, 40, 80 mg	Variable po dosages based on patient tolerance to opioids and type of conversion, e.g., from oral morphine, parenteral morphine, or other opioid analgesics. Commonly used q 12 h.
Oxymetazoline Hydrochloride	VISINE L.R.	Ocular Decongestant	Ophth Solution: 0.025%	1 - 2 drops in the affected eye(s) q 6 h.
	AFRIN, NTZ	Nasal Decongestant	Nasal Solution: 0.05% Nasal Spray: 0.05%	2 - 3 drops into each nostril bid, AM and PM. Spray 2 - 3 times into each nostril bid, AM and PM.
	DRISTAN 12-HOUR, 4-WAY LONG LASTING, NEO-SYNEPHRINE MAXIMUM STRENGTH, NOSTRILLA LONG ACTING, VICKS SINEX 12-HOUR	Nasal Decongestant	Nasal Spray: 0.05%	Same dosage as AFRIN Spray above.
Oxymorphone Hydrochloride (C-II)	NUMORPHAN	Opioid Analgesic	Inj (per mL): 1, 1.5 mg	IM or SC: 1 - 1.5 mg q 4 - 6 h, prn pain. IV: 0.5 mg q 4 - 6 h, prn pain.
			Rectal Suppos: 5 mg	Insert 1 rectally q 4 - 6 h.
Oxytetracycline (*)	TERRAMYCIN	Antibacterial	Inj (per mL): 50, 125 mg	250 mg q 24 h IM or 300 mg daily in divided doses IM at 8- to 12-hour intervals.

168

Oxytetracycline Hydrochloride (*)	TERRAMYCIN	Antibacterial	Cpsl: 250 mg	**Usual Dosage:** 250 - 500 mg q 6 h po. **Brucellosis:** 500 mg qid po with streptomycin for 3 weeks. **Gonorrhea:** Initially 1.5 g po, followed by 500 mg qid po, for a total of 9.0 g. **Syphilis:** 30 - 40 g po in equally divided doses over a period of 10 - 15 days.
Pamidronate Disodium	AREDIA	Bone Stabilizer	Powd for Inj: 30, 90 mg	**Hypercalcemia of Malignancy:** **Moderate:** 60 mg - 90 by IV infusion (given over ≥ 2 - 24 hours. **Severe:** 90 mg by IV infusion (given over 2 - 24 h. **Paget's Disease:** 30 mg daily by IV infusion (over 4 hours), on 3 consecutive days, for a total dose of 90 mg. **Osteolytic Bone Lesions of Multiple Myeloma:** 90 mg by IV infusion (over 4 hours) once monthly.
Pancuronium Bromide (*)	PAVULON	Neuromuscular Blocker	Inj (per mL): 1, 2 mg	Initially 0.04 - 0.1 mg/kg IV. Later, use incremental doses starting at 0.01 mg/kg.
Pantoprazole Sodium	PROTONIX	Gastric Acid Pump Inhibitor	Delayed-Rel. Tab: 20, 40 mg	**Erosive Esophagitis:** **Treatment:** Swallow whole 40 mg tablet once daily po for up to 8 weeks; may repeat for 8 more weeks. **Maintenance:** 40 mg once daily po. **Pathological Hypersecretory Conditions:** Initially 40 mg bid po. Maximum: 240 mg per day.
	PROTONIX I.V.		Powd for Inj: 40 mg	**Gastroesophageal Reflux Disease (GERD):** 40 mg once daily by IV infusion for 7 - 10 days; switch to tablets as soon as possible. **Pathological Hypersecretory Conditions:** 80 mg q 8 - 12 h by IV infusion. Usual maximum: 240 mg/day or 6 days of treatment.

GENERIC NAME	COMMON TRADE NAMES	THERAPEUTIC CATEGORY	PREPARATIONS	COMMON ADULT DOSAGE
Papaverine Hydrochloride (*)	PAVABID	Vasodilator	Timed-Rel. Cpsl: 150 mg	150 mg q 12 h po.
Paricalcitol	ZEMPLAR	Vitamin D Analog	Inj: 5 µg/mL	Initially 0.04 - 0.1 µg/kg (2.8 - 7 µg) IV (as a bolus injection) no more often than every other day at any time during dialysis. If a satisfactory response is not observed, the dose may be increased by 2 - 4 µg at 2- to 4-week intervals. Doses as high as 0.24 µg/kg (16.8 µg) have been safely given.
Paromomycin Sulfate	HUMATIN	Amebicide	Cpsl: 250 mg (of paromomycin base)	Intestinal Amebiasis: 25 - 35 mg/kg/day po in 3 divided doses with meals for 5 - 10 days.
Paroxetine Hydrochloride (*)	PAXIL	Antidepressant, Drug for Obsessive-Compulsive Disorder, Drug for Panic Disorder, Drug for Social Anxiety Disorder, Drug for Generalized Anxiety Disorder, Drug for Post-traumatic Stress Disorder	Tab: 10, 20, 30, 40 mg Susp: 10 mg/5 mL	**Depression:** Initially, 20 mg po once daily in the AM. May increase in 10 mg/day increments at intervals ≥ 1 week, up to a maximum of 50 mg/day. **Social Anxiety Disorder:** Initially, 20 mg po once daily in the AM. The usual dosage range is 20 - 60 mg daily po. **Generalized Anxiety Disorder:** Initially, 20 mg po once daily in the AM. The usual dosage range is 20 - 50 mg daily po. **OCD and Panic Disorder:** Initially, 20 mg po once daily in the AM. The recommended dose is 40 mg daily po. May increase in 10 mg/day increments at intervals ≥ 1 week, up to a maximum of 60 mg/day. **Post-traumatic Stress Disorder:** Initially, 20 mg po once daily in the AM. The usual dosage range is 20 - 50 mg daily. May increase in 10 mg/day increments at intervals ≥ 1 week, up to a maximum of 50 mg/day.

PAXIL CR		Antidepressant, Drug for Panic Disorder	Controlled-Rel. Tab: 12.5, 25, 37.5 mg	**Depression:** Initially, 25 mg po once daily in the AM. May increase in 12.5 mg/day increments at intervals ≥ 1 week, up to a maximum of 62.5 mg/day. **Panic Disorder:** Initially, 12.5 mg po once daily in the AM. May increase in 12.5 mg/day increments at intervals ≥ 1 week, up to a maximum of 75 mg/day.
Pegaspargase	ONCASPAR	Antineoplastic	Inj: 750 IUnits/mL	2500 IU/m² q 14 days by IM (preferred) or IV.
Peginterferon alfa-2a	PEGASYS	Antiviral	Inj: 180 μg/mL	**Chronic Hepatitis C Infection:** 180 μg SC (in the abdomen or thigh) once weekly for 48 weeks.
Pemirolast Potassium	ALAMAST	Antiallergic, Ophthalmic	Ophth Solution: 0.1%	1 - 2 drops into the affected eye(s) qid.
Pemoline (*) (C-IV)	CYLERT	CNS Stimulant	Chewable Tab: 37.5 mg Tab: 18.75, 37.5, 75 mg	**Attention Deficit Hyperactivity Disorder:** The starting dose is 37.5 mg/day po. Gradually increase daily dose by 18.75 mg at 1 week intervals until the desired response is obtained (Maximum: 112.5 mg).
Penbutolol Sulfate	LEVATOL	Antihypertensive	Tab: 20 mg	20 mg once daily po.
Penciclovir	DENAVIR	Antiviral (Topical)	Cream: 10 mg/g	Apply q 2 h while awake for 4 days. Start treatment as early as possible when lesions appear.
Penicillin G Benzathine (*)		Antibacterial	Inj (per mL): 300,000; 600,000 Units	**Streptococcal Upper Respiratory Infections (e.g., Pharyngitis):** 1,200,000 Units IM. **Syphilis (Primary, Secondary & Latent):** 2,400,000 Units IM. **Syphilis (Late):** 2,400,000 Units IM at 7-day intervals for 3 doses. **Rheumatic Fever and Glomerulonephritis (Prophylaxis):** 1,200,000 Units IM once a month or 600,000 Units IM q 2 weeks.

171

GENERIC NAME	COMMON TRADE NAMES	THERAPEUTIC CATEGORY	PREPARATIONS	COMMON ADULT DOSAGE
Penicillin G Potassium (*)	PFIZERPEN	Antibacterial	**Powd for Inj:** 5,000,000; 20,000,000 Units	5,000,000 to 80,000,000 Units daily IM or by IV drip, depending on the severity of the infection and the susceptibility of the infecting organism.
Penicillin G Procaine (*)	PFIZERPEN-AS WYCILLIN	Antibacterial	**Inj:** 300,000 Units/mL **Inj:** 600,000 Units/mL	**Usual Dosage:** 600,000 - 1,000,000 Units daily IM. **Syphilis:** 600,000 Units daily IM for 8 - 15 days. **Gonorrhea:** 4,800,000 Units IM divided into at least 2 doses and inj. at diff. sites at the same visit, with probenecid (1 g po).
Penicillin V Potassium (*)	PEN-VEE K	Antibacterial	**Tab:** 250, 500 mg **Powd for Solution (per 5 mL):** 125, 250 mg	**Streptococcal Upper Respiratory Infections:** 125 - 250 mg q 6 - 8 h po for 10 days. **Pneumococcal Infections:** 250 - 500 mg q 6 h po until afebrile for at least 48 hours. **Staphylococcal Infections:** 250 - 500 mg q 6 to 8 h po. **Vincent's Gingivitis and Pharyngitis:** 250 - 500 mg q 6 - 8 h po.
Pentamidine Isethionate	NEBUPENT PENTAM 300	Antiprotozoal	**Powd for Solution:** 300 mg **Powd for Inj:** 300 mg	300 mg once q 4 weeks, administered via a Respigard II nebulizer. 4 mg/kg once daily IV (over 60 minutes) or IM for 14 days.
Pentazocine Lactate (*) (C-IV)	TALWIN	Opioid Analgesic	**Inj:** 30 mg/mL	**Usual Dosage:** 30 mg q 3 - 4 h IM, SC or IV. **Patients in Labor:** 30 mg IM or 20 mg q 2 - 3 h IV.
Pentobarbital Sodium (*) (C-II)	NEMBUTAL SODIUM	Sedative - Hypnotic	**Cpsl:** 50, 100 mg **Elixir:** 20 mg/5 mL (18% alcohol) **Rectal Suppos:** 30, 60, 120, 200 mg	**Sedation:** Reduce hypnotic dose appropriately. **Hypnosis:** 100 mg po hs. **Sedation:** Reduce hypnotic dose appropriately. **Hypnosis:** 120 - 200 mg rectally.

		Hypnotic	Inj: 50 mg/mL	IM: 150 - 200 mg as a single dose. IV: Initially, 100 mg/70 kg. May increase in small increment to 200 - 500 mg if needed.
Pentosan Polysulfate Sodium	ELMIRON	Urinary Tract Analgesic	Cpsl: 100 mg	100 mg tid po. Take 1 h ac or 2 h pc with water.
Pentostatin	NIPENT	Antineoplastic	Powd for Inj: 10 mg	After hydration with 500 - 1000 mL of 5% Dextrose in 0.5 normal saline, give 4 mg/m² IV every other week. An additional 500 mL of 5% Dextrose should be given after the drug is administered.
Pentoxifylline (*)	TRENTAL	Hemorheologic Agent	Tab: 400 mg	400 mg tid po with meals.
Pergolide Mesylate	PERMAX	Antiparkinsonian	Tab: 0.05, 0.25, 1 mg	0.05 mg po for first 2 days; then increase the dosage by 0.1 or 0.15 mg/day every third day for the next 12 days. The dosage may then be increased by 0.25 mg/day every 3rd day until optimal response is reached. Daily dose is usually given in 3 divided doses.
Perindopril Erbumine	ACEON	Antihypertensive	Tab: 2, 4, 8 mg	Initially, 4 mg once daily po. The usual maintenance dose range is 4 - 8 mg administered as a single daily dose or in 2 divided doses.
Permethrin	ELIMITE	Scabicide	Cream: 5%	Throughly massage into skin from the head to the soles of the feet. Wash off (bath or shower) after 8 - 14 h.
	NIX		Liquid: 1%	Shampoo hair, rinse with water and towel dry. Saturate the hair and scalp; allow solution to remain for 10 minutes before rinsing off with water. If live lice are observed 7 days or more after the first application, a second treatment should be given.

GENERIC NAME	COMMON TRADE NAMES	THERAPEUTIC CATEGORY	PREPARATIONS	COMMON ADULT DOSAGE
Perphenazine (*)	TRILAFON	Antipsychotic, Antiemetic	Tab: 2, 4, 8, 16 mg Liquid Conc: 16 mg/5 mL Inj: 5 mg/mL	**Psychoses:** **Outpatients:** 4 - 8 mg tid po. **Hospitalized Patients:** 8 - 16 mg bid - qid po; or 5 mg q 6 h IM. **Nausea & Vomiting:** 8 - 16 mg daily in divided doses po; or 5 mg IM.
Phenazopyridine Hydrochloride	PYRIDIUM	Urinary Tract Analgesic	Tab: 100, 200 mg	200 mg tid po after meals.
Phendimetrazine Tartrate (*) (C-III)	BONTRIL PDM BONTRIL SLOW RELEASE PRELU-2	Anorexiant	Tab: 35 mg Slow-Rel. Cpsl: 105 mg Timed-Rel. Cpsl: 105 mg	35 mg bid - tid po, 1 h ac. 105 mg po, 30 - 60 minutes before the morning meal.
Phenelzine Sulfate (*)	NARDIL	Antidepressant	Tab: 15 mg	Initially, 15 mg tid po. Increase dosage to at least 60 mg/day at a rapid pace as patient tolerates drug. After several weeks, dosage may be reduced (over several weeks) to as low as 15 mg daily or every other day.
Phenindamine Tartrate	NOLAHIST	Antihistamine	Tab: 25 mg	25 mg q 4 - 6 h po.
Phenobarbital (*) (C-IV)		Sedative - Hypnotic, Anticonvulsant	Tab: 15, 30, 60, 100 mg Elixir: 20 mg/5 mL (alcohol)	**Sedation:** 30 - 120 mg daily po in 2 - 3 divided doses. **Hypnosis:** 100 - 200 mg hs po. **Convulsions:** 60 - 200 mg daily po.
Phenobarbital Sodium (*) (C-IV)		Sedative - Hypnotic, Anticonvulsant	Inj (per mL): 30, 60, 65, 130 mg	**Sedation:** 30 - 120 mg daily IM or IV in 2 - 3 divided doses. **Preoperative Sedation:** 100 - 200 mg IM, 60 to 90 minutes before surgery. **Hypnosis:** 100 - 320 mg IM or IV. **Acute Convulsions:** 200 - 320 mg IM or IV, repeated in 6 h prn.

174

Generic	Brand	Category	Form	Dosage
Phenoxybenzamine Hydrochloride	DIBENZYLINE	Antihypertensive	Cpsl: 10 mg	Initially, 10 bid po; increase dosage every other day, usually to 20 - 40 mg, bid - tid po.
Phentermine Hydrochloride (*) (C-IV)	PRO-FAST SA	Anorexiant	Tab: 8 mg	8 mg tid po, 30 min ac.
	PRO-FAST HS		Cpsl: 18.75 mg	18.75 mg daily po, before breakfast or 10 - 14 hours before bedtime.
	ADIPEX-P		Cpsl & Tab: 37.5 mg	37.5 mg daily po, before breakfast or 1 - 2 h after breakfast.
	PRO-FAST SR		Cpsl: 37.5 mg	37.5 mg daily po, 2 hours after breakfast.
Phentermine Resin (*) (C-IV)	IONAMIN	Anorexiant	Cpsl: 15, 30 mg	15 - 30 mg daily po, before breakfast or 10 to 14 hours before retiring.
Phentolamine Mesylate	REGITINE	Antihypertensive	Powd for Inj: 5 mg	**Preoperative:** 5 mg IM or IV, 1 - 2 h before surgery, and repeated if necessary. **During Surgery:** 5 mg IV as required.
Phenylephrine Hydrochloride	NEO-SYNEPHRINE	Sympathomimetic	Inj: 10 mg/mL (1%)	**Mild or Moderate Hypotension:** 2 - 5 mg SC; or 0.2 mg by slow IV. Repeat injections no more often than every 10 - 15 minutes. **Severe Hypotension & Shock:** Infuse a dilute solution IV (10 mg in 500 mL of Dextrose Injection) at 100 - 180 μg/min (approx. 100 to 180 drops/min). When blood pressure stabilizes, use maintenance rate of 40 - 60 μg/min (approx. 40 - 60 drops/min).
	NEO-SYNEPHRINE	Nasal Decongestant	**Nasal Spray:** 0.25% **Nasal Solution & Spray:** 0.50% **Nasal Solution & Spray:** 1.0%	2 - 3 sprays in each nostril q 4 h. 2 - 3 drops or sprays in each nostril q 4 h. 2 drops or sprays in each nostril q 4 h.
Phenytoin (*)	DILANTIN-125 DILANTIN INFATAB	Antiepileptic	**Susp:** 125 mg/5 mL **Chewable Tab:** 50 mg	Initially, 125 mg tid po; adjust dosage prn. Initially, 100 mg tid po; adjust dosage prn.

175

GENERIC NAME	COMMON TRADE NAMES	THERAPEUTIC CATEGORY	PREPARATIONS	COMMON ADULT DOSAGE
Phenytoin Sodium (*)	DILANTIN	Antiepileptic	Inj: 50 mg/mL	**Status Epilepticus:** A loading dose of 10 - 15 mg/kg slow IV (at a rate not exceeding 50 mg/min). Follow with maintenance doses of 100 mg po or IV q 6 - 8 h.
			Cpsl: 100 mg	Initially, 100 mg tid po; adjust dosage prn. For patients controlled at 100 mg tid, a single daily dose of 300 mg po may be given.
Phytonadione	AQUA-MEPHYTON	Vitamin K$_1$	Inj (per mL): 2, 10 mg	2.5 - 25 mg SC or IM. Repeat in 6 - 8 h if necessary.
Pilocarpine	OCUSERT PILO-20 OCUSERT PILO-40	Anti-Glaucoma Agent	**Ocular Therapeutic System:** releases 20 µg/h for 1 week **Ocular Therapeutic System:** releases 40 µg/h for 1 week	Place in conjunctival cul-de-sac hs; replace every 7 days. Place in conjunctival cul-de-sac hs; replace every 7 days.
Pilocarpine Hydrochloride	ISOPTO CARPINE	Anti-Glaucoma Agent	**Ophth Solution:** 0.25, 0.5, 1, 2, 3, 4, 5, 6, 8, 10%	1 or 2 drops in eye(s) up to 6 times daily. The usual range is 0.5 to 4%.
	PILOCAR, PILOSTAT		**Ophth Solution:** 0.5, 1, 2, 3, 4, 6%	1 or 2 drops in eye(s) up to 6 times daily. The usual range is 0.5 to 4%.
	PILOPINE HS GEL		**Ophth Gel:** 4%	Apply a 0.5 in. ribbon in the lower conjunctival sac of the affected eye(s) once daily hs.
Pimecrolimus	SALAGEN	Cholinomimetic	**Tab:** 5 mg	Initially, 5 mg tid po. Dosage may be increased to 10 mg tid, if necessary and tolerated.
Pimecrolimus	ELIDEL	Immunomodulator	**Cream:** 1%	Apply a thin layer bid to affected skin areas. Rub in gently and completely.
Pimozide (*)	ORAP	Antipsychotic	**Tab:** 1, 2 mg	Initially, 1 - 2 mg daily in divided doses po; may increase thereafter every other day. Most are maintained at less than 0.2 mg/kg daily or 10 mg daily, whichever is less.

Pindolol (*)	VISKEN	Antihypertensive	Tab: 5, 10 mg	Initially, 5 mg bid po. After 3 - 4 weeks dosage may be increased in increments of 10 mg/day q 2 - 4 weeks, to a maximum of 60 mg/day.
Pioglitazone Hydrochloride	ACTOS	Hypoglycemic Agent	Tab: 15, 30, 45 mg	**Monotherapy or Combination Therapy:** Usually 15 or 30 mg po once daily. For patients who do not respond adequately (as determined by fasting serum glucose), the dose may be increased to 45 mg po once daily.
Pipecuronium Bromide (*)	ARDUAN	Neuromuscular Blocker	Powd for Inj: 10 mg	**Endotracheal Intubation:** 70 - 85 μg/kg IV. **Maintenance:** 10 - 15 μg/kg IV.
Piperacillin Sodium (*)	PIPRACIL	Antibacterial	Powd for Inj: 2, 3, 4 g	**Urinary Tract Infections (Uncomplicated) and Most Community-Acquired Pneumonia:** 100 to 125 mg/kg/day IM or IV in divided doses q 6 - 12 h. **Urinary Tract Infections (Complicated):** 125 to 200 mg/kg/day IV in divided doses q 6 - 8 h. **Serious Infections:** 200 - 300 mg/kg/day IV in divided doses q 4 - 6 h. **Gonorrhea (Uncomplicated):** 2 g IM as a single dose with probenecid (1 g po).
Pirbuterol Acetate	MAXAIR	Bronchodilator	Aerosol: 200 μg/spray	2 inhalations q 4 - 6 h.
Piroxicam (*)	FELDENE	Antiinflammatory	Cpsl: 10, 20 mg	20 mg daily po.
Polyethylene Glycol 3350	MIRALAX	Saline Laxative	Powder: (with measuring cup)	Dissolve 17 g in 8 fl. oz. of water and drink once daily. May need 2 - 4 days to induce bowel movement.
Polythiazide	RENESE	Diuretic, Antihypertensive	Tab: 1, 2, 4 mg	**Diuresis:** 1 - 4 mg daily po. **Hypertension:** 2 - 4 mg daily po.

GENERIC NAME	COMMON TRADE NAMES	THERAPEUTIC CATEGORY	PREPARATIONS	COMMON ADULT DOSAGE
Potassium Chloride (*)	K-DUR	Potassium Supplement	Extended-Rel. Tab: 10, 20 mEq	Dosage must be adjusted to the individual needs of each patient. Typical dosages are given below.
	K-TAB KLOTRIX K-NORM KLOR-CON MICRO-K EXTENCAPS SLOW-K TEN-K		Extended-Rel. Tab: 10 mEq Slow-Rel. Tab: 10 mEq Extended-Rel. Cpsl: 10 mEq Extended-Rel. Tab: 8, 10 mEq Extended-Rel. Cpsl: 8, 10 mEq Extended-Rel. Tab: 8 mEq Extended-Rel. Tab: 10 mEq	Prevention of Hypokalemia: 20 - 30 mEq daily po as a single dose or in divided doses with meals and with water or other liquids. Treatment of Potassium Depletion: 40 - 100 mEq daily po in divided doses with meals and with water or other liquids.
	KLORVESS 10% LIQUID		Liquid: 20 mEq/15 mL (0.75% alcohol)	15 mL (20 mEq) diluted in 3 - 4 oz. of cold water bid - qid po.
	KLOR-CON POWDER KLOR-CON/25 POWDER		Powd for Solution: 20 mEq Powd for Solution: 25 mEq	Same dosages as shown above. Dissolve each each packet in at least 3 oz. of fluid.
	MICRO-K LS		Extended-Rel. Formulation (Powd for Susp): 20 mEq	Dissolve each packet in 2 - 6 oz. of cold water. Drink solution 1 - 5 times daily with meals.
	KLORVESS		Effervescent Powd for Solution: 20 mEq	Dissolve each packet in 3 - 4 oz. of cold water, fruit juice or other liquid. Drink solution bid to qid.
	K-LYTE/CL		Effervescent Tab: 25, 50 mEq	Dissolve 1 tablet completely in cold water (3 to 4 oz. for the 25 mEq tab and 6 to 8 oz. for the 50 mEq tab); drink solution bid - qid.
Potassium Gluconate (*)	KAON	Potassium Supplement	Elixir: 20 mEq/15 mL (5% alcohol)	15 mL (20 mEq) diluted in 3 - 4 oz. of cold water bid - qid po.

178

| Pramipexole | MIRAPEX | Antiparkinsonian | Tab: 0.125, 0.25, 0.5, 1, 1.5 mg | Increase dosage gradually from a starting dose of 0.125 mg tid po and do not increase more often than q 5 - 7 days. The table below shows a suggested ascending dosage schedule: |

Week	Oral Dosage	Total Daily Dose
1	0.125 mg tid	0.375 mg
2	0.25 mg tid	0.75 mg
3	0.5 mg tid	1.5 mg
4	0.75 mg tid	2.25 mg
5	1.0 mg tid	3.0 mg
6	1.25 mg tid	3.75 mg
7	1.5 mg tid	4.5 mg

| Pravastatin Sodium | PRAVACHOL | Antihyperlipidemic | Tab: 10, 20, 40, 80 mg | Initially 40 mg once daily po. Adjust the dosage after about 4 weeks. |

| Praziquantel | BILTRICIDE | Anthelmintic | Tab: 600 mg | **Schistomiasis:** Three 20 mg/kg doses po for 1 day only. **Clonorchiasis and Opisthorchiasis:** Three 25 mg/kg doses po for 1 day only. |

| Prazosin Hydrochloride (*) | MINIPRESS | Antihypertensive | Cpsl: 1, 2, 5 mg (as the base) | Initially, 1 mg bid - tid po. Dosage may be slowly increased to 20 mg daily, given in divided doses. |

| Prednicarbate | DERMATOP | Corticosteroid (Topical) | Cream: 0.1% | Apply a thin film to skin bid. |

| Prednisolone | PRELONE | Corticosteroid | Syrup: 15 mg/5 mL | Initial dosage varies from 5 - 60 mg daily po depending on the disease being treated and the patient's response. |

GENERIC NAME	COMMON TRADE NAMES	THERAPEUTIC CATEGORY	PREPARATIONS	COMMON ADULT DOSAGE
Prednisolone Acetate	PRED-MILD PRED FORTE	Corticosteroid (Topical)	Ophth Susp: 0.12% Ophth Susp: 1%	1 - 2 drops into affected eye(s) bid - qid. During the initial 24 - 48 h, the dosing frequency may be increased if necessary.
Prednisolone Sodium Phosphate	HYDELTRASOL	Corticosteroid	Inj: 20 mg/mL	**For IV and IM Injection:** Dose requirements are variable and must be individualized on the basis of the disease and the response of the patient. The initial dosage varies from 4 to 60 mg a day. Usually the daily parenteral dose of HYDELTRASOL is the same as the oral dose of prednisolone and the dosage interval is q 4 to 8 h. **For Intra-articular, Intralesional and Soft Tissue Injection:** Dose requirements are variable and must be individualized on the basis of the disease, the response of the patient, and the site of injection. The usual dose is from 2 to 30 mg. The frequency usually ranges from once every 3 to 5 days to once every 2 to 3 weeks.
	INFLAMASE MILD 1/8% INFLAMASE FORTE 1%	Corticosteroid (Topical)	Ophth Solution: 0.125% Ophth Solution: 1%	1 - 2 drops into affected eye(s) up to q h during the day & q 2 h at night. When a favorable response occurs, reduce dosage to 1 drop q 4 h.
Prednisone	DELTASONE	Corticosteroid	Tab: 2.5, 5, 10, 20, 50 mg	Initial dosage may vary from 5 - 60 mg daily po, depending on the disease being treated.
Primaquine Phosphate		Antimalarial	Tab: 26.3 mg (equal to 15 mg of primaquine base)	15 mg (of base) daily po for 14 days.
Primidone (*)	MYSOLINE	Antiepileptic	Susp: 250 mg/5 mL Tab: 50, 250 mg	100 - 125 mg hs po (for 3 days); 100 - 125 mg bid po (for 3 days); 100 - 125 mg tid po (for 3 days); then 250 mg tid po.

180

Probenecid	Anti-Gout Agent, Penicillin/Cephalosporin Adjunct	Tab: 500 mg	**Gout:** 250 mg bid po for 1 week, followed by 500 mg bid thereafter. **Penicillin/Cephalosporin Therapy:** The recommended dosage is 2 g po daily in divided doses. Usually 1 g po with or just before each administration of antibacterial therapy.
Procainamide Hydrochloride (*)	Antiarrhythmic	Cpsl & Tab: 250, 375, 500 mg Inj (per mL): 100, 500 mg	Up to 50 to 50 mg/kg daily in divided doses q 3 h po. **IM:** 50 mg/kg daily in divided doses given q 3 to 6 h until oral therapy is possible. **IV:** 100 mg q 5 minutes (at a rate not to exceed 50 mg/min) until the arrhythmia is suppressed or until 500 mg has been given. **IV Infusion:** Loading dose of 20 mg/mL (1 g diluted in 50 mL of 5% Dextrose Injection) at a rate of 1 mL/min for 25 - 30 min; then a maintenance dose of 2 or 4 mg/mL (1 g diluted in 500 or 250 mL of 5% Dextrose Injection) at a rate of 0.5 - 1.5 mL/min.
PROCANBID PRONESTYL-SR		Extended-Rel. Tab: 500, 1000 mg Extended-Rel. Tab: 500 mg	Up to 50 mg/kg daily in divided doses q 6 h po.
Procarbazine Hydrochloride	Antineoplastic	Cpsl: 50 mg	2 - 4 mg/kg/day po as a single dose or in divided doses for 1 week; then maintain the dosage at 4 - 6 mg/kg/day until maximum response occurs. Then give 1 - 2 mg/kg/day.
Prochlorperazine	Antiemetic	Rectal Suppos: 25 mg	**Nausea & Vomiting:** 25 mg bid rectally.

GENERIC NAME	COMMON TRADE NAMES	THERAPEUTIC CATEGORY	PREPARATIONS	COMMON ADULT DOSAGE
Prochlorperazine Edisylate (*)	COMPAZINE	Antiemetic, Antipsychotic	Syrup: 5 mg/5 mL Inj: 5 mg/mL	**Nausea & Vomiting:** 5 - 10 mg tid or qid po. **Nausea & Vomiting:** 5 - 10 mg q 3 - 4 h deep IM; or 2.5 - 10 mg by slow IV injection or IV infusion (maximum rate of 5 mg/min). **Psychosis:** Initially, 10 - 20 mg deep IM. May repeat q 2 - 4 h, if necessary, for a few doses; then switch to oral medication.
Prochlorperazine Maleate (*)	COMPAZINE	Antiemetic, Antipsychotic	Tab: 5, 10 mg Sustained-Rel. Cpsl: 10, 15 mg	**Nausea & Vomiting:** 5 - 10 mg tid or qid po. **Non-Psychotic Anxiety:** 5 mg tid or qid po. **Psychosis:** **Mild or in Outpatients:** 5 - 10 mg tid - qid po. **Moderate-to-Severe or in Hospitalized Patients:** Initially, 10 mg tid - qid po; raise the dosage slowly until symptoms are controlled. **More Severe Cases:** Optimum dosage is 100 to 150 mg daily po. **Nausea & Vomiting or Non-Psychotic Anxiety:** 15 mg po on arising or 10 mg q 12 h po.
Procyclidine Hydrochloride (*)	KEMADRIN	Antiparkinsonian	Tab: 5 mg	Initially, 2.5 mg tid po pc. If well tolerated, gradually increase to 5 mg tid pc.
Progesterone (*)	PROGESTASERT	Intrauterine Contraceptive	Intrauterine System: unit containing a reservoir of 38 mg of progesterone	Insert a single unit into the uterine cavity. Replace 1 year after insertion.
Progesterone, Micronized (*)	CRINONE 8%	Progestin	Vaginal Gel: 8% (90 mg in prefilled applicators)	**Assisted Reproductive Technology:** **Supplementation:** 1 applicatorful intra-vaginally once daily (see Note, below). **Replacement:** 1 applicatorful intravaginally bid (see Note, below). Note: if pregnancy occurs, treatment may be continued until placental autonomy is achieved (10 - 12 weeks).

182

	CRINONE 4%		Vaginal Gel: 4% (45 mg in prefilled applicators)	**Secondary Amenorrhea:** 1 applicatorful intravaginally every other day up to a total of 6 doses. For women who fail to respond, a trial of CRINONE 8% (see above) every other day for up to a total of 6 doses may be tried.
Promethazine Hydrochloride (*)	PHENERGAN	Antihistamine, Antiemetic, Sedative	**Tab:** 12.5, 25, 50 mg **Syrup:** 6.25 mg/5 mL (7% alcohol) **Inj (per mL):** 25, 50 mg **Rectal Suppos:** 12.5, 25, 50 mg	**Allergy:** 25 mg po hs, or 12.5 mg po ac & hs. By deep IM injection, 25 mg; may repeat once in 2 h, then switch to oral medication. **Motion Sickness:** 25 mg po, taken 30 - 60 min before travel; repeat once in 8 - 12 h. On succeeding days, 25 mg bid, on arising & hs. **Nausea & Vomiting:** 25 mg po, followed by 12.5 - 25 mg q 4 - 6 h po. When oral medication is not tolerated, dose by injection (deep IM) or by rectal suppositories. **Sedation:** 25 - 50 mg hs po or by deep IM.
Propafenone Hydrochloride (*)	RYTHMOL	Antiarrhythmic	**Tab:** 150, 225, 300 mg	Initiate with 150 mg q 8 h po. Dosage may be increased at a minimum of 3 - 4 day intervals to 225 mg q 8 h po, and if needed to 300 mg q 8 h po.
Propantheline Bromide	PRO-BANTHINE	Anticholinergic	**Tab:** 7.5, 15 mg	15 mg po 30 minutes ac and 30 mg hs. For mild symptoms, 7.5 mg tid po may be used.
Propoxyphene Hydrochloride (*) (C-IV)	DARVON	Opioid Analgesic	**Cpsl:** 65 mg	65 mg q 4 h po, prn pain.
Propoxyphene Napsylate (*) (C-IV)	DARVON-N	Opioid Analgesic	**Tab:** 100 mg	100 mg q 4 h po, prn pain.

183

GENERIC NAME	COMMON TRADE NAMES	THERAPEUTIC CATEGORY	PREPARATIONS	COMMON ADULT DOSAGE
Propranolol Hydrochloride (*)	INDERAL	Antihypertensive, Antianginal, Antiarrhythmic, Antimigraine Agent, Post-MI Drug	**Tab:** 10, 20, 40, 60, 80 mg	**Hypertension:** Initially, 40 mg bid po; increase dosage gradually. The usual maintenance dosage is 120 - 240 mg daily. **Angina:** 80 - 320 mg daily po in divided doses (bid to qid). **Hypertrophic Subaortic Stenosis:** 20 - 40 mg tid - qid po. ac & hs. **Arrhythmias:** 10 - 30 mg tid - qid po. ac & hs. **Migraine Headaches:** Initially, 80 mg daily po in divided doses; increase dosage gradually. The usual maintenance dosage is 160 - 240 mg daily. **Post-Myocardial Infarction:** 180 - 240 mg daily po in divided doses (bid to tid).
		Antiarrhythmic	**Inj:** 1 mg/mL	**Life-Threatening Arrhythmias:** 1 - 3 mg IV (at a rate not exceeding 1 mg/min). May repeat dose after 2 minutes, if necessary. Then no additional drug should be given for 4 h.
	INDERAL LA	Antihypertensive, Antianginal, Antimigraine Agent	**Long-Acting Cpsl:** 60, 80, 120, 160 mg	**Hypertension:** Initially, 80 mg once daily po; may increase to usual maintenance dosage of 120 - 160 mg daily. **Angina:** Initially, 80 mg once daily po; increase at 3 - 7 day intervals. The average optimal dosage is 160 mg once daily. **Hypertrophic Subaortic Stenosis:** 80 - 160 mg once daily po. **Migraine Headaches:** Initially, 80 mg once daily po; increase gradually. The usual effective dosage range is 160 - 240 mg once daily.
Propylhexedrine (*)	BENZEDREX INHALER	Nasal Decongestant	**Inhalant Tube:** delivers 0.4 to 0.5 mg/800 mL of air	2 inhalations in each nostril not more often than q 2 h.

Drug	Category	How Supplied	Dosage
Propylthiouracil (*)	Antithyroid Agent	**Tab:** 50 mg	Initial: 300 mg/day po, usually administered in 3 equal doses at 8 hour intervals. Maintenance: Usually, 100 - 150 mg daily po in 3 equal doses at 8 hour intervals.
Protamine Sulfate	Heparin Antagonist	**Inj:** 10 mg/mL	1 mg per 90 - 115 Units of heparin activity by slow IV (over 10 minutes). Maximum dose: 50 mg.
Protriptyline Hydrochloride (*) VIVACTIL	Antidepressant	**Tab:** 5, 10 mg	15 - 40 mg daily po in 3 - 4 divided doses.
Pseudoephedrine Hydrochloride (*) SUDAFED CHILDREN'S NON-DROWSY	Decongestant	**Liquid:** 15 mg/5 mL	20 mL (60 mg) q 4 - 6 h po.
SUDAFED		**Tab:** 30, 60 mg	60 mg q 4 - 6 h po.
SUDAFED NON-DROWSY 12 HOUR LONG-ACTING		**Extended-Rel. Tab:** 120 mg	120 mg q 12 h po.
SUDAFED NON-DROWSY 24 HOUR LONG-ACTING		**Controlled-Rel. Tab:** 240 mg (60 mg immediate-release, 180 mg controlled-release)	240 mg once daily po.
Pseudoephedrine Sulfate (*) DRIXORAL NON-DROWSY	Decongestant	**Extended-Rel. Tab:** 120 mg	120 mg q 12 h po.
Psyllium PERDIEM FIBER	Bulk Laxative	**Granules:** 4.03 g/rounded teaspoonful (6.0 g)	In the evening and/or before breakfast, 1 - 2 rounded teaspoonfuls should be swallowed with at least 8 oz. of a cool beverage.
SERUTAN		**Granules:** 2.5 g/heaping teaspoonful	1 - 3 heaping teaspoonfuls on cereal or other food 1 - 3 times daily po. Drink at least 8 oz. of liquid with the food.

185

GENERIC NAME	COMMON TRADE NAMES	THERAPEUTIC CATEGORY	PREPARATIONS	COMMON ADULT DOSAGE
Psyllium Hydrophilic Mucilloid	FIBERALL	Bulk Laxative	**Powder:** 3.4 g/rounded teaspoonful (5.0 - 5.9 g) **Wafer:** 3.4 g	1 rounded teaspoonful in 8 oz. of liquid 1 - 3 times daily po. 1 - 2 wafers with 8 oz. of liquid 1 - 3 times daily po.
	METAMUCIL		**Powder (Regular):** 3.4 g per rounded teaspoonful **Powder (Flavored):** 3.4 g per tablespoonful	1 rounded teaspoonful (Regular) or tablespoonful (Flavored) in 8 oz. of liquid 1 - 3 times daily po.
	SYLLACT		**Powder:** 3.3 g/rounded teaspoonful	1 rounded teaspoonful in 8 oz. of liquid 1 - 3 times daily po.
Pyrantel Pamoate	ANTIMINTH	Anthelmintic	**Susp:** 144 mg/mL (equivalent to 50 mg/mL of pyrantel)	5 mg/lb (to a maximum of 1 g) as a single dose po.
	REESE'S PINWORM MEDICINE		**Liquid:** 144 mg/mL (equivalent to 50 mg/mL of pyrantel) **Cpsl:** 180 mg (equivalent to 62.5 mg of pyrantel)	5 mg/lb (to a maximum of 1 g) as a single dose po.
Pyrazinamide		Tuberculostatic	**Tab:** 500 mg	15 - 30 mg/kg once daily po (Max: 2 g/day).
Pyridostigmine Bromide (*)	MESTINON	Cholinomimetic	**Syrup:** 60 mg/5 mL (5% alcohol) **Tab:** 60 mg	600 mg (10 tsp. or 10 tab) daily po in divided doses, spaced to provide maximum relief when maximum strength is needed.
	MESTINON TIMESPAN		**Slow-Rel. Tab:** 180 mg	1 - 3 tablets once or twice daily po.
Pyrimethamine	DARAPRIM	Antimalarial	**Tab:** 25 mg	**Chemoprophylaxis:** 25 mg once weekly po.
Quazepam (*) (C-IV)	DORAL	Hypnotic	**Tab:** 7.5, 15 mg	7.5 - 15 mg hs po.

186

Drug	Brand	Class	Forms	Dosage
Quetiapine Fumarate (*)	SEROQUEL	Antipsychotic	Tab: 25, 100, 200, 300 mg	**Over 18 yrs:** Initially 25 mg bid po. Increase in increments of 25 - 50 mg bid - tid on Days 2 and 3; by **Day 4,** dose should be in the range of 300 - 400 mg/day in 2 - 3 divided doses. Make further dosage adjustments prn at intervals of at least 2 days in increments or decrements of 25 - 50 mg bid. Usual dose range: 150 - 750 mg/day.
Quinapril Hydrochloride (*)	ACCUPRIL	Antihypertensive, Heart Failure Drug	Tab: 5, 10, 20, 40 mg	**Hypertension:** **Initial:** 10 mg once daily po. Adjust dosage at intervals of at least 2 weeks. **Maintenance:** Most patients require 20 - 80 mg daily po as a single dose or in 2 equally divided doses. **Heart Failure:** Used in conjunction with other conventional therapies including diuretics or digoxin. Initially, give 5 mg bid po. Titrate patients at weekly intervals until an effective dose is attained, usually 10 - 20 mg bid.
Quinidine Gluconate (*)	QUINAGLUTE	Antiarrhythmic	Extended-Rel. Tab: 324 mg	324 - 648 mg q 8 - 12 h po.
Quinidine Sulfate (*)	QUINIDEX EXTENTABS	Antiarrhythmic	Extended-Rel. Tab: 300 mg	Initially 300 mg q 8 - 12 h po. If tolerated and the serum level is well within the therapeutic range, the dose may be increased cautiously.
Quinine Sulfate (*)		Antimalarial	Cpsl: 200, 260, 325 mg Tab: 260 mg	260 - 650 mg tid po for 6 - 12 days.

GENERIC NAME	COMMON TRADE NAMES	THERAPEUTIC CATEGORY	PREPARATIONS	COMMON ADULT DOSAGE
Rabeprazole Sodium	ACIPHEX	Gastric Acid Pump Inhibitor, Anti-Ulcer Agent	Delayed-Rel. Tab: 20 mg	**Healing of Duodenal Ulcers:** 20 mg once daily po after the morning meal for ≤ 4 weeks. **Healing of Erosive or Ulcerative GERD:** 20 mg once daily po for 4 - 8 weeks. **Maintenance of Healing of Erosive or Ulcerative GERD:** 20 mg once daily po. **Treatment of Pathological Hypersecretory Conditions, including Zollinger-Ellison Syndrome:** Initially, 60 mg once daily po. Adjust dosage to patient needs and continue for as long as clinically indicated.
Raloxifene Hydrochloride	EVISTA	Antiosteoporotic	Tab: 60 mg	60 mg once daily po.
Ramipril (*)	ALTACE	Antihypertensive, Heart Failure Drug	Cpsl: 1.25, 2.5, 5, 10 mg	**Hypertension:** Initially, 2.5 mg once daily po. The usual maintenance dosage range is 2.5 to 20 mg daily administered as a single dose or in two equally divided doses. **Heart Failure Post-M.I.:** Initially 2.5 mg bid po. If hypotension occurs, reduce dosage to 1.25 mg bid po, but all patients should be titrated toward a target dosage of 5 mg bid. **Reduction in Risk of M.I., Stroke, and Death From Cardiovascular Causes:** 2.5 mg once daily po for 1 week, 5 mg once daily po for the next 3 weeks, then increase as tolerated to a maintenance dose of 10 mg daily.
Ranitidine Hydrochloride (*)	ZANTAC 75	Histamine H₂-Blocker	Tab: 84 mg (equivalent to 75 mg of ranitidine)	**Heartburn, Acid Indigestion, Sour Stomach:** 75 mg once or twice daily po.
	ZANTAC	Histamine H₂-Blocker, Anti-Ulcer Agent	Syrup: 15 mg/mL (7.5% alcohol) Cpsl & Tab: 150, 300 mg Effervescent Tab: 150 mg Effervescent Granules: 150 mg/packet	**Active Duodenal Ulcer:** 150 mg bid po; or 300 mg once daily po hs. **Maintenance Therapy:** 150 mg daily po hs. **Pathological Hypersecretory Conditions:** 150 mg bid po, or more frequently if needed.

188

				Gastroesophageal Reflux and Benign Gastric Ulcer: 150 mg bid po. **Erosive Esophagitis:** 150 mg qid po.
			Inj: 25 mg/mL	**IM:** 50 mg q 6 - 8 h. **Intermittent IV:** 50 mg q 6 - 8 h as a bolus (diluted solution) or as an infusion (at a rate not greater than 5 - 7 mL/min). **Continuous IV Infusion:** 6.25 mg/h.
Repaglinide	PRANDIN	Hypoglycemic Agent	**Tab:** 0.5, 1, 2 mg	There is no fixed dosage regimen for the management of type 2 diabetes with this drug. **Starting Dose:** **For patients not previously treated or whose HbA_{1C} is < 8%:** 0.5 mg po ac. **For patients previously treated with blood glucose lowering drugs or whose HbA_{1C} is > 8%:** 1 - 2 mg po ac. Dosage adjustments should be determined by blood glucose response. The recommended dose range is 0.5 - 4 mg po with meals and the drug may be given bid - qid ac.
Reserpine		Antihypertensive	**Tab:** 0.1, 0.25 mg	Initially, 0.5 mg daily po for 1 - 2 weeks; for maintenance, reduce to 0.1 - 0.25 mg daily.
Reteplase, Recombinant	RETAVASE	Thrombolytic	**Powd for Inj:** 18.8 mg (10.8 IUnits)	10 IU by bolus IV injection (given over 2 min), followed by a second 10 IU bolus IV injection (over 2 min) 30 minutes after the initiation of the first injection.
Rifabutin (*)	MYCOBUTIN	Tuberculostatic	**Cpsl:** 150 mg	300 mg once daily po.
Rifampin (*)	RIFADIN RIFADIN I.V.	Tuberculostatic	**Cpsl:** 150, 300 mg **Powd for Inj:** 600 mg	10 mg/kg daily in a single administration, po (1 hour before or 2 hours after a meal) or IV, not to exceed 600 mg daily.

GENERIC NAME	COMMON TRADE NAMES	THERAPEUTIC CATEGORY	PREPARATIONS	COMMON ADULT DOSAGE
Rifapentine	PRIFTIN	Tuberculostatic	Tab: 150 mg	**Intensive Phase:** 600 mg twice weekly po with an interval of ≥ 3 days between doses continued for 2 months. Administer in combination as part of an appropriate drug regimen that includes daily companion drugs. **Continuation Phase:** Continue treatment once weekly for 4 months in combination with isoniazid or an appropriate drug for susceptible organisms.
Riluzole	RILUTEK	Drug for Amyotrophic Lateral Sclerosis	Tab: 50 mg	50 mg q 12 h po, taken at least 1 h ac or 2 h pc.
Rimantadine Hydrochloride	FLUMADINE	Antiviral	Syrup: 50 mg/5 mL Tab: 100 mg	**Prophylaxis:** 100 mg bid po. **Treatment:** 100 mg bid po. Start therapy within 48 h of symptoms; continue for 7 days from initial onset of symptoms.
Rimexolone	VEXOL	Corticosteroid (Topical)	Ophth Susp: 1%	**Post-Operative Inflammation:** 1 - 2 drops into the affected eye(s) qid beginning 24 h after surgery & continuing for 2 weeks. **Anterior Uveitis:** 1 - 2 drops into the affected eye(s) q 1 h during waking hours for the first week, 1 drop q 2 h during waking hours of the second week, and then taper off until the uveitis is resolved.
Risedronate Sodium	ACTONEL	Bone Stabilizer	Tab: 5, 30, 35 mg	**Prevention / Treatment of Postmenopausal & Glucocorticoid-induced Osteoporosis:** 5 mg once daily po or one 35 mg tablet once weekly po. **Paget's Disease:** 30 mg once daily po for 2 months. Take ≥ 30 min. before the first food or drink of the day other than water. Take while in an upright position with a full glass (6 - 8 oz.) of plain water and avoid lying down for 30 min. to minimize the possibility of GI side effects.

Risperidone (*)	RISPERDAL	Antipsychotic	**Tab:** 0.25, 0.5, 1, 2, 3, 4 mg **Oral Solution:** 1 mg/mL	Initially, 1 mg bid po. Increase in increments of 1 mg bid on 2nd & 3rd day, as tolerated, to a target dose of 3 mg bid. Further dosage adjustements should be made at intervals of ≥ 1 week.
Ritonavir	NORVIR	Antiviral	**Oral Solution:** 80 mg/mL **Cpsl:** 100 mg	600 mg bid po with food. For patients who experience nausea, initiate therapy with 300 mg bid po for 1 day, 400 mg bid for 2 days, 500 mg bid for 1 day, then 600 mg bid po thereafter.
Rivastigmine Tartrate	EXELON	Drug for Alzheimer's Disease	**Cpsl:** 1.5, 3, 4.5, 6 mg **Solution:** 2 mg/mL	1.5 mg bid po. After 2 weeks the dose may be increased to 3 mg bid. Subsequent increases to 4.5 and 6 mg bid should be attempted after a minimum of 2 weeks at the previous dose. Take with food in divided doses in the AM and PM.
Rizatriptan Benzoate	MAXALT	Antimigraine Agent	**Tab:** 5, 10 mg	5 - 10 mg po. For redosing, doses should be separated by at least 2 h. Maximum: 30 mg within 24 h.
	MAXALT-MLT		**Oral Disintegrating Tab:** 5, 10 mg	5 - 10 mg placed on the tongue where it will dissolve. For redosing, doses should be separated by at least 2 h. Maximum: 30 mg within 24 h.
Rofecoxib	VIOXX	Antiinflammatory, Non-Opioid Analgesic	**Tab:** 12.5, 25, 50 mg **Susp (per 5 mL):** 12.5, 25 mg	**Osteoarthritis:** Initially 12.5 mg once daily po. Some patients may benefit by an increase to the maximum of 25 mg once daily po. **Rheumatoid Arthritis:** 25 mg once daily po. **Acute Pain & Primary Dysmenorrhea:** Initially 50 mg once daily po for up to 5 days.

GENERIC NAME	COMMON TRADE NAMES	THERAPEUTIC CATEGORY	PREPARATIONS	COMMON ADULT DOSAGE
Ropinirole Hydrochloride	REQUIP	Antiparkinsonian	Tab: 0.25, 0.5, 1, 2, 4, 5 mg	The recommended initial dose is 0.25 mg tid po. Based on patient response titrate the dosage in weekly increments as follows: **Week 1:** 0.25 mg tid po. **Week 2:** 0.5 mg tid po. **Week 3:** 0.75 mg tid po. **Week 4:** 1.0 mg tid po. After week 4, if necessary, the dosage may be increased by 1.5 mg/day on a weekly basis up to a dose of 9 mg/day, and then by ≤ 3 mg/day weekly to a total dose of 24 mg/day.
Rosiglitazone Maleate	AVANDIA	Hypoglycemic Agent	Tab: 2, 4, 8 mg	**Monotherapy or With Metformin:** Usually 4 mg po as a single dose once daily or in divided doses bid. For patients who do not respond adequately after 12 weeks of therapy (as determined by fasting serum glucose), the dose may be increased to 8 mg po as a single daily dose or in divided doses bid.
Salmeterol	SEREVENT	Bronchodilator	Aerosol: 25 µg base/spray (as the xinafoate salt)	**Asthma and Bronchospasm:** 2 inhalations bid, approximately q 12 h. **Prevention of Exercise-Induced Bronchospasm:** 2 inhalations at least 30 - 60 min. before exercise.
	SEREVENT DISKUS		Powder: 50 µg base (as the xinafoate salt) in a blister strip	**Asthma:** 1 inhalation (50 µg) orally via the inhalation device bid (AM & PM, approximately 12 h apart).
Salsalate	DISALCID	Antiinflammatory	Cpsl: 500 mg Tab: 500, 750 mg	3000 mg daily po, given in divided doses as 1500 mg bid or 1000 mg tid.
	SALFLEX		Tab: 500, 750 mg	Same dosage as for DISALCID above.
Saquinavir	FORTOVASE	Antiviral	Cpsl: 200 mg	1200 mg po tid po taken within 2 h after a meal in combination with a nucleoside analog.

Scopolamine (*)	TRANSDERM-SCOP	Anticholinergic, Antiemetic	Transdermal: 1.5 mg/patch	Apply 1 patch to the area behind one ear at least 4 hours before the antiemetic effect is required. Effective for 3 days.
Scopolamine Hydrobromide	ISOPTO HYOSCINE	Mydriatic - Cycloplegic	Ophth Solution: 0.25%	**Refraction:** Instill 1 - 2 drops in the eye(s) 1 hour before refracting. **Uveitis:** Instill 1 - 2 drops in the eye(s) up to qid.
Secobarbital Sodium (*) (C-II)		Sedative - Hypnotic	Inj: 50 mg/mL	**Hypnotic:** 100 - 200 mg IM or 50 - 250 mg IV. **Preoperative Sedation:** 1 mg/kg IM, 10 - 15 minutes before the procedure.
Selegiline Hydrochloride (*)	ELDEPRYL	Antiparkinsonian	Cpsl: 5 mg	5 mg bid po, at breakfast and lunch.
Selenium Sulfide	EXSEL, SELSUN Rx	Antiseborrheic, Antifungal	Lotion: 2.5%	**Seborrheic Dermatitis & Dandruff: Massage** 5 to 10 mL into wet scalp; let stand for 2 - 3 minutes. Rinse & repeat. Apply twice a week for 2 weeks; then may be used once weekly or once every 2 - 4 weeks. **Tinea Versicolor:** Apply to affected areas and lather with water; leave on skin for 10 minutes, then rinse. Repeat once daily for 7 days.
Sennosides	EX-LAX EX-LAX CHOCOLATED	Irritant Laxative	**Tab:** 15 mg **Tab:** 15 mg	2 tabs once daily or bid with water. 2 tabs once daily or bid with water.
	EX-LAX, MAXIMUM RELIEF		**Tab:** 25 mg	2 tabs once daily or bid with water.
	SENOKOT	Irritant Laxative	**Syrup:** 8.8 mg/5 mL **Tab:** 8.6 mg **Granules:** 15 mg/tsp.	10 - 15 mL daily po, preferably hs. (Maximum: 15 mL bid po). 2 tablets daily po, preferably hs. (Maximum: 2 bid po). 1 teaspoonful daily po, preferably hs. (Maximum: 2 teaspoonfuls bid po).
	SENOKOTXTRA		**Tab:** 17 mg	1 tablet daily po, preferably hs. (Maximum: 2 tablets bid po).

GENERIC NAME	COMMON TRADE NAMES	THERAPEUTIC CATEGORY	PREPARATIONS	COMMON ADULT DOSAGE
Sertraline Hydrochloride (*)	ZOLOFT	Antidepressant, Drug for Obsessive-Compulsive Disorder, Drug for Panic Disorder, Drug for Post-Traumatic Stress Disorder	Tab: 25, 50, 100 mg Oral Solution: 20 mg/mL (12% alcohol)	**Depression and OCD:** Initially, 50 mg once daily po, either in the morning or evening. The dosage may be increased, at intervals of not less than 1 week, up to a maximum of 200 mg daily. **Panic Disorder and PTSD:** Initially, 25 mg once daily po, either in the morning or evening. The dosage may be increased, at intervals of not less than 1 week, to 50 mg once daily.
Sibutramine (*)	MERIDIA	Anorexiant	Cpsl: 5, 10, 15 mg	Initially, 10 mg once daily po. If there is inadequate weight loss after 4 weeks, the dose may be titrated to a total of 15 mg once daily.
Sildenafil Citrate (*)	VIAGRA	Agent for Impotence	Tab: 25, 50, 100 mg	50 mg po, taken prn approximately 1 h prior to sexual activity. May be taken between 30 min and 4 h before sexual activity and dose may be decreased to 25 mg or increased to 100 mg. The maximum dosing frequency is once per day.
Silver Sulfadiazine	SSD	Burn Preparation	Cream: 1%	Apply to a thickness of 1/16 inch once or twice daily.
Simethicone	GAS-X	Antigas Drug	Chewable Tab: 80 mg	Chew 80 - 160 mg prn pc or hs.
	GAS-X, EXTRA STRENGTH		Chewable Tab: 125 mg Liquid: 50 mg/5 mL	Chew 125 - 250 mg prn pc or hs. 10 - 20 mL (100 - 200 mg) po prn pc or hs.
	GAS-X, MAXIMUM STENGTH		Softgel: 166 mg	166 - 332 mg po prn pc or hs.
	MYLICON		Solution (Drops): 40 mg/0.6 mL	0.6 mL (40 mg) qid po pc and hs.
	MYLANTA GAS		Gelcap: 62.5 mg Chewable Tab: 80, 125 mg	62.5 mg qid, po, pc and hs. Chew 80 - 125 mg qid, pc and hs.

PHAZYME		**Solution (Drops):** 40 mg/0.6 mL **Tab:** 60 mg	1.2 mL (80 mg) qid po pc and hs.
PHAZYME-95		**Tab:** 95 mg	60 mg qid po, pc and hs.
PHAZYME-125		**Softgel:** 125 mg **Liquid:** 62.5 mg/5 mL	95 mg qid po, pc and hs.
			125 mg qid po, pc and hs. 10 mL qid po, pc and hs.
PHAZYME-166		**Softgel & Chewable Tab:** 166 mg	166 mg tid po, pc and hs.
Simvastatin	Antihyperlipidemic	**Tab:** 5, 10, 20, 40, 80 mg	**Usual Dosage:** Initially 20 mg once daily po in the evening. Dosage range: 5 - 80 mg once daily po in the evening. Adjust dose at intervals of ≥ 4 weeks. **Homozygous Familial Hypercholesterolemia:** 40 mg once daily po in the evening or 80 mg daily in 3 divided doses po (20 mg bid + 40 mg in the evening).
ZOCOR			
Sodium Chloride	Nasal Moisturizer	**Nasal Solution:** 0.64%	2 - 6 sprays into each nostril prn.
AFRIN SALINE EXTRA MOISTURIZING			
AYR SALINE, NASAL	Nasal Moisturizer	**Nasal Solution & Spray:** 0.65%	2 - 4 drops or 2 sprays into each nostril prn.
Sodium Nitroprusside (*)	Antihypertensive, Heart Failure Drug	**Inj:** 50 mg (in 1 L D₅W)	**Acute Hypertension:** The average effective IV infusion rate is about 3 μg/kg/min. At this rate, some patients will become dangerously hypotensive. Begin IV infusion at a very low rate (0.3 μg/kg/min), with gradual upward titration every few minutes until the desired effect is achieved or the maximum infusion rate (10 μg/kg/min) has been reached.

195

[Continued on the next page]

GENERIC NAME	COMMON TRADE NAMES	THERAPEUTIC CATEGORY	PREPARATIONS	COMMON ADULT DOSAGE
Sodium Nitroprusside [Continued]				**Congestive Heart Failure**: Titrate by increasing the infusion rate until measured cardiac output is no longer increasing, systemic blood pressure cannot be further reduced without compromising the perfusion of vital organs, or the maximum recommended infusion rate (10 μg/kg/min) has been reached, whichever comes first.
Sodium Polystyrene Sulfonate	KAYEXALATE	Potassium-Removing Resin	Powder: 10 - 12 g/heaping teaspoonful	Average daily dose is 15 - 60 g po. Usually, 15 g mixed in liquid 1 - 4 times daily po.
	SODIUM POLYSTYRENE SULFONATE SUSP.		Susp: 15 g/60 mL (0.1% alcohol)	Same dosage as for KAYEXALATE above.
Sotalol Hydrochloride (*)	BETAPACE	Antiarrhythmic	Tab: 80, 120, 160, 240 mg	**Treatment of Ventricular Arrhythmias**: Initially, 80 mg bid po. Dosage may be increased at 2 - 3 day intervals up to 320 mg/day po given in 2 or 3 divided doses.
Sparfloxacin (*)	ZAGAM	Antibacterial	Tab: 200 mg	400 mg po as a loading dose, followed by 200 mg once daily for a total of 10 days (i.e., 11 tablets).
Spectinomycin Hydrochloride	TROBICIN	Antibacterial	Powd for Inj: 2, 4 g	2 g as a single deep IM injection.
Spironolactone	ALDACTONE	Antihypertensive, Diuretic	Tab: 25, 50, 100 mg	**Diuresis**: Initially, 100 mg po, as a single dose or in divided doses, for at least 5 days. **Hypertension**: Initially 50 - 100 mg po as a single dose or in divided doses.
Stanozolol (C-III)	WINSTROL	Anabolic Steroid	Tab: 2 mg	Initially, 2 mg tid po. After a favorable response, decrease dosage at intervals of 1 to 3 months to a maintenance dosage of 2 mg once daily.

196

Stavudine	ZERIT	Antiviral	Cpsl: 15, 20, 30, 40 mg Powd for Solution: 1 mg/mL	**Initial Dosage:** < 60 kg: 30 mg twice daily (q 12 h) po. ≥ 60 kg: 40 mg twice daily (q 12 h) po. **Dosage Adjustment: Monitor patients for the development of peripheral neuropathy. If symptoms develop, stop the drug. If the symptoms resolve completely, consider resumption of therapy with half of the above mg dosages.**
Streptokinase	STREPTASE	Thrombolytic	Powd for Inj: 250,000 IUnits, 750,000 IUnits, and 1,500,000 IUnits	250,000 IU IV (over 30 minutes), followed by 100,000 IU/h by IV infusion. Length of therapy determined by condition (see below). **Pulmonary Embolism:** 24 h (72 h if concurrent deep vein thrombosis is suspected). **Deep Vein Thrombosis:** 72 h. **Arterial Thrombosis or Embolism:** 24 - 72 h.
Streptomycin Sulfate (*)		Antibacterial, Tuberculostatic	Inj: 1 g/2.5 mL	**Tuberculosis:** any of the following regimens may be used. Generally no more than 120 g is given over the course of therapy. 15 mg/kg daily IM (Maximum: 1 g). 25 - 30 mg/kg bid IM (Maximum 1.5 g). 25 - 30 mg/kg two or three times weekly IM (Maximum: 1.5 g). **Tularemia:** 1 - 2 g daily IM in divided doses for 7 - 14 days until afebrile for 5 - 7 days. **Plague:** 2 g daily IM in 2 divided doses for a minimum of 10 days. **Bacterial Endocarditis:** **Streptococcal Endocarditis:** 1 g bid IM for the 1st week, followed by 500 mg bid IM for the 2nd week. **Enterococcal Endocarditis:** 1 g bid IM for 2 weeks, followed by 500 mg bid IM for an additional 4 weeks (with penicillin).

GENERIC NAME	COMMON TRADE NAMES	THERAPEUTIC CATEGORY	PREPARATIONS	COMMON ADULT DOSAGE
Streptozocin	ZANOSAR	Antineoplastic	Powd for Inj: 1 g	**Daily Schedule:** 500 mg/m² IV for 5 consecutive days q 6 weeks. **Weekly Schedule:** 1000 mg/m² IV weekly for the first 2 weeks. Dosage may be increased in selected patients to a maximum of 1500 mg/m² IV once a week.
Succinylcholine Chloride	ANECTINE	Neuromuscular Blocker	Inj: 20 mg/mL Powd for IV Infusion: 500, 1000 mg	**Short Surgical Procedures:** 0.6 mg/kg IV. **Long Surgical Procedures:** 2.5 - 4.3 mg/min by IV infusion; or 0.3 - 1.1 mg/kg initially by IV injection followed, at appropriate intervals, by 0.04 - 0.07 mg/kg.
Sucralfate	CARAFATE	Anti-Ulcer Agent	Tab: 1 g Susp: 1 g/10 mL	**Active Duodenal Ulcer:** 1 g qid po on an empty stomach. **Maintenance:** 1 g bid po.
Sulconazole Nitrate	EXELDERM	Antifungal (Topical)	Cream & Solution: 1 %	Gently massage a small amount into the skin once or twice daily.
Sulfacetamide Sodium	SODIUM SULAMYD	Antibacterial (Topical)	Ophth Solution: 10% Ophth Oint: 10%	1 - 2 drops into the affected eye(s) q 2 - 3 h during the day, less often at night. Apply a small amount to affected eye(s) q 3 - 4 h and hs.
	SODIUM SULAMYD		Ophth Solution: 30%	**Conjunctivitis or Corneal Ulcer:** 1 drop into the affected eye(s) q 2 h or less frequently. **Trachoma:** 2 drops into eye(s) q 2 h.
	BLEPH-10		Ophth Solution: 10%	**Conjunctivitis and other Superficial Ocular Infections:** 1 - 2 drops into the affected eye(s) q 2 - 3 h initially. Dosage may be reduced as the condition responds. The usual duration of therapy is 7 to 10 days. **Trachoma:** 2 drops into eye(s) q 2 h.

		Ophth Oint: 10%	**Conjunctivitis and other Superficial Ocular Infections:** Apply a small amount (approx. 1/2 inch) into the affected eye(s) q 3 - 4 h and hs. Dosage may be reduced as the condition responds. The usual duration of therapy is 7 to 10 days.
Sulfasalazine (*)	KLARON	Anti-Acne Agent	Lotion: 10%	Apply a thin film to affected areas bid.
	AZULFIDINE-EN	Bowel Antiinflammatory Agent, Antirheumatic	Enteric-Coated Tab: 500 mg	**Ulcerative Colitis:** **Initial:** 3 - 4 g daily po in evenly divided doses. **Maintenance:** 2 g daily po. **Rheumatoid Arthritis:** Initially 0.5 - 1 g daily po; then 2 g daily po in evenly divided doses.
Sulfinpyrazone	ANTURANE	Anti-Gout Agent	**Tab:** 100 mg **Cpsl:** 200 mg	**Initial:** 200 - 400 mg po in 2 divided doses with meals or milk. **Maintenance:** 400 mg daily po in 2 divided doses with meals or milk.
Sulfisoxazole (*)		Antibacterial	**Tab:** 500 mg	Initially 2 - 4 g po, then 4 - 8 g/day divided in 4 - 6 doses.
Sulindac (*)	CLINORIL	Antiinflammatory	**Tab:** 150, 200 mg	**Osteoarthritis, Rheumatoid Arthritis, and Ankyl. Spondylitis:** 150 mg bid po with food. **Acute Painful Shoulder:** 200 mg bid po with food for 7 - 14 days. **Acute Gouty Arthritis:** 200 mg bid po with food for 7 days.

199

GENERIC NAME	COMMON TRADE NAMES	THERAPEUTIC CATEGORY	PREPARATIONS	COMMON ADULT DOSAGE
Sumatriptan Succinate (*)	IMITREX	Antimigraine Agent	**Inj:** 12 mg/mL	6 mg SC. A second 6 mg dose may be given in patients who failed to respond to the first dose. Maximum: two 6 mg doses in 24 h, separated by ≥ 1 h.
			Tab: 25, 50, 100 mg	25 - 100 mg po taken with fluids as early as possible after the onset of attack. If a suitable response does not occur within 2 h, a second dose of up to 100 mg may be given. If headache returns, additional doses may be taken at 2 h intervals, not to exceed 200 mg per day.
			Nasal Spray (per 0.1 mL): 5, 20 mg	5, 10, or 20 mg administered in one nostril as a single dose. (A 10 mg dose is achieved by administering 5 mg in each nostril).
Suprofen	PROFENAL	Antiinflammatory (Topical)	**Ophth Solution:** 1 %	On the day of surgery, instill 2 drops into the conjunctival sac at 3, 2, and 1 hour prior to surgery. Two drops may be instilled into the conjunctival sac q 4 h, while awake, the day preceding surgery.
Tacrine Hydrochloride (*)	COGNEX	Drug for Alzheimer's Disease	**Cpsl:** 10, 20, 30, 40 mg	**Initial:** 10 mg qid po. Maintain this dose for ≥ 4 weeks, every other week monitoring transaminase levels beginning at week 4 of therapy. **Titration:** After 4 weeks, increase to 20 mg qid po providing there are no significant transaminase elevations and the patient is tolerating treatment. Titrate to higher doses (30 and 40 mg qid po) at 4 week intervals on the basis of tolerance and transaminase levels during monitoring.

Tacrolimus (*)	PROGRAF	Immunosuppressant	Cpsl: 0.5, 1, 5 mg	Liver Transplantation: 0.15 - 0.3 mg/kg/day po in 2 divided doses (q 12 h). Administer the initial dose no sooner than 6 h after transplantation. If IV therapy was initiated, begin 8 - 12 h after discontinuing IV therapy. Kidney Transplantation: 0.2 mg/kg/day po in 2 divided doses (q 12 h). Administer the initial dose within 24 h of transplantation, but should be delayed until renal function has recovered.
			Inj: 5 mg/mL	0.05 - 0.1 mg/kg/day as a continuous IV infusion. Administer initial dose no sooner than 6 h after transplantation. Convert to oral therapy as soon as the patient can tolerate oral dosing.
	PROTOPIC	Immunomodulator	Oint: 0.03, 0.1%	Apply a thin layer bid to affected areas of dry skin. Rub in gently and completely.
Tamoxifen Citrate	NOLVADEX	Antineoplastic	Tab: 10, 20 mg	Breast Cancer: 20 - 40 mg daily po. Give doses over 20 mg daily in divided doses (morning and evening). Reduction in Breast Cancer Incidence in High-Risk Women and Ductal Carcinoma in situ: 20 mg daily po for 5 years.
Tamsulosin Hydrochloride	FLOMAX	Benign Prostatic Hyperplasia Drug	Cpsl: 0.4 mg	Initially 0.4 mg once daily po; take dose 30 min. after the same meal each day. May increase dose to 0.8 mg once daily po after 2 - 4 weeks if the response is inadequate. If therapy is interrupted, resume at 0.4 mg once daily and re-titrate.
Tazarotene	TAZORAC	Anti-Acne Agent, Anti-Psoriasis Agent	Cream & Gel: 0.05, 0.1%	After the skin is clean and dry, apply a thin film once daily, in the evening, to the acne or psoriatic lesions. Use enough to cover the entire lesion.

GENERIC NAME	COMMON TRADE NAMES	THERAPEUTIC CATEGORY	PREPARATIONS	COMMON ADULT DOSAGE
Telmisartan	MICARDIS	Antihypertensive	Tab: 20, 40, 80 mg	Initially, 40 mg daily po. The usual dosage range is 20 - 80 mg daily.
Temazepam (*) (C-IV)	RESTORIL	Hypnotic	Cpsl: 7.5, 15, 30 mg	7.5 - 30 mg po hs.
Tenofovir Disoproxil Fumarate	VIREAD	Antiviral	Tab: 300 mg	300 mg once daily po with food.
Terazosin Hydrochloride	HYTRIN	Antihypertensive, Benign Prostatic Hyperplasia Drug	Cpsl: 1, 2, 5, 10 mg (as the base)	**Hypertension:** Initially, 1 mg po hs. Dosage may be slowly increased to the suggested dosage range of 1 - 5 mg once daily po. **Benign Prostatic Hyperplasia:** Initially, 1 mg po hs. Increase the dose in a stepwise fashion to 2, 5, or 10 mg daily to achieved desired effect. Doses of 10 mg once daily are generally required and may require 4 - 6 weeks of therapy to assess benefits.
Terbinafine Hydrochloride	LAMISIL AT	Antifungal (Topical)	Cream & Solution: 1%	**Interdigital *Tinea pedis:*** Apply to affected and surrounding areas bid for at least 1 week. ***Tinea cruris* or *T. corporis:*** Apply to affected and surrounding areas once daily or bid for at least 1 week.
			Tab: 250 mg	**Onychomycosis:** Fingernail: 250 mg daily po for 6 weeks. Toenail: 250 mg daily po for 12 weeks.
Terbutaline Sulfate (*)	BRETHINE	Bronchodilator	Tab: 2.5, 5 mg Inj: 1 mg/mL	**12-15 yrs:** 2.5 mg tid (q 6 h) po. **Over 15 yrs:** 5 mg tid (q 6 h) po. 0.25 mg SC; may repeat once in 15 - 30 min.
Terconazole	TERAZOL 3	Antifungal (Topical)	Vaginal Cream: 0.8% Vaginal Suppos: 80 mg	1 applicatorful intravaginally hs for 3 days. Insert 1 vaginally hs for 3 days.
	TERAZOL 7		Vaginal Cream: 0.4%	1 applicatorful intravaginally hs for 7 days.
Testolactone	TESLAC	Antineoplastic	Tab: 50 mg	250 mg qid po.

202

Drug	Class	Formulation	Dosage
Testosterone (C-III)	Androgen, Antineoplastic	Inj (per mL): 25, 50, 100 mg (aqueous suspension)	**Replacement Therapy**: 25 - 50 mg 2 - 3 times a week by deep IM injection. **Breast Cancer**: 50 - 100 mg 3 times a week by deep IM injection.
ANDRODERM	Androgen	Transdermal: rate = 2.5, 5 mg/day	**Replacement Therapy**: Apply one 5 mg patch or two 2.5 mg patches nightly for 24 h to intact clean, dry skin of the back, abdomen, thighs, or upper arms. Increase to 7.5 mg or decrease to 2.5 mg daily as per morning serum testosterone levels.
TESTODERM	Androgen	Transdermal: rate = 4, 6 mg/24 hr	**Replacement Therapy**: Start with a 6 mg/day system applied daily on clean, dry scrotal skin for up to 8 weeks; if scrotal area is inadequate, use a 4 mg/day system.
TESTODERM TTS	Androgen	Transdermal: rate = 5 mg/24 hr	**Replacement Therapy**: Apply once daily (at about the same time each day) to a dry area of the arm, back, or upper buttocks.
ANDROGEL	Androgen	Gel: 1% (2.5 g/packette to deliver 25 mg). 1% (5.0 g/packette to deliver 50 mg)	**Replacement Therapy**: Apply to clean, intact, dry skin of the upper arms, shoulders, and/or abdomen; do not apply to the scrotum. Use 5 g once daily in the AM; may increase dose by 2.5 g every 2 weeks. Wash hands after each application.
Testosterone Cypionate (C-III) DEPO-TESTOSTERONE	Androgen, Antineoplastic	Inj (per mL): 100, 200 mg (in oil)	**Male Hypogonadism**: 50 - 400 mg q 2 - 4 weeks IM. **Breast Cancer**: 200 - 400 mg q 2 - 4 weeks IM.
Testosterone Enanthate (C-III) DELATESTRYL	Androgen, Antineoplastic	Inj: 200 mg/mL (in oil)	Same dosages as for DEPO-TESTOSTERONE above.
Tetracaine Hydrochloride PONTOCAINE	Local Anesthetic	Cream: 1%	Apply to the affected area prn.
PONTOCAINE HCL PONTOCAINE EYE		Ophth Solution: 0.5% Ophth Oint: 0.5%	1 - 2 drops into eye(s). Apply 0.5 - 1 inch to lower conjunctival fornix.

GENERIC NAME	COMMON TRADE NAMES	THERAPEUTIC CATEGORY	PREPARATIONS	COMMON ADULT DOSAGE
Tetracycline Hydrochloride (*)	SUMYCIN	Antibacterial	Cpsl & Tab: 250, 500 mg Syrup: 125 mg/5 mL	**Usual Dosage:** 1 - 2 g po divided into 2 or 4 equal doses. **Brucellosis:** 500 mg qid po for 3 weeks with streptomycin. **Syphilis:** 30 - 40 g po in equally divided doses over a period of 10 - 15 days. **Gonorrhea:** Initially, 1.5 g po followed by 500 mg q 6 h for 4 days (total dose of 9 g). **Uncomplicated Urethral, Endocervical or Rectal Infections due to *Chlamydia trachomatis*:** 500 mg qid po for at least 7 days.
	TOPICYCLINE	Antibacterial (Topical)	**Powd for Solution:** 150 mg [with 70 mL of liquid]	Apply generously bid to the entire affected area until the skin is wet.
Tetrahydrozoline Hydrochloride	TYZINE	Nasal Decongestant	**Nasal Solution:** 0.1%	2 - 4 drops in each nostril q 4 - 6 h.
	VISINE	Ocular Decongestant	**Ophth Solution:** 0.05%	1 - 2 drops in affected eye(s) up to qid.
Theophylline, Anhydrous (*)	ELIXOPHYLLIN	Bronchodilator	**Elixir:** 80 mg/15 mL (20% alcohol) **Cpsl:** 100, 200 mg	See Oral Theophylline Doses Table, p. 312.
	RESPBID		**Sustained-Rel. Tab:** 250, 500 mg	See Oral Theophylline Doses Table, p. 313.
	SLO-BID		**Extended-Rel. Cpsl:** 50, 75, 100, 125, 200, 300 mg	See Oral Theophylline Doses Table, p. 313.
	SLO-PHYLLIN		**Syrup:** 80 mg/15 mL **Tab:** 100, 200 mg **Extended-Rel. Cpsl:** 60, 125, 250 mg	See Oral Theophylline Doses Table, p. 312. See Oral Theophylline Doses Table, p. 313.
	THEO-24		**Extended-Rel. Cpsl:** 100, 200, 300, 400 mg	See Oral Theophylline Doses Table, p. 314.

204

Generic	Brand	Class	Dosage Forms	Dosing
	THEO-DUR		**Extended-Rel. Tab:** 100, 200, 300, 450 mg.	See Oral Theophylline Doses Table, p. 313.
	THEOLAIR		**Liquid:** 80 mg/15 mL **Tab:** 125, 250 mg	See Oral Theophylline Doses Table, p. 312.
	THEOLAIR-SR		**Sustained-Rel Tab:** 200, 250, 300, 500 mg	See Oral Theophylline Doses Table, p. 313.
	T-PHYL		**Controlled-Rel. Tab:** 200 mg	See Oral Theophylline Doses Table, p. 313.
	UNIPHYL		**Controlled-Rel. Tab:** 400, 600 mg	400 - 600 mg po once daily in the morning or in the evening.
Thiabendazole (*)	MINTEZOL	Anthelmintic	**Susp:** 500 mg/5 mL **Chewable Tab:** 500 mg	**Strongyloidiasis, Intestinal Roundworms and Cutaneous Larva Migrans:** 2 doses/day (as below) po for 2 successive days. **Trichinosis:** 2 doses/day (as below) po for 2 - 4 successive days. **Visceral Larva Migrans:** 2 doses/day (as below) po for 7 successive days. Each Dose: 10 mg/lb.
Thiethylperazine Maleate	TORECAN	Antiemetic	**Tab:** 10 mg **Inj:** 10 mg/2 mL	10 mg once daily to tid po. 10 mg once daily to tid IM.
Thioguanine		Antineoplastic	**Tab:** 40 mg	Initially, 2 mg/kg daily po. If no improvement occurs after 4 weeks, the dosage may be increased to 3 mg/kg/day.
Thioridazine (*)	MELLARIL-S	Antipsychotic	**Susp (per 5 mL):** 25, 100 mg	Initially 50 - 100 mg tid po, with a gradual increment to a maximum of 800 mg daily if necessary. The maintenance dosage varies from 200 - 800 mg daily, divided into 2 or 4 doses.

205

GENERIC NAME	COMMON TRADE NAMES	THERAPEUTIC CATEGORY	PREPARATIONS	COMMON ADULT DOSAGE
Thioridazine Hydrochloride (*)	MELLARIL	Antipsychotic	**Liquid Conc (per mL):** 30, (3% alcohol), 100 mg (4.2% (alcohol) **Tab:** 10, 15, 25, 50, 100, 150, 200 mg	Same dosage as for MELLARIL-S above.
Thiothixene (*)	NAVANE	Antipsychotic	**Cpsl:** 1, 2, 5, 10, 20 mg	**Mild Psychoses:** Initially 2 mg tid po; dosage may be increased to 15 mg/day if needed. **More Severe Psychoses:** Initially 5 mg bid po; the usual optimal dosage is 20 - 30 mg daily. Dosage may be increased to 60 mg/day.
Thiothixene Hydrochloride (*)	NAVANE	Antipsychotic	**Liquid Conc:** 5 mg/mL (7% alcohol) **Inj (per mL):** 2, 5 mg	Same dosages as for NAVANE Capsules above. 4 mg bid to qid IM.
Thyroid Dessicated	ARMOUR THYROID	Thyroid Hormone	**Tab:** 15, 30, 60, 90, 120, 180, 240, 300 mg	Initial: 30 mg daily po, with increments of 15 mg q 2 - 3 weeks. **Maintenance:** Usually 60 - 120 mg daily po.
Tiagabine Hydrochloride (*)	GABITRIL	Antiepileptic	**Tab:** 2, 4, 12, 16 mg	**12-18 yrs:** 4 mg once daily po for 1 week. May increase to 4 mg bid po for 1 week; then may increase by 4 - 8 mg weekly to the clinical response or up to 32 mg/day in 2 - 4 divided doses. Take with food. **Over 18 yrs:** 4 mg once daily po. May increase by 4 - 8 mg weekly to the clinical response or up to 56 mg/day in 2 - 4 divided doses. Take with food.
Ticarcillin Disodium (*)	TICAR	Antibacterial	**Powd for Inj:** 1, 3, 6 g	**Urinary Tract Infections:** **Uncomplicated:** 1 g IM or direct IV q 6 h. **Complicated:** 150 - 200 mg/kg/day by IV infusion in divided doses q 4 or 6 h. **Most Other Infections:** 200 - 300 mg/kg/day by IV infusion in divided doses q 4 or 6 h.

206

Ticlopidine Hydrochloride	TICLID	Platelet Aggregation Inhibitor	**Tab: 250 mg**	250 mg bid po, taken with food.
Tiludronate Sodium	SKELID	Bone Stabilizer	**Tab: 240 mg** (equivalent to 200 mg of tiludronic acid)	400 mg (acid) po daily with 6 - 8 oz. of water for 3 mos. Do not take within 2 h of food.
Timolol Hemihydrate	BETIMOL	Anti-Glaucoma Agent	**Ophth Solution: 0.25, 0.5%**	1 drop (0.25%) into affected eye(s) bid.
Timolol Maleate (*)	BLOCADREN	Antihypertensive, Post-MI Drug, Antimigraine Agent	**Tab: 5, 10, 20 mg**	**Hypertension:** Initially 10 mg po. The usual maintenance dosage is 20 - 40 mg daily. **Myocardial Infarction:** 10 mg bid po. **Migraine Headaches:** 10 mg bid po. The 20 mg daily dosage may be given as a single dose during maintenance therapy.
	TIMOPTIC TIMOPTIC-XE	Anti-Glaucoma Agent	**Ophth Solution: 0.25, 0.5% Ophth Gel: 0.25, 0.5%**	1 drop into affected eye(s) bid. Apply to affected eye(s) once daily.
Tinzaparin Sodium	INNOHEP	Anticoagulant	**Inj: 40000 IUnits/2 mL**	175 IU/kg SC once daily for ≥ 6 days and until the patient is adequately anticoagulated with warfarin.
Tioconazole	VAGISTAT-1	Antifungal (Topical)	**Vaginal Oint: 6.5%**	Insert 1 applicatorful intravaginally hs.
Tizanidine Hydrochloride	ZANAFLEX	Skeletal Muscle Relaxant	**Tab: 2, 4 mg**	Initially, 4 mg po. May increase by 2 - 4 mg prn q 6 - 8 h to a maximum of 3 doses in 24 h. Maximum: 36 mg per day.
Tobramycin	TOBREX	Antibacterial	**Ophth Oint: 3 mg/g (0.3%)**	**Mild to Moderate Infections:** Apply 1/2 inch ribbon into the affected eye(s) q 4 h. **Severe Infections:** Apply 1/2 inch ribbon into the affected eye(s) q 3 - 4 h until condition improves; reduce dosage prior to stopping.
			Ophth Solution: 3 mg/mL (0.3%)	**Mild to Moderate Infections:** 1 - 2 drops into the affected eye(s) q 4 h. **Severe Infections:** 2 drops into the affected eye(s) hourly until improvement occurs; reduce dosage prior to discontinuation.

GENERIC NAME	COMMON TRADE NAMES	THERAPEUTIC CATEGORY	PREPARATIONS	COMMON ADULT DOSAGE
Tobramycin Sulfate (*)	NEBCIN	Antibacterial	Inj (per mL): 10, 40 mg Powd for Inj: 30 mg	**Serious Infections:** 3 mg/kg/day IM or IV in 3 equal doses q 8 h. **Life-Threatening Infections:** Up to 5 mg/kg/day may be given IM or IV in 3 or 4 equal doses.
Tocainide Hydrochloride	TONOCARD	Antiarrhythmic	Tab: 400, 600 mg	Initially 400 mg q 8 h po. The usual dosage is 1200 - 1800 mg/day in 3 divided doses.
Tolazamide	TOLINASE	Hypoglycemic Agent	Tab: 100, 250, 500 mg	Initial: 100 - 250 mg daily po, administered with breakfast or the first main meal. Dosage adjustments are made in increments of 100 to 250 mg at weekly intervals. Maintenance: Usually 250 - 500 mg daily po.
Tolbutamide	ORINASE	Hypoglycemic Agent	Tab: 500 mg	Initial: 1 - 2 g daily po, as a single dose in the AM or in divided doses throughout the day. Maintenance: Usually 0.25 - 2 g daily po, as a single dose in the AM or in divided doses throughout the day.
Tolcapone (*)	TASMAR	Antiparkinsonian	Tab: 100, 200 mg	Initially 100 or 200 mg tid po always as an adjunct to levodopa/carbidopa therapy.
Tolmetin Sodium (*)	TOLECTIN 200 TOLECTIN DS TOLECTIN 600	Antiinflammatory	Tab: 200 mg Cpsl: 400 mg Tab: 600 mg	Initially 400 mg tid po, preferably including a dose on arising and a dose hs; adjust dosage after 1 - 2 weeks. Control is usually achieved at 600 - 1800 mg daily in divided doses (generally tid).
Tolnaftate	AFTATE	Antifungal (Topical)	Gel, Powder, Spray Powder & Liquid Spray: 1 %	Apply a thin layer over affected area morning and night for 2 - 3 weeks.
	TINACTIN		Cream, Solution, Powder, Spray Powder & Spray Liquid: 1 %	Apply to affected areas morning and night for 2 - 4 weeks.

Tolterodine Tartrate	DETROL	Urinary Antispasmodic	**Tab:** 1, 2 mg	Initially 2 mg bid po. The dosage may be reduced to 1 mg bid po based on individual response and tolerability.
	DETROL LA		**Extended-Rel. Cpsl:** 2, 4 mg	4 mg po, taken once daily with liquids and swallowed whole.
Topiramate	TOPAMAX	Antiepileptic	**Tab:** 25, 100, 200 mg **Sprinkle Cpsl:** 15, 25 mg	Initially, 25 - 50 mg/day po followed by titration to an effective dose (400 mg/day) in increments of 25 - 50 mg per week. Sprinkle Capsules may be swallowed whole or the contents may be sprinkled onto soft food.
Torsemide	DEMADEX	Diuretic, Antihypertensive	**Tab:** 5, 10, 20, 100 mg **Inj:** 10 mg/mL	**Hypertension:** 5 mg once daily po. After 4 - 6 weeks, the dose may be increased to 10 mg once daily po. **Diuresis in:** **Congestive Heart Failure:** Initially, 10 or 20 mg once daily po or slow IV (over 2 min). If the response is inadequate, titrate dose upward by approximately doubling. Maximum dose: 200 mg. **Chronic Renal Failure:** Initially, 20 mg once daily po or IV (over 2 min). If the response is inadequate, titrate dose upward by approximately doubling. Max.: 200 mg. **Hepatic Cirrhosis:** Initially, 5 or 10 mg once daily po or IV (over 2 min), together with a potassium-spraing diuretic. If the response is inadequate, titrate dose upward by approx. doubling. Maximum dose: 40 mg.
Tramadol Hydrochloride (*)	ULTRAM	Opioid Analgesic	**Tab:** 50 mg	50 - 100 mg q 4 - 6 h po, not to exceed 400 mg/day.

GENERIC NAME	COMMON TRADE NAMES	THERAPEUTIC CATEGORY	PREPARATIONS	COMMON ADULT DOSAGE
Trandolapril	MAVIK	Antihypertensive, Heart Failure Drug	**Tab:** 1, 2, 4 mg	**Hypertension:** **African-American Patients:** Initially, 2 mg once daily po. **Other Patients:** Initially, 1 mg once daily po. **Heart Failure Post-MI:** Initially 1 mg daily po, then titrate patient (as tolerated) toward a target dose of 4 mg daily.
Tranexamic Acid	CYKLOKAPRON	Systemic Hemostatic	**Inj:** 100 mg/mL **Tab:** 500 mg	10 mg/kg IV immediat. before dental surgery. After surgery, give 25 mg/kg po tid - qid for 2 to 8 days. In patients unable to take oral medication, give 10 mg/kg tid - qid. 25 mg/kg po tid - qid beginning 1 day prior to dental surgery.
Tranylcypromine Sulfate (*)	PARNATE	Antidepressant	**Tab:** 10 mg	30 mg/day po in divided doses. Adjust dosage in approximately 2 weeks in 10 mg increments at intervals of 1 - 3 weeks to a maximum of 60 mg per day.
Travoprost	TRAVATAN	Anti-Glaucoma Agent	**Ophth Solution:** 0.004%	1 drop into the affected eye(s) once daily in the evening.
Trazodone Hydrochloride (*)	DESYREL	Antidepressant	**Tab:** 50, 100, 150, 300 mg	Initially 150 mg/day po in divided doses. The dose may be increased by 50 mg/day q 3 - 4 days to a maximum of 400 mg/day (for outpatients) or 600 mg/day (for more severely-depressed inpatients).
Tretinoin (*)	RETIN-A	Anti-Acne Agent	**Cream:** 0.025, 0.05, 0.1% **Gel:** 0.01, 0.025% **Liquid:** 0.05%	Cover the entire affected area once daily hs.
	AVITA		**Cream:** 0.025%	Cover the entire affected area once daily hs.
	RENOVA		**Cream:** 0.02%, 0.05%	Apply to face once daily hs, using only enough (i.e., "pea-size" amount) to cover the affected area lightly.

Triamcinolone	ARISTOCORT	Corticosteroid	**Tab:** 1, 2, 4, 8 mg	Initial dose may vary from 4 to 48 mg po per day. Dose requirements are variable and must be individualized based on the disease and the patient's response.
Triamcinolone Acetonide	KENALOG-10	Corticosteroid	**Inj:** 10 mg/mL	**Intra-articular or Intrabursal Injection and Injection into Tendon Sheaths:** Initially, 2.5 to 5 mg (for smaller joints) and 5 - 15 mg (for larger joints). **Intradermal Injection:** Varies depending on the disease, but should be limited to 1.0 mg per injection site.
	KENALOG-40	Corticosteroid	**Inj:** 40 mg/mL	**IM (deep):** Usual initial dose is 60 mg. Dosage is usually adjusted from 40 - 80 mg, depending on the patient response and the duration of relief. **Intra-articular or Intrabursal Injection and Injection into Tendon Sheaths:** Initially, 2.5 to 5 mg (for smaller joints) and 5 - 15 mg (for larger joints).
	ARISTOCORT A	Corticosteroid (Topical)	**Cream:** 0.025, 0.1, 0.5% **Oint:** 0.1%	Apply to affected area as a thin film tid - qid depending on the severity of the condition.
	KENALOG	Corticosteroid (Topical)	**Oint:** 0.025, 0.1, 0.5% **Cream:** 0.025, 0.1, 0.5% **Lotion:** 0.025, 0.1% **Spray:** 0.2%	Apply a thin film to the affected area bid - qid (of the 0.025%) or bid - tid (of the 0.1% or 0.5%). Rub in gently. Apply to the affected area bid - qid (of the 0.025%) or bid - tid (of the 0.1 or 0.5%). Rub in gently. Apply to the affected area bid - qid (of the 0.025%) or bid - tid (of the 0.1%). Rub in. Spray onto affected area tid - qid.
	AZMACORT	Corticosteroid (Topical)	**Aerosol:** 100 μg/spray	2 inhalations tid or qid.
	NASACORT NASACORT AQ	Corticosteroid (Topical)	**Aerosol:** 55 μg/spray **Aerosol:** 55 μg/spray	2 sprays in each nostril once a day. If needed, the dose may be doubled, either as a once a day dosage or divided up to 4 times daily.

211

GENERIC NAME	COMMON TRADE NAMES	THERAPEUTIC CATEGORY	PREPARATIONS	COMMON ADULT DOSAGE
Triamcinolone Diacetate	ARISTOCORT FORTE	Corticosteroid	Inj (per mL): 25, 40 mg	Initial dosage may vary from 3 - 48 mg daily, depending on the specific disease being treated. The average dose is 40 mg IM once a week or 5 - 40 mg intra-articularly or intrasynovially.
Triamcinolone Hexacetonide	ARISTOSPAN	Corticosteroid	Inj (per mL): 5, 20 mg	Initial dosage may vary from 2 - 48 mg daily, depending on the specific disease being treated. The average dose is 2 - 20 mg intra-articularly (depending on the size of the joint), repeated q 3 - 4 weeks. Up to 0.5 mg/square inch of skin may be given by intralesional or sublesional injection.
Triamterene	DYRENIUM	Diuretic	Cpsl: 50, 100 mg	100 mg bid po pc.
Triazolam (*) (C-IV)	HALCION	Hypnotic	Tab: 0.125, 0.25 mg	0.25 mg hs po.
Trichlormethiazide	NAQUA	Diuretic, Antihypertensive	Tab: 2, 4 mg	**Diuresis:** 1 - 4 mg daily po. **Hypertension:** 2 - 4 mg daily po.
Trifluoperazine Hydrochloride (*)	STELAZINE	Antipsychotic	Tab: 1, 2, 5, 10 mg Inj: 2 mg/mL	Initially, 2 - 5 mg bid po. Most show optimum response on 15 - 20 mg daily po. 1 - 2 mg by deep IM q 4 - 6 h prn.
Trifluridine	VIROPTIC	Antiviral (Topical)	Ophth Solution: 1%	1 drop into affected eye(s) q 2 h while awake for a maximum of 9 drops daily until the cornea has re-epithelialized. Then use 1 drop q 4 h while awake for 7 days.

Trihexyphenidyl Hydrochloride (*)	Antiparkinsonian	**Tab:** 2, 5 mg	Initially 1 mg po on the first day. The dose may be increased by 2 mg increments at intervals of 3 - 5 days to a maximum of 6 - 10 mg daily.
Trimethobenzamide Hydrochloride (*)	Antiemetic	**Cpsl:** 100, 250, 300 mg **Rectal Suppos:** 200 mg **Inj:** 100 mg/mL	250 mg tid or qid po. 200 mg tid or qid rectally. 200 mg tid or qid IM.
TIGAN			
Trimethoprim (*)	Antibacterial	**Tab:** 100, 200 mg	100 mg q 12 h po for 10 days, or 200 mg q 24 h po for 10 days.
PROLOPRIM			
Trimethoprim Hydrochloride (*)	Antibacterial	**Solution:** 50 mg/5 mL	100 mg bid po for 10 days, or 200 mg once daily po for 10 days.
PRIMSOL			
Trimetrexate Glucuronate	Antiparasitic	**Powd for Inj:** 25 mg	**Must be administ. with concurrent leucovorin.** 45 mg/m^2 once daily by IV infusion over 60 to 90 minutes. Leucovorin must be given daily during treatment with NEUTREXIN and for 72 h past the last dose of NEUTREXIN. Leucovorin may be given IV at a dose of 20 mg/m^2 over 5 - 10 minutes q 6 h for a total daily dose of 80 mg/m^2 or orally as 4 doses of 20 mg/m^2 spaced equally during the day. Recommended course of therapy is 21 days of NEUTREXIN and 24 days of leucovorin.
NEUTREXIN			
Trimipramine Maleate (*)	Antidepressant	**Cpsl:** 25, 50, 100 mg	**Outpatients:** Initially, 75 mg/day po in divided doses. Maintenance doses range from 50 to 150 mg/day po. **Hospitalized Patients:** Initially, 100 mg/day po in divided doses. May gradually increase in a few days to 200 mg/day. If no improvement occurs in 2 - 3 weeks, dose may be raised to a maximum dose of 250 - 300 mg/day.
SURMONTIL			
Trolamine Salicylate	Analgesic (Topical)	**Cream:** 10%	Apply to affected area not more than tid to qid. Affected areas may be wrapped loosely prn.
MYOFLEX			
Troleandomycin	Antibacterial	**Cpsl:** 250 mg	250 - 500 mg qid po.
TAO			

GENERIC NAME	COMMON TRADE NAMES	THERAPEUTIC CATEGORY	PREPARATIONS	COMMON ADULT DOSAGE
Tropicamide	MYDRIACYL	Mydriatic - Cycloplegic	Ophth Solution: 0.5, 1.0%	**Refraction**: Instill 1 - 2 drops of the 1% solution in the eye(s); repeat in 5 minutes if the patient is not seen in 20 - 30 minutes. **Fundus Examination**: Instill 1 - 2 drops of the 0.5% solution 15 - 20 minutes prior to the examination.
Trovafloxacin Mesylate (*)	TROVAN	Antibacterial	Tab: 100, 200 mg Inj: 5 mg/mL (as alatrofloxacin mesylate)	**Community-Acquired Pneumonia and Skin and Skin Structure Infections (Complicated)**: 200 mg once daily po or by IV infusion, followed by 200 mg once daily po for 7 - 14 days. **Nosocomial Pneumonia**: 300 mg by IV infusion, followed by 200 mg once daily po for 10 - 14 days. **Gynecologic and Pelvic Infections and Intra-Abdominal Infections (Complicated)**: 300 mg by IV infusion, followed by 200 mg once daily po for 7 - 14 days.
Tubocurarine Chloride (*)		Neuromuscular Blocker	Inj: 3 mg (20 Units)/mL	**Usual Effective IV Doses (General Reference)**: **Paresis of Limb Muscles**: 0.1 - 0.2 mg/kg. **Abdominal Relaxation**: 0.4 - 0.5 mg/kg. **Endotracheal Intubation**: 0.5 - 0.6 mg/kg. In prolonged procedures, repeat incremental doses in 40 - 60 minutes, as required.
Unoprostone Isopropyl	RESCULA	Anti-Glaucoma Agent	Ophth Solution: 0.15%	1 drop into the affected eye(s) bid.
Urea	UREAPHIL	Osmotic Diuretic	Inj: 40 g/150 mL	1 - 1.5 g/kg by slow IV infusion, at a rate not to exceed 4 mL/min (Maximum: 120 g/day).

Urokinase	ABBOKINASE	Thrombolytic	Powd for Inj: 250,000 IUnits	**Pulmonary Embolism:** A priming dose of 2,000 IU/lb IV (at a rate of 90 mL/h over 10 min), followed by an IV infusion of 2,000 IU/lb/h (at a rate of 15 mL/h) for 12 h. **Lysis of Coronary Artery Thrombosis: After an** IV bolus of heparin (2,500 - 10,000 IU), infuse into occluded artery at a rate of 4 mL/min (6,000 IU/min) for periods up to 2 h.
Valacyclovir Hydrochloride	VALTREX	Antiviral	**Tab:** 500 mg, 1 g	**Herpes zoster:** 1000 mg tid po for 7 days. **Genital Herpes:** **Initial Episodes:** 1000 mg bid po for 10 days. **Recurrent Episodes:** 500 mg bid po for 5 days. **Herpes labialis:** 2000 mg bid po for 1 day, taken about 12 h apart.
Valdecoxib	BEXTRA	Antiinflammatory, Non-Opioid Analgesic	**Tab:** 10, 20 mg	**Osteoarthritis & Adult Rheumatoid Arthritis:** 10 mg once daily po. **Primary Dysmenorrhea:** 20 mg bid po, prn.
Valganciclovir Hydrochloride	VALCYTE	Antiviral	**Tab:** 450 mg	**Induction:** 900 mg bid po with food for 21 days. **Maintenance:** 900 mg once daily po with food.
Valproate Sodium	DEPACON	Antiepileptic	**Inj:** 100 mg/mL	Administer as an IV infusion over 60 min. (≤ 20 mg/min) with the same frequency as the oral products (Divalproex sodium (DEPAKOTE) and Valproic acid (DEPAKENE)).
Valproic Acid (*)	DEPAKENE	Antiepileptic	**Syrup:** 250 mg/5 mL **Cpsl:** 250 mg	Initially 15 mg/kg/day po in 2 or 3 divided doses, increasing at 1 week intervals by 5 to 10 mg/kg/day (Maximum: 60 mg/kg/day).
Valsartan	DIOVAN	Antihypertensive, Heart Failure Drug	**Tab:** 40, 80, 160, 320 mg	**Hypertension:** Initially, 80 mg daily po. The dosage range is 80 - 320 mg once daily po. **Heart Failure:** Initially, 40 mg bid po. Titrate to 80 and 160 mg bid to the highest dose tolerated.

215

GENERIC NAME	COMMON TRADE NAMES	THERAPEUTIC CATEGORY	PREPARATIONS	COMMON ADULT DOSAGE
Vancomycin Hydrochloride (*)	VANCOCIN HCL	Antibacterial	**Powd for Solution:** 1, 10 g **Cpsl:** 125, 250 mg	**Pseudomembranous Colitis:** 500 mg - 2 g daily po in 3 or 4 divided doses for 7 - 10 days.
			Powd for Inj: 500 mg; 1, 10 g	2 g daily, divided either as 500 mg q 6 h or 1 g q 12 h, by IV infusion (at a rate no more than 10 mg/min) over at least 60 minutes.
Vasopressin	PITRESSIN	Posterior Pituitary Hormone	**Inj:** 20 pressor Units/mL	**Diabetes Insipidus:** 5 - 10 Units bid - tid IM or SC prn. **Abdominal Distention:** Initially, 5 Units IM; increase to 10 Units at subsequent injections if necessary. Repeat at 3 - 4 hour intervals.
Vecuronium Bromide	NORCURON	Neuromuscular Blocker	**Powd for Inj:** 10, 20 mg	Initially 0.08 - 0.1 mg/kg as an IV bolus. Maintenance doses of 0.010 - 0.015 mg/kg are recommended and are usually required within 25 - 40 minutes.
Venlafaxine (*)	EFFEXOR	Antidepressant	**Tab:** 25, 37.5, 50, 75, 100 mg	Initially, 75 mg/day po, given in 2 or 3 divided doses, with food. Dose may be increased to 150 mg/day and then to 225 mg/day at intervals of ≥ 4 days.
	EFFEXOR XR		**Extended-Rel. Cpsl:** 37.5, 75, 150 mg	Transferring from EFFEXOR, give total daily dose on a once a day basis. Initially, 75 mg once daily po, with food. May start at 37.5 mg once daily po, with food, for 4 - 7 days. May increase by increments of up to 75 mg daily at intervals of at least 4 days. Usual maximum is 225 mg/day.

216

Verapamil Hydrochloride (*)	CALAN	Antianginal, Antiarrhythmic, Antihypertensive	**Tab:** 40, 80, 120 mg	**Angina:** 80 - 120 mg tid po. **Arrhythmias:** **Digitalized Patients with Chronic Atrial Fibrillation:** 240 - 320 mg/day po in 3 or 4 divided doses. **Prophylaxis of PSVT (Non-Digitalized Patients):** 240 - 480 mg/day po in 3 or 4 divided doses. **Hypertension:** 80 mg tid po. Adjust dosage up to 360 mg daily.
	COVERA-HS	Antianginal, Antihypertensive	**Extended-Rel. Tab:** 180, 240 mg	**Angina & Hypertension:** Initially, 180 mg once daily po hs. The dose may be increased in the following manner: 240 mg po each evening, 360 mg po each evening (2 x 180 mg), or 480 mg po each evening (2 x 240 mg).
	CALAN SR ISOPTIN SR	Antihypertensive	**Sustained-Rel. Cplt:** 120, 180, 240 mg **Sustained-Rel. Tab:** 120, 180, 240 mg	**Hypertension:** Initially 180 mg po in the AM with food. Adjust doses upward at weekly intervals, until therapeutic goal is reached as follows: (a) 240 mg each AM; (b) 180 mg bid, AM & PM, or 240 mg each AM and 120 mg each PM; (c) 240 mg q 12 h.
	VERELAN	Antihypertensive	**Sustained-Rel. Cpsl:** 120, 180, 240, 360 mg	**Hypertension:** Initially 240 mg po in the AM with food. Adjust doses upward until the therapeutic goal is reached as follows: (a) 240 mg each AM; (b) 360 mg each AM; (c) 480 mg each AM.
		Antiarrhythmic	**Inj:** 2.5 mg/mL	5 - 10 mg IV (over at least 2 minutes). Repeat with 10 mg after 30 minutes if response is not adequate.
Vidarabine Monohydrate	VIRA-A	Antiviral (Topical)	**Ophth Oint:** 3%	Apply 1/2 inch into lower conjunctival sac 5 times daily at 3 h intervals.

217

GENERIC NAME	COMMON TRADE NAMES	THERAPEUTIC CATEGORY	PREPARATIONS	COMMON ADULT DOSAGE
Vinblastine Sulfate	VELBAN	Antineoplastic	Powd for Inj: 10 mg	Dose at weekly intervals as follows: 1st dose- 3.7 mg/m² IV; 2nd dose- 5.5 mg/m² IV; 3rd dose- 7.4 mg/m² IV; 4th dose- 9.25 mg/m² IV; 5th dose- 11.1 mg/m² IV. The dose should not be increased after that dose which reduces the WBC to approx. 3,000 cell/mm².
Vincristine Sulfate (*)	ONCOVIN	Antineoplastic	Inj: 1 mg/mL	1.4 mg/m² IV (at weekly intervals).
Vinorelbine Tartrate	NAVELBINE	Antineoplastic	Inj: 10 mg/mL	Initially, 30 mg/m² weekly by IV injection (over 6 - 10 minutes). If granulocyte counts fall to 1000 - 1499 cells/mm², reduce dose to 15 mg/m²; below 100, do not administer.
Warfarin Sodium (*)	COUMADIN	Anticoagulant	Tab: 1, 2, 2.5, 3, 4, 5, 6, 7.5, 10 mg	Must be individualized for each patient based on the prothrombin time. Maintenance dosage for most patients is 2 - 10 mg daily po.
			Powd for Inj: 5 mg	Individualize dosage. Give as an IV bolus dose over 1 - 2 min into a peripheral vein.
Xylometazoline Hydrochloride	OTRIVIN	Nasal Decongestant	Nasal Solution: 0.1% Nasal Spray: 0.1%	2 -3 drops into each nostril q 8 - 10 h. 2 - 3 sprays into each nostril q 8 - 10 h.
	NATRU-VENT		Nasal Spray: 0.1%	1 spray into each nostril q 8 - 10 h.
Zafirlukast (*)	ACCOLATE	Drug for Asthma	Tab: 10, 20 mg	20 mg bid po. Take at least 1 h ac or 2 h pc.
Zalcitabine	HIVID	Antiviral	Tab: 0.375, 0.750 mg	Monotherapy: 0.750 mg q 8 h po. Combination Therapy: 0.750 mg po, given concomitantly with 200 mg of zidovudine, q 8 h.
Zaleplon	SONATA	Hypnotic	Cpsl: 5, 10 mg	5 - 10 mg hs po.

Zanamivir	RELENZA	Antiviral	Powd for Inhalation: 5 mg	2 inhalations (5 mg per inhalation; total dose of 10 mg) bid (at an interval of at least 2 h) on the 1st day; then 2 inhalations (total dose of 10 mg) bid (12 h apart AM and PM) for a total of 5 days.
Zidovudine (*)	RETROVIR	Antiviral	Syrup: 50 mg/5 mL Cpsl: 100 mg Tab: 300 mg	Symptomatic HIV Infection: 100 mg q 4 h po (600 mg total daily dose). Asymptomatic HIV Infection: 100 mg q 4 h po while awake (500 mg/day).
	RETROVIR I.V. INFUSION		Inj: 10 mg/mL	1 - 2 mg/kg infused IV over 1 hour at a constant rate; administer q 4 h around the clock (6 times daily).
Zileuton (*)	ZYFLO	Drug for Asthma	Tab: 600 mg	600 mg qid po.
Zinc Oxide		Skin Protectant	Oint: 20%	Apply topically prn.
Ziprasidone Hydrochloride	GEODON	Antipsychotic	Cpsl: 20, 40, 60, 80 mg	Initially, 20 mg bid po with food. Adjust the dosage at intervals of ≥ 2 days up to a maximum of 80 mg bid po.
Ziprasidone Mesylate	GEODON for INJECTION	Antipsychotic	Powd for Inj: 20 mg/mL (after reconstitution)	10 - 20 mg IM prn up to a maximum of 40 mg daily (10 mg q 2 h IM or 20 mg q 4 h IM). Use for a maximum of 3 days; switch to oral ziprasidone as soon as possible.
Zoledronic Acid	ZOMETA	Bone Stabilizer	Powd for Inj: 4.264 mg (as the monohydrate equiv. to 4 mg of the anhydrous acid)	Hypercalcemia of Malignancy: The maximum recommended dose is 4 mg. This dose must be given as a single dose by IV infusion over ≥ 15 min. Adequately rehydrate the patient prior to drug administration. Multiple Myeloma & Metastatic Bone Lesions from Solid Tumors: 4 mg by IV infusion over 15 min q 3 - 4 weeks.

GENERIC NAME	COMMON TRADE NAMES	THERAPEUTIC CATEGORY	PREPARATIONS	COMMON ADULT DOSAGE
Zolmitriptan (*)	ZOMIG ZOMIG ZMT	Antimigraine Agent	**Tab**: 2.5, 5 mg **Oral Disintegrating** **Tab**: 2.5 mg	Initially, 2.5 mg or lower po. If the headache returns, the dose may be repeated after 2 h. Do not exceed 10 mg within a 24 h period.
Zolpidem Tartrate (*) (C-IV)	AMBIEN	Hypnotic	**Tab**: 5, 10 mg	10 mg po hs.
Zonisamide (*)	ZONEGRAN	Antiepileptic	**Cpsl**: 100 mg	≥ **16 yrs**: Initially 100 mg once daily po; may increase at intervals of at least 2 weeks by 100 mg per day in 1 or 2 divided doses. Usual dosage range: 100 - 400 mg/day po in 1 or 2 divided doses.

C-II: Controlled Substance, Schedule II
C-III: Controlled Substance, Schedule III
C-IV: Controlled Substance, Schedule IV

(*): indictes that there is information on therapeutic, toxic and/or lethal blood concentrations of the drug in the **DRUG LEVELS** section (pp. 269 to 306).

SELECTED

COMBINATION

DRUG

PREPARATIONS

C-II: Controlled Substance, Schedule II
C-III: Controlled Substance, Schedule III
C-IV: Controlled Substance, Schedule IV
C-V: Controlled Substance, Schedule V

TRADE NAME	THERAPEUTIC CATEGORY	DOSAGE FORMS AND COMPOSITION	COMMON ADULT DOSAGE
A-200	Pediculicide	**Shampoo:** pyrethrum extract (0.33%), piperonyl butoxide (4%)	Apply to affected area until all the hair is thoroughly wet. Allow product to remain on the area for 10 minutes but no longer. Add sufficient warm water to form a lather and shampoo as usual. Rinse thoroughly. Remove dead lice and eggs from the hair with a fine-toothed comb. Repeat treatment in 7 - 10 days to kill any newly hatched lice.
ACCURETIC 10/12.5 ACCURETIC 20/12.5 ACCURETIC 20/25	Antihypertensive	**Tab:** quinapril HCl (10 mg), hydrochlorothiazide (12.5 mg) **Tab:** quinapril HCl (20 mg), hydrochlorothiazide (12.5 mg) **Tab:** quinapril HCl (20 mg), hydrochlorothiazide (25 mg)	1 tab once daily po. 1 tab once daily po. Use only to increase the HCTZ component after 2 - 3 weeks of oral therapy with ACCURETIC 20/12.5; then, 1 tab once daily po.
ACNOMEL	Anti-Acne Agent	**Cream:** sulfur (8%), resorcinol (2%), alcohol (11%)	Apply a thin coating once or twice daily.
ACTIFED COLD & ALLERGY	Decongestant-Antihistamine	**Tab:** pseudoephedrine HCl (60 mg), triprolidine HCl (2.5 mg)	1 tab q 4 - 8 h po.
ACTIFED COLD & SINUS	Decongestant-Antihistamine-Analgesic	**Tab & Cplt:** pseudoephedrine HCl (30 mg), chlorpheniramine maleate (2 mg), acetaminophen (500 mg)	2 tab (or cplt) q 6 h po.

| ADDERALL 5 mg (C-II) | CNS Stimulant | **Tab:** dextroamphetamine sulfate (1.25 mg), dextroamphetamine saccharate (1.25 mg), amphetamine aspartate (1.25 mg), amphetamine sulfate (1.25 mg) | **Narcolepsy:** Initially, 10 mg daily po in the AM. Increase in increments of 10 mg/day at weekly intervals. Give the first dose on awakening and additional doses at intervals of 4 - 6 h. |

ADDERALL 7.5 mg (C-II)
Tab: dextroamphetamine sulfate (1.875 mg), dextroamphetamine saccharate (1.875 mg), amphetamine aspartate (1.875 mg), amphetamine sulfate (1.875 mg)

ADDERALL 10 mg (C-II)
Tab: dextroamphetamine sulfate (2.5 mg), dextroamphetamine saccharate (2.5 mg), amphetamine aspartate (2.5 mg), amphetamine sulfate (2.5 mg)

ADDERALL 12.5 mg (C-II)
Tab: dextroamphetamine sulfate (3.125 mg), dextroamphetamine saccharate (3.125 mg), amphetamine aspartate (3.125 mg), amphetamine sulfate (3.125 mg)

ADDERALL 15 mg (C-II)
Tab: dextroamphetamine sulfate (3.75 mg), dextroamphetamine saccharate (3.75 mg), amphetamine aspartate (3.75 mg), amphetamine sulfate (3.75 mg)

ADDERALL 20 mg (C-II)
Tab: dextroamphetamine sulfate (5 mg), dextroamphetamine saccharate (5 mg), amphetamine aspartate (5 mg), amphetamine sulfate (5 mg)

ADDERALL 30 mg (C-II)
Tab: dextroamphetamine sulfate (7.5 mg), dextroamphetamine saccharate (7.5 mg), amphetamine aspartate (7.5 mg), amphetamine sulfate (7.5 mg)

TRADE NAME	THERAPEUTIC CATEGORY	DOSAGE FORMS AND COMPOSITION	COMMON ADULT DOSAGE
ADVAIR DISKUS	Corticosteroid-Bronchodilator	Powder for Inhalation: fluticasone propionate (100 μg), salmeterol (50 μg) Powder for Inhalation: fluticasone propionate (250 μg), salmeterol (50 μg) Powder for Inhalation: fluticasone propionate (500 μg), salmeterol (50 μg)	1 inhalation bid (approximately 12 h apart). **For the Recommended Starting Strengths, see the Table below.**

For Patients Not Currently on an Inhaled Corticosteroid, it is recommended that the 100 μg / 50 μg strength be used to start.

For Patients Currently on an Inhaled Corticosteroid, the recommended strengths to start with are:

Current Daily Dose of Inhaled Corticosteroid		Recommended Strength of ADVAIR DISKUS
Beclomethasone Dipropionate	≤ 420 μg 462 to 840 μg	100 μg / 50 μg Strength (Use bid.) 250 μg / 50 μg Strength (Use bid.)
Budesonide	≤ 400 μg 800 to 1200 μg 1600 μg	100 μg / 50 μg Strength (Use bid.) 250 μg / 50 μg Strength (Use bid.) 500 μg / 50 μg Strength (Use bid.)
Flunisolide	≤ 1000 μg 1250 to 2000 μg	100 μg / 50 μg Strength (Use bid.) 250 μg / 50 μg Strength (Use bid.)
Fluticasone Propionate Inhalation Aerosol	≤ 176 μg 440 μg 660 to 880 μg	100 μg / 50 μg Strength (Use bid.) 250 μg / 50 μg Strength (Use bid.) 500 μg / 50 μg Strength (Use bid.)
Fluticasone Propionate Inhalation Powder	≤ 200 μg 500 μg 1000 μg	100 μg / 50 μg Strength (Use bid.) 250 μg / 50 μg Strength (Use bid.) 500 μg / 50 μg Strength (Use bid.)
Triamcinolone Acetonide	≤ 1000 μg 1100 to 1600 μg	100 μg / 50 μg Strength (Use bid.) 250 μg / 50 μg Strength (Use bid.)

ADVICOR 500/20	Antihyperlipidemic	Tab: niacin (extended-release) (500 mg), lovastatin (20 mg)	1 tab once daily po hs with a low-fat snack.
ADVICOR 750/20		Tab: niacin (extended-release) (750 mg), lovastatin (20 mg)	1 tab once daily po hs with a low-fat snack.
ADVICOR 1000/20		Tab: niacin (extended-release) (1000 mg), lovastatin (20 mg)	1 tab once daily po hs with a low-fat snack.

ADVIL COLD & SINUS	Decongestant-Analgesic	**Cplt:** pseudoephedrine HCl (30 mg), ibuprofen (200 mg).	1 - 2 cplt q 4 - 6 h po.
AGGRENOX	Platelet Aggregation Inhibitor	**Cpsl:** aspirin (25 mg) [immediate-release], dipyridamole (200 mg) [extended-release]	1 cpsl bid po (1 in the AM and 1 in the PM). Swallow whole; do not chew or crush.
ALDACTAZIDE	Diuretic, Antihypertensive	**Tab:** spironolactone (25 mg), hydrochlorothiazide (25 mg) **Tab:** spironolactone (50 mg), hydrochlorothiazide (50 mg)	**Diuresis:** The usual maintenance dose is 100 mg of each component daily po, as a single dose or in divided doses, but may range from 25 to 200 mg of each component daily. **Hypertension:** Usually 50 - 100 mg of each component daily po, as a single dose or in divided doses.
ALDOCLOR-250	Antihypertensive	**Tab:** chlorothiazide (250 mg), methyldopa (250 mg)	1 tab bid or tid po.
ALDORIL-15 ALDORIL-25 ALDORIL D30 ALDORIL D50	Antihypertensive	**Tab:** hydrochlorothiazide (15 mg), methyldopa (250 mg) **Tab:** hydrochlorothiazide (25 mg), methyldopa (250 mg) **Tab:** hydrochlorothiazide (30 mg), methyldopa (500 mg) **Tab:** hydrochlorothiazide (50 mg), methyldopa (500 mg)	1 tab bid or tid po. 1 tab bid or tid po. 1 tab bid or tid po. 1 tab bid or tid po.
ALESSE	Oral Contraceptive (Combination Monophasic)	**Tab:** ethinyl estradiol (20 μg), levonorgestrel (0.10 mg) in 21-Day and 28-Day Minipacks (contains 7 inert tabs)	21-Day regimen po or 28-Day regimen po.
ALEVE COLD & SINUS	Decongestant-Analgesic	**Cplt:** pseudoephedrine HCl (120 mg), naproxen sodium (220 mg)	1 cplt q 12 h po.
ALLEGRA-D	Decongestant-Antihistamine	**Extended-Rel. Tab:** pseudoephedrine HCl (120 mg), fexofenadine HCl (60 mg)	1 tab bid po.
ALLEREST ALLERGY & SINUS RELIEF	Decongestant-Analgesic	**Tab:** pseudoephedrine HCl (30 mg), acetaminophen (325 mg)	2 tab q 4 - 6 h po.
ALLEREST MAXIMUM STRENGTH	Decongestant-Antihistamine	**Tab:** pseudoephedrine HCl (30 mg), chlorpheniramine maleate (2 mg)	2 tab q 4 - 6 h po.

TRADE NAME	THERAPEUTIC CATEGORY	DOSAGE FORMS AND COMPOSITION	COMMON ADULT DOSAGE
ANALPRAM-HC	Corticosteroid-Local Anesthetic	**Cream:** hydrocortisone acetate (1%), pramoxine HCl (1%), pramoxine HCl (2.5%). **Cream & Lotion:** hydrocortisone acetate (1%), pramoxine HCl (1%)	Apply to the affected area as a thin film tid or qid.
ANEXSIA 5/500 (C-III) ANEXSIA 7.5/650 (C-III) ANEXSIA 10/660 (C-III)	Analgesic	**Tab:** hydrocodone bitartrate (5 mg), acetaminophen (500 mg) **Tab:** hydrocodone bitartrate (7.5 mg), acetaminophen (650 mg) **Tab:** hydrocodone bitartrate (10 mg), acetaminophen (660 mg)	1 - 2 tab q 4 - 6 h po, prn pain. 1 tab q 4 - 6 h po, prn pain. 1 tab q 4 - 6 h po, prn pain.
ANUSOL	Antihemorrhoidal	**Oint:** pramoxine HCl (1%), mineral oil (46.7%), zinc oxide (12.5%)	Apply externally to the affected area up to 5 times daily.
APRESAZIDE 25/25 APRESAZIDE 50/50 APRESAZIDE 100/50	Antihypertensive	**Cpsl:** hydralazine HCl (25 mg), hydrochlorothiazide (25 mg) **Cpsl:** hydralazine HCl (50 mg), hydrochlorothiazide (50 mg) **Cpsl:** hydralazine HCl (100 mg), hydrochlorothiazide (50 mg)	1 cpsl bid po. 1 cpsl bid po. 1 cpsl bid po.
APRI	Oral Contraceptive (Combination Monophasic)	**Tab:** ethinyl estradiol (30 μg), desogestrel (0.15 mg) in 21-Day and 28-Day Dialpaks (contains 7 inert tabs)	21-Day regimen po or 28-Day regimen po.
ARTHROTEC 50	Antiinflammatory	**Enteric-Coated Tab:** diclofenac sodium (50 mg), misoprostol (200 μg)	**Osteoarthritis:** 1 tab tid po. **Rheumatoid Arthritis:** 1 tab tid to qid po.
ARTHROTEC 75	Antiinflammatory	**Enteric-Coated Tab:** diclofenac sodium (75 mg), misoprostol (200 μg)	**Osteoarthritis and Rheumatoid Arthtis:** 1 tab bid po.
ATACAND HCT 16-12.5	Antihypertensive	**Tab:** candesartan cilexetil (16 mg), hydrochlorothiazide (12.5 mg)	1 tab daily po.
ATACAND HCT 32-12.5		**Tab:** candesartan cilexetil (32 mg), hydrochlorothiazide (12.5 mg)	1 tab daily po.

226

AUGMENTIN 125

Antibacterial

Powd for Susp (per 5 mL): amoxicillin (125 mg), clavulanic acid (31.25 mg)
Chewable Tab: amoxicillin (125 mg), clavulanic acid (31.25 mg)

Usual Dosage: 1 AUGMENTIN 250 tablet q 8 h po or 1 AUGMENTIN 500 tablet q 12 h po. The 125 mg/5 mL or 250 mg/5 mL suspension may be given in place of the 500 mg tablet.

AUGMENTIN 200

Powd for Susp (per 5 mL): amoxicillin (200 mg), clavulanic acid (28.5 mg)
Chewable Tab: amoxicillin (200 mg), clavulanic acid (28.5 mg)

AUGMENTIN 250

Powd for Susp (per 5 mL): amoxicillin (250 mg), clavulanic acid (62.5 mg)
Chewable Tab: amoxicillin (250 mg), clavulanic acid (62.5 mg)
Tab: amoxicillin (250 mg), clavulanic acid (125 mg)

Severe Infections & Respiratory Infections: 1 AUGMENTIN 500 tablet q 8 h po or 1 AUGMENTIN 875 tablet q 12 h po. The 200 mg/5 mL or 400 mg/5 mL suspension may be given in place of the 875 mg tablet.

AUGMENTIN 400

Powd for Susp (per 5 mL): amoxicillin (400 mg), clavulanic acid (57 mg)
Chewable Tab: amoxicillin (400 mg), clavulanic acid (57 mg)

**AUGMENTIN 500
AUGMENTIN 875**

Tab: amoxicillin (500 mg), clavulanic acid (125 mg)
Tab: amoxicillin (875 mg), clavulanic acid (125 mg)

AUGMENTIN XR

Antibacterial

Extended-Rel. Tab: amoxicillin (1000 mg), clavulanic acid (62.5 mg)

Acute Bacterial Sinusitis: 2 tabs q 12 h po for 10 days.
Community-acquired Pneumonia: 2 tabs q 12 h po for 7 - 10 days.

AURALGAN OTIC

Analgesic (Topical)

Otic Solution (per mL): benzocaine (14 mg = 1.4%), antipyrine (54 mg = 5.4%), glycerin

Instill in ear canal until filled, then insert a cotton pledget moistened with solution into meatus. Repeat q 1 - 2 h.

**AVALIDE 150/12.5
AVALIDE 300/12.5**

Antihypertensive

Tab: irbesartan (150 mg), hydrochlorothiazide (12.5 mg)
Tab: irbesartan (300 mg), hydrochlorothiazide (12.5 mg)

1 tab (150/12.5) daily po.
[Used to titrate after the above].

TRADE NAME	THERAPEUTIC CATEGORY	DOSAGE FORMS AND COMPOSITION	COMMON ADULT DOSAGE
AVANDAMET 1 mg/500 mg AVANDAMET 2 mg/500 mg AVANDAMET 4 mg/500 mg	Hypoglycemic Agent- Antihyperglycemic Agent	Tab: rosiglitazone maleate (1 mg), metformin HCl (500 mg) Tab: rosiglitazone maleate (2 mg), metformin HCl (500 mg) Tab: rosiglitazone maleate (4 mg), metformin HCl (500 mg)	**Previously on Metformin Alone:** Add rosiglitazone 4 mg/day po to the current metformin dose. May increase after 8 to 12 weeks. **Previously on Rosiglitazine Alone:** Add metformin 1000 1000 mg/day po to the current rosiglitazone dose. May increase after 1 to 2 weeks. **Previously on Rosiglitazine plus Metformin:** Switch on a mg to mg basis. May increase by rosiglitazone 4 mg and/or metformin 500 mg per day. For all of the above - give in divided doses. Maximum is 8 mg of rosiglitazone and 2000 mg of metformin daily.
BACTRIM	Antibacterial	Susp (per 5 mL): sulfamethoxazole (200 mg), trimethoprim (40 mg) Tab: sulfamethoxazole (400 mg), trimethoprim (80 mg)	**Urinary Tract Infections:** 1 BACTRIM DS tab, 2 BACTRIM tab or 20 mL of Suspension q 12 h po for 10 - 14 days.
BACTRIM DS		Tab: sulfamethoxazole (800 mg), trimethoprim (160 mg)	**Shigellosis:** 1 BACTRIM DS tab, 2 BACTRIM tab or 20 mL of Suspension q 12 h for 5 days. **Acute Exacerbations of Chronic Bronchitis:** 1 BACTRIM DS tab, 2 BACTRIM tab or 20 mL of Suspension q 12 h po for 14 days. ***P. carinii* Pneumonia Treatment:** 20 mg/kg trimethoprim and 100 mg/kg sulfamethoxazole per 24 h in equally divided doses q 6 h for 14 days.

Name	Class	Composition	Dosage
BACTRIM I.V. INFUSION	Antibacterial	Inj (per 5 mL): sulfamethoxazole (400 mg), trimethoprim (80 mg)	**P. carinii Pneumonia Prophylax.:** 1 BACTRIM DS tab, 2 BACTRIM tab or 20 mL of Suspension q 24 h po. **Travelers' Diarrhea:** 1 BACTRIM DS tab, 2 BACTRIM tab or 20 mL of Suspension q 12 h po for 5 days. **Severe Urinary Tract Infections and Shigellosis:** 8 - 10 mg/kg daily (based on trimethoprim) in 2 - 4 equally divided doses q 6, 8 or 12 h by IV infusion for up to 14 days for UTI and 5 days for shigellosis. **P. carinii Pneumonia:** 15 - 20 mg/kg daily (based on trimethoprim) in 3 - 4 equally divided doses q 6 - 8 h by IV infusion for up to 14 days.
BANCAP HC (C-III)	Analgesic	Cpsl: hydrocodone bitartrate (5 mg), acetaminophen (500 mg)	1 cpsl q 6 h po, prn pain. Maximum: 2 cpsl q 6 h po.
BAYER PLUS, EXTRA-STRENGTH	Analgesic	Cplt: aspirin (500 mg), calcium carbonate	1 - 2 cplt q 4 - 6 h po. Max. of 8 cplt in 24 h.
BAYER PM, EXTRA-STRENGTH	Analgesic-Sedative	Cplt: aspirin (500 mg), diphenhydramine HCl (25 mg)	2 cplt hs po.
BENADRYL ALLERGY / COLD	Decongestant-Antihistamine-Analgesic	Tab: pseudoephedrine HCl (30 mg), diphenhydramine HCl (12.5 mg), acetaminophen (500 mg)	2 tab q 6 h po while symptoms persist.
BENADRYL ALLERGY & SINUS	Decongestant-Antihistamine	Liquid (per 5 mL): pseudoephedrine HCl (30 mg), diphenhydramine HCl (12.5 mg)	10 mL q 4 - 6 h po. Maximum: 40 mL/day.
BENADRYL ALLERGY / CONGESTION	Decongestant-Antihistamine	Tab: pseudoephedrine HCl (60 mg), diphenhydramine HCl (25 mg)	1 tab q 4 - 6 h po. Maximum: 4 tabs daily.

TRADE NAME	THERAPEUTIC CATEGORY	DOSAGE FORMS AND COMPOSITION	COMMON ADULT DOSAGE
BENADRYL ALLERGY SINUS HEADACHE	Decongestant-Antihistamine-Analgesic	Cplt & Gelcap: pseudoephedrine HCl (30 mg), diphenhydramine HCl (12.5 mg), acetaminophen (500 mg)	2 cplt (or gelcap) q 6 h po.
BENADRYL ITCH STOPPING Original Strength	Antihistamine	Cream & Spray: diphenhydramine HCl (1%), zinc acetate (0.1%)	Apply to affected areas not more than tid or qid.
Extra Strength		Cream & Spray: diphenhydramine HCl (2%), zinc acetate (0.1%)	Apply to affected areas not more than tid or qid.
BENADRYL SEVERE ALLERGY & SINUS HEADACHE	Decongestant-Antihistamine-Analgesic	Cplt: pseudoephedrine HCl (30 mg), diphenhydramine HCl (25 mg), acetaminophen (500 mg)	2 cplt q 6 h po.
BENYLIN EXPECTORANT	Antitussive-Expectorant	Liquid (per 5 mL): dextromethorphan HBr (5 mg), guaifenesin (100 mg)	20 mL q 6 - 8 h po, not to exceed 80 mL in 24 h.
BENZACLIN	Anti-Acne Agent	Gel: benzoyl peroxide (5%), clindamycin phosphate (1%)	Apply to clean, dry skin bid (AM and PM).
BENZAMYCIN	Anti-Acne Agent	Gel: benzoyl peroxide (5%), erythromycin (3%)	Apply topically bid, AM and PM.
BICILLIN C-R	Antibacterial	Inj (per mL): penicillin G benzathine (150,000 Units), penicillin G procaine (150,000 Units) Inj (per mL): penicillin G benzathine (300,000 Units), penicillin G procaine (300,000 Units)	**Streptococcal Infections:** 2,400,000 Units by deep IM injection (multiple sites). **Pneumococcal Infections (except Meningitis):** 1,200,000 Units by deep IM injection, repeated q 2 - 3 days until the temperature is normal for 48 hours.
BLEPHAMIDE	Antibacterial-Corticosteroid	Ophth Susp: sulfacetamide sodium (10%), prednisolone acetate (0.2%) Ophth Oint: sulfacetamide sodium (10%), prednisolone acetate (0.2%)	1 drop into affected eye(s) bid to qid. Apply to affected eye(s) tid - qid and once or twice at night.
BREVICON	Oral Contraceptive (Combination Monophasic)	Tab: ethinyl estradiol (35 μg), norethindrone (0.5 mg) in 21-Day and 28-Day Wallettes (contains 7 inert tabs)	21-Day regimen po or 28-Day regimen po.

Brand	Class	Composition	Dosage
BRONKAID DUAL ACTION	Decongestant-Expectorant	**Tab:** ephedrine sulfate (25 mg), guaifenesin (400 mg)	1 tab q 4 h po.
CAFERGOT	Antimigraine Agent	**Tab:** ergotamine tartrate (1 mg), caffeine (100 mg) **Rectal Suppos:** ergotamine tartrate (2 mg), caffeine (100 mg)	2 tab stat po, then 1 tab q 0.5 h if needed (maximum of 6 tab per attack). Insert 1 rectally stat, then 1 suppos. after 1 h if needed.
CAPOZIDE 25/15 CAPOZIDE 25/25 CAPOZIDE 50/15 CAPOZIDE 50/25	Antihypertensive	**Tab:** captopril (25 mg), hydrochlorothiazide (15 mg) **Tab:** captopril (25 mg), hydrochlorothiazide (25 mg) **Tab:** captopril (50 mg), hydrochlorothiazide (15 mg) **Tab:** captopril (50 mg), hydrochlorothiazide (25 mg)	1 CAPOZIDE 25/15 tab bid po, 1 h ac. Increased captopril dosage may be obtained by utilizing CAPOZIDE 50/15 bid, or higher hydrochlorothiazide dosage may be obtained by utilizing CAPOZIDE 25/25 bid. CAPOZIDE 25/15 and 50/15 may also be used tid po.
CHERACOL (C-V)	Antitussive-Expectorant	**Syrup (per 5 mL):** codeine phosphate (10 mg), guaifenesin (100 mg), alcohol (4.75%)	10 mL q 4 - 6 h po.
CHERACOL D	Antitussive-Expectorant	**Liquid (per 5 mL):** dextromethorphan HBr (10 mg), guaifenesin (100 mg), alcohol (4.75%)	10 mL q 4 h po.
CHLOR-TRIMETON ALLERGY-D 4 HOUR	Decongestant-Antihistamine	**Tab:** pseudoephedrine sulfate (60 mg), chlorpheniramine maleate (4 mg)	1 tab q 4 - 6 h po, up to 4 tabs per day.
CHLOR-TRIMETON ALLERGY-D 12 HOUR	Decongestant-Antihistamine	**Sustained-Rel. Tab:** pseudoephedrine sulfate (120 mg), chlorpheniramine maleate (8 mg)	1 tab q 12 h po.
CIPRO HC OTIC	Antibacterial-Corticosteroid	**Otic Susp (per mL):** ciprofloxacin HCl (equivalent to 2 mg of ciprofloxacin base), hydrocortisone (10 mg)	Instill 3 drops into the affected ear(s) bid for 7 days.
CLARITIN-D 12-HOUR	Decongestant-Antihistamine	**Extended-Rel. Tab:** pseudoephedrine sulfate (120 mg), loratidine (5 mg)	1 tab q 12 h po.
CLARITIN-D 24-HOUR	Decongestant-Antihistamine	**Extended-Rel. Tab:** pseudoephedrine sulfate (240 mg), loratidine (10 mg)	1 tab q 24 h po.

TRADE NAME	THERAPEUTIC CATEGORY	DOSAGE FORMS AND COMPOSITION	COMMON ADULT DOSAGE
COLY-MYCIN S OTIC	Antibacterial-Corticosteroid	**Otic Susp (per mL):** neomycin sulfate (4.71 mg, equivalent to 3.3 mg neomycin base), colistin sulfate (3 mg), hydrocortisone acetate (10 mg = 1%)	5 instilled drops into the affected ear(s) tid - qid.
COMBIPRES 0.1 COMBIPRES 0.2 COMBIPRES 0.3	Antihypertensive	**Tab:** clonidine HCl (0.1 mg), chlorthalidone (15 mg) **Tab:** clonidine HCl (0.2 mg), chlorthalidone (15 mg) **Tab:** clonidine HCl (0.3 mg), chlorthalidone (15 mg)	1 tab once daily or bid po. 1 tab once daily or bid po. 1 tab once daily or bid po.
COMBIVENT	Drug for COPD	**Aerosol:** ipratropium bromide (18 μg), albuterol sulfate (103 μg) per spray	2 inhalations qid.
COMBIVIR	Antiviral	**Tab:** lamivudine (150 mg), zidovudine (300 mg)	1 tab bid po.
COMTREX ACUTE HEAD COLD	Decongestant-Antihistamine-Analgesic	**Tab:** pseudoephedrine HCl (30 mg), brompheniramine maleate (2 mg), acetaminophen (500 mg)	2 tab q 6 h po, not to exceed 8 tab in 24 h.
COMTREX ALLERGY-SINUS	Decongestant-Antihistamine-Analgesic	**Tab:** pseudoephedrine HCl (30 mg) chlorpheniramine maleate (2 mg), acetaminophen (500 mg)	2 tab q 6 h po, not to exceed 8 tab in 24 h.
COMTREX COUGH & COLD RELIEF	Antitussive-Decongestant-Antihistamine-Analgesic	**Cplt & Tab:** dextromethorphan HBr (15 mg), pseudoephedrine HCl (30 mg), chlorpheniramine maleate (2 mg), acetaminophen (500 mg)	2 cplt (or tab) q 6 h po, not to exceed 8 cplt (or tab) in 24 h.
COMTREX DAY & NIGHT	Decongestant-Analgesic-Antihistamine	**Daytime Cplt:** pseudoephedrine HCl (30 mg), acetaminophen (500 mg) **Nighttime Cplt:** pseudoephedrine HCl (30 mg), acetaminophen (500 mg), chlorpheniramine maleate (2 mg)	2 Daytime cplts q 6 h po during waking hours. 2 Nighttime cplts hs po, prn.
COMTREX DEEP CHEST COLD	Decongestant-Analgesic-Antitussive-Expectorant	**Softgel:** pseudoephedrine HCl (30 mg), acetaminophen (250 mg), dextromethorphan HBr (10 mg), guaifenesin (100 mg)	2 softgel q 4 h po, not to exceed 12 softgel in 24 h.
CORICIDIN D	Decongestant-Antihistamine-Analgesic	**Tab:** pseudoephedrine sulfate (30 mg), chlorpheniramine maleate (2 mg), acetaminophen (325 mg)	2 tab q 4 h po.
CORICIDIN HBP COLD & FLU	Antihistamine-Analgesic	**Tab:** chlorpheniramine maleate (2 mg), acetaminophen (325 mg)	2 tab q 4 - 6 h po.

Drug	Category	Composition	Dosage
CORICIDIN HBP COUGH & COLD	Antihistamine-Antitussive	**Tab:** chlorpheniramine maleate (4 mg), dextromethorphan HBr (30 mg)	1 tab q 6 h po.
CORICIDIN HBP MAXIMUM STRENGTH FLU	Antihistamine-Analgesic-Antitussive	**Tab:** chlorpheniramine maleate (2 mg), acetaminophen (500 mg), dextromethorphan HBr (15 mg)	2 tab q 6 h po while symptoms persist.
CORICIDIN HBP NIGHT-TIME COLD & FLU	Antihistamine-Analgesic	**Tab:** diphenhydramine HCl (25 mg), acetaminophen (325 mg)	1 - 2 tab q 4 - 6 h po.
CORTISPORIN	Antibacterial-Corticosteroid	**Ophth Susp (per mL):** polymyxin B sulfate (10,000 Units), neomycin sulfate (equal to 3.5 mg of neomycin base), hydrocortisone (10 mg = 1%)	1 - 2 drops into the affected eye(s) q 3 - 4 h, depending on the severity of the condition.
CORTISPORIN OTIC	Antibacterial-Corticosteroid	**Otic Solution & Susp (per mL):** polymyxin B sulfate (10,000 Units), neomycin sulfate (equal to 3.5 mg of neomycin base), hydrocortisone (10 mg = 1%)	4 drops instilled in the affected ear(s) tid to qid.
CORZIDE 40/5 CORZIDE 80/5	Antihypertensive	**Tab:** nadolol (40 mg), bendroflumethiazide (5 mg) **Tab:** nadolol (80 mg), bendroflumethiazide (5 mg)	1 tab daily po. 1 tab daily po.
COSOPT	Anti-Glaucoma Agent	**Ophth Solution:** dorzolamide HCl (2%), timolol maleate (0.5%)	1 drop in the affected eye(s) bid.
CYCLESSA	Oral Contraceptive (Combination Triphasic)	**Tab:** 7 tabs: ethinyl estradiol (25 μg), desogestrel (0.1 mg); 7 tabs: ethinyl estradiol (25 μg), desogestrel (0.125 mg); 7 tabs: ethinyl estradiol (25 μg), desogestrel (0.15 mg) in 28-Day Pilpaks (contains 7 inert tabs)	28-Day regimen po.
DARVOCET-N 50 (C-IV)	Analgesic	**Tab:** propoxyphene napsylate (50 mg), acetaminophen (325 mg)	2 tab q 4 h prn pain po.
DARVOCET-N 100 (C-IV)	Analgesic	**Tab:** propoxyphene napsylate (100 mg), acetaminophen (650 mg)	1 tab q 4 h prn pain po.
DARVON COMPOUND-65 (C-IV)	Analgesic	**Cpsl:** propoxyphene HCl (65 mg), aspirin (389 mg), caffeine (32.4 mg)	1 cpsl q 4 h po, prn pain.

TRADE NAME	THERAPEUTIC CATEGORY	DOSAGE FORMS AND COMPOSITION	COMMON ADULT DOSAGE
DECADRON W/XYLOCAINE	Corticosteroid-Local Anesthetic	**Inj (per mL):** dexamethasone sodium phosphate (4 mg), lidocaine HCl (10 mg)	Initial dose ranges from 0.1 to 0.75 mL by injection. Some patients respond to a single injection; in others, additional doses may be needed, usually at 4 - 7 day intervals.
DECONAMINE	Decongestant-Antihistamine	**Syrup (per 5 mL):** pseudoephedrine HCl (30 mg), chlorpheniramine maleate (2 mg) **Tab:** pseudoephedrine HCl (60 mg), chlorpheniramine maleate (4 mg)	5 - 10 mL tid - qid po. 1 tab tid - qid po.
DECONAMINE SR	Decongestant-Antihistamine	**Sustained-Rel. Cpsl:** pseudoephedrine HCl (120 mg), chlorpheniramine maleate (8 mg)	1 cpsl q 12 h po.
DEMULEN 1/35 DEMULEN 1/50	Oral Contraceptive (Combination Monophasic)	**Tab:** ethinyl estradiol (35 μg), ethynodiol diacetate (1 mg) in 21-Day and 28-Day Compaks (contains 7 inert tabs) **Tab:** ethinyl estradiol (50 μg), ethynodiol diacetate (1 mg) in 21-Day and 28-Day Compaks (contains 7 inert tabs)	21-Day regimen po or 28-Day regimen po. 21-Day regimen po or 28-Day regimen po.
DESENEX (Original)	Antifungal (Topical)	**Oint, Cream, & Powder:** total undecylenate = 25% as undecylenic acid and zinc undecylenate	Cleanse the skin with soap and water and dry thoroughly. Apply to the affected skin areas morning and night.
DESOGEN	Oral Contraceptive (Combination Monophasic)	**Tab:** ethinyl estradiol (30 μg), desogestrel (0.15 mg) in 28-Day packs (contains 7 inert tabs)	28-Day regimen po.
DEXACIDIN	Antibacterial-Corticosteroid	**Ophth Oint (per g):** neomycin sulfate (equal to 3.5 mg of neomycin base), polymyxin B sulfate (10,000 Units), dexamethasone (1 mg)	Apply a small amount (about 0.5 in.) into the conjunctival sac tid - qid.
DIMETANE-DX	Antitussive-Decongestant-Antihistamine	**Syrup (per 5 mL):** dextromethorphan HBr (10 mg), pseudoephedrine HCl (30 mg), brompheniramine maleate (2 mg), alcohol (0.95%)	10 mL q 4 h po.
DIMETAPP COLD & ALLERGY	Decongestant-Antihistamine	**Elixir (per 5 mL):** pseudoephedrine HCl (15 mg), brompheniramine maleate (1 mg)	20 mL q 4 h po.

DIMETAPP NIGHTTIME FLU	Decongestant-Antihistamine-Antitussive-Analgesic	**Syrup (per 5 mL):** pseudoephedrine HCl (15 mg), brompheniramine maleate (1 mg), dextromethorphan HBr (5 mg), acetaminophen (160 mg)	20 mL q 4 h po.
DIMETAPP NON-DROWSY FLU	Decongestant-Antitussive-Analgesic	**Syrup (per 5 mL):** pseudoephedrine HCl (15 mg), dextromethorphan HBr (5 mg), acetaminophen (160 mg)	20 mL q 4 h po.
DIMETAPP DM COLD & COUGH	Decongestant-Antihistamine-Antitussive	**Elixir (per 5 mL):** pseudoephedrine HCl (15 mg), brompheniramine maleate (1 mg), dextromethorphan HBr (5 mg)	20 mL q 4 h po.
DIOVAN HCT 80/12.5 DIOVAN HCT 160/12.5 DIOVAN HCT 160/25	Antihypertensive Antihypertensive Antihypertensive	**Tab:** valsartan (80 mg), hydrochlorothiazide (12.5 mg). **Tab:** valsartan (160 mg), hydrochlorothiazide (12.5 mg) **Tab:** valsartan (160 mg), hydrochlorothiazide (25 mg)	1 tab daily po. 1 tab daily po. 1 tab daily po.
DOMEBORO	Astringent	**Powder (per packet):** aluminum sulfate (1191 mg), calcium acetate (938 mg) **Effervescent Tab:** aluminum sulfate (878 mg), calcium acetate (604 mg)	**As a Compress:** Dissolve 1 or 2 packets (or tabs) in 16 fl. oz. of warm water. Saturate a clean dressing in the sol'n, gently squeeze and apply loosely to the affected area. Remove, remoisten and reapply q 15 - 30 minutes prn. **As a Soak:** Dissolve 1 or 2 packets (or tablets) in 16 fl. oz. of warm water. Soak the affected area for 15 - 30 minutes. Repeat tid.
DOXIDAN	Irritant Laxative-Stool Softener	**Cpsl:** casanthranol (30 mg), docusate sodium (100 mg)	1 - 3 cpsl daily po.
DRIXORAL ALLERGY SINUS	Decongestant-Antihistamine-Analgesic	**Extended-Rel. Tab:** pseudoephedrine sulfate (60 mg), dexbrompheniramine maleate (3 mg), acetaminophen (500 mg)	2 tab q 12 h po.
DRIXORAL COLD & ALLERGY	Decongestant-Antihistamine	**Sustained-Rel. Tab:** pseudoephedrine sulfate (120 mg), dexbrompheniramine maleate (6 mg)	1 tab q 12 h po.

235

TRADE NAME	THERAPEUTIC CATEGORY	DOSAGE FORMS AND COMPOSITION	COMMON ADULT DOSAGE
DURATUSS	Decongestant-Expectorant	**Sustained-Rel. Tab:** pseudoephedrine HCl (120 mg), guaifenesin (600 mg)	1 tab q 12 h po.
DURATUSS HD (C-III)	Antitussive-Decongestant-Expectorant	**Elixir (per 5 mL):** hydrocodone bitartrate (2.5 mg), pseudoephedrine HCl (30 mg), guaifenesin (100 mg), alcohol (5%)	10 mL q 4 - 6 h po.
DYAZIDE	Diuretic, Antihypertensive	**Cpsl:** triamterene (37.5 mg), hydrochlorothiazide (25 mg)	1 - 2 cpsl once daily po.
ELIXOPHYLLIN-GG	Drug for COPD	**Liquid (per 15 mL):** theophylline anhydrous (100 mg), guaifenesin (100 mg)	Dose based on theophylline; see Oral Theophylline Doses Table, p. 312. **Initial:** 6 mg/kg po; then reduce to 3 mg/kg q 6 h for 2 doses. **Maintenance:** 3 mg/kg q 8 h po.
ELIXOPHYLLIN-KI	Drug for COPD	**Elixir (per 15 mL):** theophylline anhydrous (80 mg), potassium iodide (130 mg), alcohol (10%)	Dose based on theophylline; see Oral Theophylline Doses Table, p. 312. **Initial:** 6 mg/kg po; then reduce to 3 mg/kg q 6 h for 2 doses. **Maintenance:** 3 mg/kg q 8 h po.
EMETROL	Antiemetic	**Solution (per 5 mL):** dextrose (1.87 g), levulose (1.87 g), phosphoric acid (21.5 g)	15 - 30 mL po. Repeat q 15 min. until distress subsides.
EMLA	Local Anesthetic	**Cream:** lidocaine (2.5%), prilocaine (2.5%)	**Minor Dermal Procedures:** Apply 2.5 g over 20 - 25 cm² of the skin surface, cover with an occlusive dressing, and allow to remain for at least 1 h. **Major Dermal Procedures:** Apply 2 g per 10 cm² of the skin surface, cover with an occlusive dressing, and allow to remain for at least 2 h.

EMPIRIN W/CODEINE #3 (C-III) #4 (C-III)	Analgesic	**Tab:** aspirin (325 mg), codeine phosphate (30 mg) **Tab:** aspirin (325 mg), codeine phosphate (60 mg)	1 - 2 tab q 4 h po, prn. 1 tab q 4 h po, prn.
ENLON-PLUS	Cholinomimetic- Anticholinergic	**Inj (per mL):** edrophonium chloride (10 mg), atropine sulfate (0.14 mg)	Dosages range from 0.05 - 1 mL/kg IV given slowly over 45 to 60 seconds at a point of at least 5% recovery of twitch response to neuromuscular stimulation (95% block). The dosage delivered is 0.5 to 1 mg/kg edrophonium and 7 to 14 μg/kg atropine. A total dosage of 1 mg/kg of edrophonium should rarely be exceeded.
ENTEX LA	Decongestant-Expectorant	**Sustained-Rel. Tab:** phenylephrine HCl (30 mg), guaifenesin (600 mg)	1 tab bid (q 12 h) po.
ENTEX PSE	Decongestant-Expectorant	**Long-Acting Tab:** pseudoephedrine HCl (120 mg), guaifenesin (600 mg)	1 tab bid (q 12 h) po.
EPIFOAM	Corticosteroid-Local Anesthetic	**Aerosolized Foam:** hydrocortisone acetate (1%), pramoxine HCl (1%)	Apply to affected area tid to qid.
E-PILO-1	Anti-Glaucoma Agent	**Ophth Solution:** epinephrine bitartrate (1%), pilocarpine HCl (1%)	1 - 2 drops into affected eye(s) up to qid.
E-PILO-2		**Ophth Solution:** epinephrine bitartrate (1%), pilocarpine HCl (2%)	1 - 2 drops into affected eye(s) up to qid.
E-PILO-4		**Ophth Solution:** epinephrine bitartrate (1%), pilocarpine HCl (4%)	1 - 2 drops into affected eye(s) up to qid.
E-PILO-6		**Ophth Solution:** epinephrine bitartrate (1%), pilocarpine HCl (6%)	1 - 2 drops into affected eye(s) up to qid.
ESGIC	Analgesic	**Cpsl & Tab:** acetaminophen (325 mg), butalbital (50 mg), caffeine (40 mg)	1 - 2 cpsls (or tab) q 4 h po, prn pain.
ESGIC-PLUS		**Cpsl & Tab:** acetaminophen (500 mg), butalbital (50 mg), caffeine (40 mg)	1 cpsl (or tab) q 4 h po, prn pain.

237

TRADE NAME	THERAPEUTIC CATEGORY	DOSAGE FORMS AND COMPOSITION	COMMON ADULT DOSAGE
ESIMIL	Antihypertensive	**Tab:** guanethidine monosulfate (10 mg), hydrochlorothiazide (25 mg)	2 tab daily po. Dosage may be increased at weekly intervals.
ESTRATEST	Estrogen-Androgen	**Tab:** esterified estrogens (1.25 mg), methyltestosterone (2.5 mg)	1 tab daily po. Administration should be cyclic: 3 weeks on and 1 week off.
ESTRATEST H.S.	Estrogen-Androgen	**Tab:** esterified estrogens (0.625 mg), methyltestosterone (1.25 mg)	1 -2 tab daily po. Administration should be cyclic: 3 weeks on and 1 week off.
ESTROSTEP 21	Oral Contraceptive (Combination Estrophasic)	**Tab:** 5 triangular tabs: ethinyl estradiol (20 µg), norethindrone acetate (1 mg); 7 square tabs: ethinyl estradiol (30 µg), norethindrone acetate (1 mg); 9 round tabs: ethinyl estradiol (35 µg), norethindrone acetate (1 mg)	21-Day regimen po.
ESTROSTEP FE	Oral Contraceptive (Combination Estrophasic)	**Tab:** 5 triangular tabs: ethinyl estradiol (20 µg), norethindrone acetate (1 mg); 7 square tabs: ethinyl estradiol (30 µg), norethindrone acetate (1 mg); 9 round tabs: ethinyl estradiol (35 µg), norethindrone acetate (1 mg); 7 (brown) tabs: ferrous fumarate (75 mg)	28-Day regimen po.
ETRAFON ETRAFON 2-10 ETRAFON-FORTE	Antipsychotic-Antidepressant	**Tab:** perphenazine (2 mg), amitriptyline HCl (25 mg) **Tab:** perphenazine (2 mg), amitriptyline HCl (10 mg) **Tab:** perphenazine (4 mg), amitriptyline HCl (25 mg)	1 tab tid or qid po. 1 tab tid or qid po. 1 tab tid or qid po.
EXCEDRIN, ASPIRIN FREE	Analgesic	**Cplt & Geltab:** acetaminophen (500 mg), caffeine (65 mg)	2 cplt (or geltabs) q 6 h po while symptoms persist.
EXCEDRIN EXTRA-STRENGTH	Analgesic	**Tab, Cplt & Geltab:** acetaminophen (250 mg), aspirin (250 mg), caffeine (65 mg)	2 tabs (cplt or geltabs) q 6 h po while symptoms persist.
EXCEDRIN MIGRAINE	Analgesic	**Tab & Cplt:** acetaminophen (250 mg), aspirin (250 mg), caffeine (65 mg)	2 tabs (or cplts) q 6 h po while symptoms persist.
EXCEDRIN PM	Analgesic-Sedative	**Tab, Cplt & Geltab:** acetaminophen (500 mg), diphenhydramine citrate (38 mg)	2 tabs (cplts or geltabs) hs po.

EXCEDRIN QUICK TABS	Analgesic	**Tab (Quick-dissolving):** acetaminophen (500 mg), caffeine (65 mg)	Allow 2 tabs to dissolve fully on the tongue q 6 h.
EX-LAX GENTLE STRENGTH	Irritant Laxative-Stool Softener	**Cplt:** sennosides (10 mg), docusate sodium (65 mg)	2 cplts once or twice daily po.
EXTENDRYL	Decongestant-Antihistamine-Anticholinergic	**Syrup (per 5 mL):** phenylephrine HCl (10 mg), chlorpheniramine maleate (2 mg), methscopolamine nitrate (1.25 mg) **Chewable Tab:** phenylephrine HCl (10 mg), chlorpheniramine maleate (2 mg), methscopolamine nitrate (1.25 mg)	10 mL q 4 h po. 2 tab q 4 h po.
EXTENDRYL SR	Decongestant-Antihistamine-Anticholinergic	**Sustained-Rel. Cpsl:** phenylephrine HCl (20 mg), chlorpheniramine maleate (8 mg), methscopolamine nitrate (2.5 mg)	1 cpsl q 12 h po.
FANSIDAR	Antimalarial	**Tab:** sulfadoxine (500 mg), pyrimethamine (25 mg)	**Acute Malarial Attack:** 2 - 3 tab po alone or with quinine. **Malaria Prophylaxis:** 1 tab po once weekly or 2 tab po q 2 weeks 1 to 2 days before departure to an endemic area; continue during stay and for 4 to 6 weeks after return.
FEMHRT 1/5	Progestin-Estrogen	**Tab:** norethindrone acetate (1 mg), ethinyl estradiol (5 µg)	1 tablet daily po.
FERO-FOLIC-500	Hematinic	**Controlled-Rel. Tab:** ferrous sulfate (525 mg), folic acid (800 µg), sodium ascorbate (500 mg)	1 tab daily po.
FERO-GRAD-500	Hematinic	**Controlled-Rel. Tab:** ferrous sulfate (525 mg), sodium ascorbate (500 mg)	1 tab daily po.
FIORICET	Analgesic	**Tab:** acetaminophen (325 mg), butalbital (50 mg), caffeine (40 mg)	1 - 2 tab q 4 h po. Maximum of 6 tabs daily.
FIORICET W/CODEINE (C-III)	Analgesic	**Cpsl:** acetaminophen (325 mg), butalbital (50 mg), caffeine (40 mg), codeine phosphate (30 mg)	1 - 2 cpsl q 4 h po. Maximum of 6 cpsls daily.

TRADE NAME	THERAPEUTIC CATEGORY	DOSAGE FORMS AND COMPOSITION	COMMON ADULT DOSAGE
FIORINAL (C-III)	Analgesic	**Cpsl & Tab:** aspirin (325 mg), caffeine (40 mg), butalbital (50 mg)	1 - 2 cpsl (or tab) q 4 h po. Maximum of 6 daily.
FIORINAL W/CODEINE (C-III)	Analgesic	**Cpsl:** aspirin (325 mg), caffeine (40 mg), butalbital (50 mg), codeine phosphate (30 mg)	1 - 2 cpsl q 4 h po. Maximum of 6 cpsls daily.
FML-S	Antibacterial-Corticosteroid	**Ophth Susp:** sulfacetamide sodium (10%), fluorometholone (0.1%)	1 drop in affected eye(s) qid.
GLUCOVANCE 1.25MG/250MG	Hypoglycemic Agent-Antihyperglycemic Agent	**Tab:** glyburide (1.25 mg), metformin (250 mg)	**First-Line:** 1.25mg/250mg once daily po with a meal. May take 1.25mg/250mg bid po (AM & PM) if HbA$_{1c}$ is > 9% or the fasting plasma glucose (FPG) is > 200 mg/dL. **Second-Line (Previously-treated with Sulfonylurea and/or Metformin):** 2.5mg/500mg or 5mg/500mg bid po (AM and PM). May increase by up to 5mg/500mg q 2 weeks (do not exceed daily doses of the individual components previously taken). Maximum: 20mg/2000mg per day.
2.5MG/500MG		**Tab:** glyburide (2.5 mg), metformin (500 mg)	
5MG/500MG		**Tab:** glyburide (5 mg), metformin (500 mg)	
HALEY'S M-O	Emollient Laxative-Saline Laxative	**Liquid (per 5 mL):** mineral oil (1.25 mL), magnesium hydroxide (304 mg)	15 - 30 mL po in the morning and hs.
HUMIBID DM	Antitussive-Expectorant	**Sustained-Rel. Tab:** dextromethorphan HBr (30 mg), guaifenesin (600 mg)	1 or 2 tablets q 12 h po.
HYCODAN (C-III)	Antitussive-Anticholinergic	**Syrup (per 5 mL):** hydrocodone bitartrate (5 mg), homatropine methylbromide (1.5 mg) **Tab:** hydrocodone bitartrate (5 mg), homatropine methylbromide (1.5 mg)	5 mL q 4 - 6 h po. 1 tab q 4 - 6 h po.

Drug	Category	Composition	Dosage
HYCOTUSS EXPECTORANT (C-III)	Antitussive-Expectorant	**Syrup (per 5 mL):** hydrocodone bitartrate (5 mg), guaifenesin (100 mg), alcohol (10%)	5 mL q 4 h po, pc & hs.
HYDROCET (C-III)	Analgesic	**Cpsl:** hydrocodone bitartrate (5 mg), acetaminophen (500 mg)	1 - 2 cpsl q 4 - 6 h po, prn pain.
HYDROPRES-50	Antihypertensive	**Tab:** hydrochlorothiazide (50 mg), reserpine (0.125 mg)	1 tab daily po.
HYZAAR 50-12.5 HYZAAR 100-25	Antihypertensive	**Tab:** losartan potassium (50 mg), hydrochlorothiazide (12.5 mg) **Tab:** losartan potassium (100 mg), hydrochlorothiazide (25 mg)	1 tab daily po. 1 tab daily po.
IMODIUM ADVANCED	Antidiarrheal-Anti Gas Drug	**Chewable Tab:** loperamide HCl (2 mg), simethicone (125 mg)	Chew 1 tab and take with water after each loose stool. Do not take more than 4 tab per day.
INDERIDE-40/25 INDERIDE-80/25	Antihypertensive	**Tab:** propranolol HCl (40 mg), hydrochlorothiazide (25 mg) **Tab:** propranolol HCl (80 mg), hydrochlorothiazide (25 mg)	1 tab bid po. 1 tab bid po.
JENEST-28	Oral Contraceptive (Combination Biphasic)	**Tab:** 7 tabs: norethindrone (0.5 mg), ethinyl estradiol (35 μg); 14 tabs: norethindrone (1 mg), ethinyl estradiol (35 μg); + 7 placebos in 28-Day Compaks	28-Day regimen po.
KALETRA	Antiviral	**Cpsl:** lopinavir (133.3 mg), ritonavir (33.3 mg) **Solution (per mL):** lopinavir (80 mg), ritonavir (20 mg), alcohol (42.4%)	**Alone:** 400 mg/100 mg (3 capsules or 5 mL) bid po with food. **Concomitant Therapy with Efavirenz or Nevirapine:** An increase to 533 mg/133 mg (4 capsules or 6.5 mL) bid po with food may be considered.
LEVLEN	Oral Contraceptive (Combination Monophasic)	**Tab:** ethinyl estradiol (30 μg), levonorgestrel (0.15 mg) in 21-Day and 28-Day Slidecases (contains 7 inert tabs)	21-Day regimen po or 28-Day regimen po.
LEVLITE	Oral Contraceptive (Combination Monophasic)	**Tab:** ethinyl estradiol (20 μg), levonorgestrel (0.10 mg) in 21-Day and 28-Day Slidecases (contains 7 inert tabs)	21-Day regimen po or 28-Day regimen po.
LEVORA 0.15/30	Oral Contraceptive (Combination Monophasic)	**Tab:** levonorgestrel (0.15 mg), ethinyl estradiol (30 μg) in 21-Day and 28-Day Dispensers (contains 7 inert tabs)	21-Day regimen po or 28-Day regimen po.

241

TRADE NAME	THERAPEUTIC CATEGORY	DOSAGE FORMS AND COMPOSITION	COMMON ADULT DOSAGE
LEXXEL	Antihypertensive	**Extended-Rel. Tab:** enalapril maleate (5 mg), felodipine (2.5 mg) **Extended-Rel. Tab:** enalapril maleate (5 mg), felodipine (5 mg)	1 tab once daily po. 1 tab once daily po.
LIBRAX	Anticholinergic-Antianxiety	**Cpsl:** clidinium bromide (2.5 mg), chlordiazepoxide HCl (5 mg)	1 - 2 cpsl qid po, ac & hs.
LIMBITROL DS (C-IV)	Antianxiety Agent-Antidepressant	**Tab:** chlordiazepoxide (10 mg), amitriptyline HCl (25 mg)	1 tab tid or qid po.
LOESTRIN 21 1/20	Oral Contraceptive (Combination Monophasic)	**Tab:** ethinyl estradiol (20 μg), norethindrone acetate (1 mg) in 21-Day Petipacs	21-Day regimen po.
LOESTRIN 21 1.5/30		**Tab:** ethinyl estradiol (30 μg), norethindrone acetate (1.5 mg) in 21-Day Petipacs	21-Day regimen po.
LOESTRIN FE 1/20	Oral Contraceptive (Combination Monophasic)	**Tab:** 21 tabs: ethinyl estradiol (20 μg), norethindrone acetate (1 mg) + 7 tabs: ferrous fumarate (75 mg) in 28-Day Petipacs	28-Day regimen po.
LOESTRIN FE 1.5/30		**Tab:** 21 tabs: ethinyl estradiol (30 μg), norethindrone acetate (1.5 mg) + 7 tabs: ferrous fumarate (75 mg) in 28-Day Petipacs	28-Day regimen po.
LOMOTIL (C-V)	Antidiarrheal	**Liquid (per 5 mL):** diphenoxylate HCl (2.5 mg), atropine sulfate (0.025 mg), alcohol (15%) **Tab:** diphenoxylate HCl (2.5 mg), atropine sulfate (0.025 mg)	10 mL qid po until control of diarrhea is achieved. 2 tab qid po until control of diarrhea is achieved.
LO/OVRAL	Oral Contraceptive (Combination Monophasic)	**Tab:** ethinyl estradiol (30 μg), norgestrel (0.3 mg) in 21-Day Pilpaks	28-Day regimen po.
LOPRESSOR HCT 50/25	Antihypertensive	**Tab:** metoprolol tartrate (50 mg), hydrochlorothiazide (25 mg)	2 tab daily po as a single dose or in divided doses.
LOPRESSOR HCT 100/25		**Tab:** metoprolol tartrate (100 mg), hydrochlorothiazide (25 mg)	1 - 2 tab daily po as a single dose or in divided doses.
LOPRESSOR HCT 100/50		**Tab:** metoprolol tartrate (100 mg), hydrochlorothiazide (50 mg)	1 tab daily po as a single dose or in divided doses.

Drug	Class	Composition	Dosage
LORTAB (C-III)	Analgesic	**Elixir (per 5 mL):** hydrocodone bitartrate (2.5 mg), acetaminophen (120 mg), alcohol (7%).	15 mL q 4 h po, prn pain.
LORTAB 2.5/500 (C-III) LORTAB 5/500 (C-III) LORTAB 7.5/500 (C-III) LORTAB 10/500 (C-III)		**Tab:** hydrocodone bitartrate (2.5 mg), acetaminophen (500 mg) **Tab:** hydrocodone bitartrate (5 mg), acetaminophen (500 mg) **Tab:** hydrocodone bitartrate (7.5 mg), acetaminophen (500 mg) **Tab:** hydrocodone bitartrate (10 mg), acetaminophen (500 mg)	1 - 2 tab q 4 - 6 h po, prn pain. 1 - 2 tab q 4 - 6 h po, prn pain. 1 tab q 4 - 6 h po, prn pain. 1 tab q 4 - 6 h po, prn pain.
LORTAB ASA (C-III)	Analgesic	**Tab:** hydrocodone bitartrate (5 mg), aspirin (500 mg)	1 - 2 tab q 4 - 6 h po, prn pain.
LOTENSIN HCT 5/6.25 LOTENSIN HCT 10/12.5 LOTENSIN HCT 20/12.5 LOTENSIN HCT 20/25	Antihypertensive	**Tab:** benazepril HCl (5 mg), hydrochlorothiazide (6.25 mg) **Tab:** benazepril HCl (10 mg), hydrochlorothiazide (12.5 mg) **Tab:** benazepril HCl (20 mg), hydrochlorothiazide (12.5 mg) **Tab:** benazepril HCl (20 mg), hydrochlorothiazide (25 mg)	1 tab daily po. 1 tab daily po. 1 tab daily po. 1 tab daily po.
LOTREL	Antihypertensive	**Cpsl:** amlodipine besylate (2.5 mg), benazepril HCl (10 mg) **Cpsl:** amlodipine besylate (5 mg), benazepril HCl (10 mg) **Cpsl:** amlodipine besylate (5 mg), benazepril HCl (20 mg)	1 cpsl daily po. 1 cpsl daily po. 1 cpsl daily po.
LOTRISONE	Antifungal-Corticosteroid	**Cream & Lotion:** clotrimazole (1%), betamethasone dipropionate (0.05%)	Massage into affected skin areas bid for up to 4 weeks.
LUFYLLIN-EPG	Drug for COPD	**Elixir (per 10 mL):** dyphylline (100 mg), guaifenesin (200 mg), ephedrine HCl (16 mg), phenobarbital (16 mg), alcohol (5.5%) **Tab:** dyphylline (100 mg), guaifenesin (200 mg), ephedrine HCl (16 mg), phenobarbital (16 mg)	10 - 20 mL q 6 h po. 1 - 2 tab q 6 h po.
LUFYLLIN-GG	Drug for COPD	**Elixir (per 15 mL):** dyphylline (100 mg), guaifenesin (100 mg), alcohol (17%) **Tab:** dyphylline (200 mg), guaifenesin (200 mg)	30 mL qid po. 1 tab qid po.
LUNELLE MONTHLY CONTRACEPTIVE	Injectable Contraceptive	**Inj:** estradiol cypionate (5 mg), medroxyprogesterone acetate (25 mg)/0.5 mL	0.5 mL once monthly IM.
MAALOX	Antacid-Antigas Drug	**Liquid (per 5 mL):** magnesium hydroxide (200 mg), aluminum hydroxide (200 mg), simethicone (20 mg)	10 - 20 mL qid po.
MAALOX MAX MAXIMUM STRENGTH	Antacid-Antigas Drug	**Liquid (per 5 mL):** magnesium hydroxide (400 mg), aluminum hydroxide (400 mg), simethicone (40 mg)	10 - 20 mL qid po.

TRADE NAME	THERAPEUTIC CATEGORY	DOSAGE FORMS AND COMPOSITION	COMMON ADULT DOSAGE
MALARONE	Antimalarial	**Tab:** atovaquone (250 mg), proguanil HCl (100 mg).	Take at the same time each day with food or a milky drink. Repeat dose if vomiting occurs within 1 hour. **Prophylaxis:** 1 tab daily po starting 1 - 2 days before entering endemic area, during stay, and for 7 days after returning. **Treatment:** 4 tabs daily po for 3 consecutive days.
MARAX	Drug for COPD	**Tab:** theophylline (130 mg), ephedrine sulfate (25 mg), hydroxyzine HCl (10 mg).	1 tab bid - qid po. Some patients are adequately controlled with 1/2 - 1 tab hs.
MAXITROL	Antibacterial-Corticosteroid	**Ophth Suspension (per mL):** polymyxin B sulfate (10,000 Units), neomycin sulfate (equal to 3.5 mg of neomycin base), dexamethasone (0.1%) **Ophth Oint (per g):** polymyxin B sulfate (10,000 Units), neomycin sulfate (equal to 3.5 mg of neomycin base), dexamethasone (0.1%)	1 or 2 drops into the affected eye(s) q 1 h in severe disease; in mild cases, 1 - 2 drops 4 to 6 times daily. Apply a small amount into the conjunctival sac tid to qid.
MAXZIDE MAXZIDE-25 MG	Antihypertensive, Diuretic	**Tab:** triamterene (75 mg), hydrochlorothiazide (50 mg) **Tab:** triamterene (37.5 mg), hydrochlorothiazide (25 mg)	1 tab daily po. 1 - 2 tab daily po.
METIMYD	Antibacterial-Corticosteroid	**Ophth Susp:** sulfacetamide sodium (10%), prednisolone acetate (0.5%) **Ophth Oint:** sulfacetamide sodium (10%), prednisolone acetate (0.5%)	2 - 3 drops into the affected eye(s) q 1 - 2 h during the day and hs. Apply to affected eye(s) tid or qid and hs.
MICARDIS HCT 40/12.5 MICARDIS HCT 80/12.5	Antihypertensive	**Tab:** telmisartan (40 mg), hydrochlorothiazide (12.5 mg) **Tab:** telmisartan (80 mg), hydrochlorothiazide (12.5 mg)	1 tab daily po. 1 tab daily po.

MIDRIN	Analgesic, Antimigraine Agent	**Cpsl:** isometheptene mucate (65 mg), dichloralphenazone (100 mg), acetaminophen (325 mg)	**Tension Headache:** 1 - 2 cpsl q 4 h po, up to 8 cpsl daily. **Migraine Headache:** 2 cpsl stat, then 1 cpsl q h po until relieved, up to 5 cpsl within a 12-hour period.
MINIZIDE 1 MINIZIDE 2 MINIZIDE 5	Antihypertensive	**Cpsl:** prazosin HCl (1 mg), polythiazide (0.5 mg) **Cpsl:** prazosin HCl (2 mg), polythiazide (0.5 mg) **Cpsl:** prazosin HCl (5 mg), polythiazide (0.5 mg)	1 cpsl bid - tid po, the strength depending upon individual requirement after titration.
MIRCETTE	Oral Contraceptive (Combination Biphasic)	**Tab:** 21 white tabs: ethinyl estradiol (20 μg), desogestrel (0.15 mg); 2 green inert tabs; 5 yellow tabs: ethinyl estradiol (10 μg) in 28-Day Dispensers	28-Day regimen po.
MODICON	Oral Contraceptive (Combination Monophasic)	**Tab:** ethinyl estradiol (35 μg), norethindrone (0.5 mg) in 21-Day and 28-Day Dialpaks (contains 7 inert tabs)	21-Day regimen po or 28-Day regimen po.
MODURETIC	Diuretic	**Tab:** amiloride HCl (5 mg), hydrochlorothiazide (50 mg)	Initially 1 tab daily po. Dosage may be raised to 2 tab daily as a single dose or in divided doses.
MOTOFEN (C-IV)	Antidiarrheal	**Tab:** difenoxin HCl (1 mg), atropine sulfate (0.025 mg)	2 tab po (1st dose), then 1 tab after each loose stool or 1 tab q 3 - 4 h prn. Maximum: 8 tab per 24 hours.
MOTRIN SINUS / HEADACHE	Decongestant-Analgesic	**Cplt:** pseudoephedrine HCl (30 mg), ibuprofen (200 mg)	1 - 2 cplt q 4 - 6 h po.
NALDECON SENIOR DX	Antitussive-Expectorant	**Liquid (per 5 mL):** dextromethorphan HBr (10 mg), guaifenesin (200 mg)	10 mL q 4 h po.
NAPHCON-A	Ocular Decongestant-Antihistamine	**Ophth Solution:** naphazoline HCl (0.025%), pheniramine maleate (0.3%)	1 - 2 drops in the affected eye(s) up to qid.
NECON 0.5/35	Oral Contraceptive (Combination Monophasic)	**Tab:** norethindrone (0.5 mg), ethinyl estradiol (35 μg) in 21-Day and 28-Day Dispensers (contains 7 inert tabs)	21-Day regimen po or 28-Day regimen po.

TRADE NAME	THERAPEUTIC CATEGORY	DOSAGE FORMS AND COMPOSITION	COMMON ADULT DOSAGE
NECON 1/35	Oral Contraceptive (Combination Monophasic)	Tab: norethindrone (1 mg), ethinyl estradiol (35 μg) in 21-Day and 28-Day Dispensers (contains 7 inert tabs)	21-Day regimen po or 28-Day regimen po.
NECON 1/50	Oral Contraceptive (Combination Monophasic)	Tab: norethindrone (1 mg), mestranol (50 μg) in 21-Day and 28-Day Dispensers (contains 7 inert tabs)	21-Day regimen po or 28-Day regimen po.
NECON 10/11	Oral Contraceptive (Combination Biphasic)	Tab: 10 tabs: norethindrone (0.5 mg), ethinyl estradiol (35 μg); 11 tabs: norethindrone (1 mg), ethinyl estradiol (35 μg) in 21-Day and 28-Day Dispensers (contains 7 inert tabs)	21-Day regimen po or 28-Day regimen po.
NEODECADRON	Antibacterial-Corticosteroid	Ophth Solution: neomycin sulfate (equal to 0.35% of neomycin base), dexamethasone sodium phosphate (0.1%)	1 - 2 drops into eye(s) every h during the day and q 2 h at night. When a favorable response occurs, reduce the dosage to 1 drop q 4 h.
		Ophth Oint: neomycin sulfate (equal to 0.35% of neomycin base), dexamethasone sodium phosphate (0.05%)	Apply a thin coating to eye(s) tid - qid. When a favorable response occurs, reduce the dosage to bid.
		Topical Cream: neomycin sulfate (equal to 0.35% of base), dexamethasone sodium phosphate (0.1%)	Apply topically to the affected area as a thin film tid - qid.
NEOSPORIN	Antibacterial	Ophth Solution (per mL): polymyxin B sulfate (10,000 Units), neomycin sulfate (equal to 1.75 mg of neomycin base), gramicidin (0.025 mg)	1 - 2 drops in the affected eye(s) bid - qid for 7 - 10 days.
		Ophth Oint (per g): polymyxin B sulfate (10,000 Units), neomycin sulfate (equal to 3.5 mg of neomycin base), bacitracin zinc (400 Units)	Apply to eye(s) q 3 - 4 h for 7 - 10 days.
		Oint (per g): polymyxin B sulfate (5,000 Units), neomycin sulfate (equal to 3.5 mg of neomycin base), bacitracin zinc (400 Units)	Apply topically 1 - 3 times daily.
NEOSPORIN PLUS PAIN RELIEF MAXIMUM STRENGTH	Antibacterial-Local Anesthetic	Cream (per g): polymyxin B sulfate (10,000 Units), neomycin sulfate (equal to 3.5 mg of neomycin base), pramoxine HCl (10 mg)	Apply topically 1 - 3 times daily.
		Oint (per g): polymyxin B sulfate (10,000 Units), neomycin sulfate (equal to 3.5 mg of neomycin base), bacitracin zinc (500 Units), pramoxine HCl (10 mg)	Apply topically 1 - 3 times daily.

NORDETTE	Oral Contraceptive (Combination Monophasic)	**Tab:** ethinyl estradiol (30 μg), levonorgestrel (0.15 mg) in 21-Day and 28-Day Pilpaks (contains 7 inert tabs)	21-Day regimen po or 28-Day regimen po.
NORGESIC	Skeletal Muscle Relaxant-Analgesic	**Tab:** orphenadrine citrate (25 mg), aspirin (385 mg), caffeine (30 mg)	1 - 2 tab tid or qid po.
NORGESIC FORTE		**Tab:** orphenadrine citrate (50 mg), aspirin (770 mg), caffeine (60 mg)	1 tab tid or qid po.
NORINYL 1 + 35	Oral Contraceptive (Combination Monophasic)	**Tab:** ethinyl estradiol (35 μg), norethindrone (1 mg) in 21-Day and 28-Day Wallettes (contains 7 inert tabs)	21-Day regimen po or 28-Day regimen po.
NORINYL 1 + 50	Oral Contraceptive (Combination Monophasic)	**Tab:** mestranol (50 μg), norethindrone (1 mg) in 21-Day and 28-Day Wallettes (contains 7 inert tabs)	21-Day regimen po or 28-Day regimen po.
NOVACET LOTION	Anti-Acne Agent	**Lotion:** sulfacetamide sodium (10%), sulfur (5%)	Apply a thin film to affected areas 1 to 3 times daily.
NUCOFED (C-III)	Decongestant-Antitussive	**Syrup (per 5 mL):** pseudoephedrine HCl (60 mg), codeine phosphate (20 mg)	5 mL q 6 h po.
		Cpsl: pseudoephedrine HCl (60 mg), codeine phosphate (20 mg)	1 cpsl q 6 h po.
NUCOFED EXPECTORANT (C-III)	Decongestant-Expectorant-Antitussive	**Syrup (per 5 mL):** pseudoephedrine HCl (60 mg), guaifenesin (200 mg), codeine phosphate (20 mg), alcohol (12.5%)	5 mL q 6 h po.
NUCOFED PEDIATRIC EXPECTORANT (C-III)	Decongestant-Expectorant-Antitussive	**Syrup (per 5 mL):** pseudoephedrine HCl (30 mg), guaifenesin (100 mg), codeine phosphate (10 mg), alcohol (6%)	10 mL q 6 h po.
NUVA-RING	Intrauterine Contraceptive	**Vaginal Ring:** ethinyl estradiol (0.015 mg/day), etonogestrel (0.12 mg/day)	Insert into the vagina & leave in place for 3 weeks; remove for 1 week. Insert a new ring 1 week after the old one was removed & repeat (as above).
ORNEX NO DROWSINESS	Decongestant-Analgesic	**Cplt:** pseudoephedrine HCl (30 mg), acetaminophen (325 mg)	2 cplt q 4 h po, not to exceed 8 cplt in 24 h.
ORNEX NO DROWSINESS MAXIMUM STRENGTH	Decongestant-Analgesic	**Cplt:** pseudoephedrine HCl (30 mg), acetaminophen (500 mg)	2 cplt q 6 h po, not to exceed 8 cplt in 24 h.

247

TRADE NAME	THERAPEUTIC CATEGORY	DOSAGE FORMS AND COMPOSITION	COMMON ADULT DOSAGE
ORTHO-CEPT	Oral Contraceptive (Combination Monophasic)	Tab: ethinyl estradiol (30 μg), desogestrel (0.15 mg) in 21-Day and 28-Day Dialpaks (contains 7 inert tabs)	21-Day regimen po or 28-Day regimen po.
ORTHO-CYCLEN	Oral Contraceptive (Combination Monophasic)	Tab: ethinyl estradiol (35 μg), norgestimate (0.25 mg) in 21-Day and 28-Day Dialpaks (contains 7 inert tabs)	21-Day regimen po or 28-Day regimen po.
ORTHO EVRA	Oral Contraceptive (Transdermal)	Transdermal Patch (release per 24 h): ethinyl estradiol (20 μg), norelgestromin (0.15 mg) in cycles (3 patches) and a single patch	This system uses of 28-day (4-week) cycle. Apply a new patch each week for 3 weeks (21 days total). Week 4 is patch-free. Wear only 1 patch at a time.
ORTHO-NOVUM 1/35	Oral Contraceptive (Combination Monophasic)	Tab: ethinyl estradiol (35 μg), norethindrone (1 mg) in 21-Day and 28-Day Dialpaks (contains 7 inert tabs)	21-Day regimen po or 28-Day regimen po.
ORTHO-NOVUM 1/50	Oral Contraceptive (Combination Monophasic)	Tab: mestranol (50 μg), norethindrone (1 mg) in 21-Day and 28-Day Dialpaks (contains 7 inert tabs)	21-Day regimen po or 28-Day regimen po.
ORTHO-NOVUM 7/7/7	Oral Contraceptive (Combination Triphasic)	Tab: 7 tabs: ethinyl estradiol (35 μg), norethindrone (0.5 mg); 7 tabs: ethinyl estradiol (35 μg), norethindrone (0.75 mg); 7 tabs: ethinyl estradiol (35 μg), norethindrone (1 mg) in 21-Day and 28-Day Dialpaks (contains 7 inert tabs)	21-Day regimen po or 28-Day regimen po.
ORTHO-NOVUM 10/11	Oral Contraceptive (Combination Biphasic)	Tab: 10 tabs: ethinyl estradiol (35 μg), norethindrone (0.5 mg); 11 tabs: ethinyl estradiol (35 μg), norethindrone (1 mg) in 21-Day and 28-Day Dialpaks (with 7 inert tabs)	21-Day regimen po or 28-Day regimen po.
ORTHO-PREFEST	Estrogen-Progestin	30 Tab Pkg: estradiol (1 mg) [pink] tabs; estradiol (1 mg) + norgestimate (90 μg) [white] tabs: in an alternating sequence of 3 tablets each	One pink tablet daily for 3 days, followed by 1 white tablet daily for 3 days. Repeat without interruption.
ORTHO TRI-CYCLEN	Oral Contraceptive (Combination Triphasic)	Tab: 7 tabs: ethinyl estradiol (35 μg), norgestimate (0.18 mg); 7 tabs: ethinyl estradiol (35 μg), norgestimate (0.215 mg); 7 tabs: ethinyl estradiol (35 μg), norgestimate (0.25 mg) in 21-Day and 28-Day Dialpaks (contains 7 inert tabs)	21-Day regimen po or 28-Day regimen po.

ORTHO TRI-CYCLEN LO	Oral Contraceptive (Combination Triphasic)	**Tab:** 7 tabs: ethinyl estradiol (25 μg), norgestimate (0.18 mg); 7 tabs: ethinyl estradiol (25 μg), norgestimate (0.215 mg); 7 tabs: ethinyl estradiol (25 μg), norgestimate (0.25 mg) in 28-Day Dialpaks (contains 7 inert tabs)	28-Day regimen po.
OTOBIOTIC	Antibacterial-Corticosteroid	**Otic Solution (per mL):** polymyxin B sulfate (10,000 Units), hydrocortisone (0.5%)	4 drops into ear(s) tid or qid.
OVCON-35	Oral Contraceptive (Combination Monophasic)	**Tab:** ethinyl estradiol (35 μg), norethindrone (0.4 mg) in 28-Day dispensers (contains 7 inert tabs)	28-Day regimen po.
OVCON-50	Oral Contraceptive (Combination Monophasic)	**Tab:** ethinyl estradiol (50 μg), norethindrone (1 mg) in 28-Day dispensers (contains 7 inert tabs)	28-Day regimen po.
OVRAL-28	Oral Contraceptive (Combination Monophasic)	**Tab:** ethinyl estradiol (50 μg), norgestrel (0.5 mg) in 28-Day Pilpaks (contains 7 inert tabs)	28-Day regimen po.
P_1E_1	Anti-Glaucoma Agent	**Ophth Solution:** pilocarpine HCl (1%), epinephrine bitartrate (1%)	1 - 2 drops into affected eye(s) up to qid.
P_2E_1		**Ophth Solution:** pilocarpine HCl (2%), epinephrine bitartrate (1%)	1 - 2 drops into affected eye(s) up to qid.
P_4E_1		**Ophth Solution:** pilocarpine HCl (4%), epinephrine bitartrate (1%)	1 - 2 drops into affected eye(s) up to qid.
P_6E_1		**Ophth Solution:** pilocarpine HCl (6%), epinephrine bitartrate (1%)	1 - 2 drops into affected eye(s) up to qid.
PAZO	Antihemorrhoidal	**Oint:** camphor (2%), ephedrine sulfate (0.2%), zinc oxide (5%)	Apply to affected areas up to qid.
		Rectal Suppos: ephedrine sulfate (3.86 mg), zinc oxide (96.5 mg)	Insert 1 rectally up to qid.
PEDIOTIC	Antibacterial-Corticosteroid	**Otic Susp (per mL):** polymyxin B sulfate (10,000 Units), neomycin sulfate (equal to 3.5 mg of neomycin base), hydrocortisone (10 mg = 1%)	4 drops into the affected ear(s) tid to qid.
PEPCID COMPLETE	Histamine H_2 Blocker-Antacid	**Chewable Tab:** famotidine (10 mg), calcium carbonate (800 mg), magnesium hydroxide (165 mg)	Chew 1 tab once daily. Do not exceed 2 tabs in 24 h.

249

TRADE NAME	THERAPEUTIC CATEGORY	DOSAGE FORMS AND COMPOSITION	COMMON ADULT DOSAGE
PERCOCET 2.5/325 (C-II) PERCOCET 5/325 (C-II) PERCOCET 7.5/325 (C-II) PERCOCET 7.5/500 (C-II) PERCOCET 10/325 (C-II) PERCOCET 10/650 (C-II)	Analgesic	**Tab:** oxycodone HCl (2.5 mg), acetaminophen (325 mg) **Tab:** oxycodone HCl (5 mg), acetaminophen (325 mg) **Tab:** oxycodone HCl (7.5 mg), acetaminophen (325 mg) **Tab:** oxycodone HCl (7.5 mg), acetaminophen (500 mg) **Tab:** oxycodone HCl (10 mg), acetaminophen (325 mg) **Tab:** oxycodone HCl (10 mg), acetaminophen (650 mg)	2 tabs q 6 h po, prn pain. 1 tab q 6 h po, prn pain. 1 tab q 6 h po, prn pain. 1 tab q 6 h po, prn pain. 1 tab q 6 h po, prn pain. 1 tab q 6 h po, prn pain.
PERCODAN (C-II)	Analgesic	**Tab:** oxycodone HCl (4.5 mg), oxycodone terephthalate (0.38 mg), aspirin (325 mg)	1 tab q 6 h po, prn pain.
PERCODAN-DEMI (C-II)	Analgesic	**Tab:** oxycodone HCl (2.25 mg), oxycodone terephthalate (0.19 mg), aspirin (325 mg)	1 - 2 tab q 6 h po, prn pain.
PERCOGESIC	Analgesic-Antihistamine	**Cplt:** acetaminophen (325 mg), phenyltoloxamine citrate (30 mg)	2 cplt q 4 h po.
PERCOGESIC EXTRA-STRENGTH	Analgesic-Antihistamine	**Cplt:** acetaminophen (500 mg), diphenhydramine HCl (12.5 mg)	2 cplt q 6 h po.
PERDIEM OVERNIGHT RELIEF	Bulk Laxative-Irritant Laxative	**Granules (per rounded teaspoonful):** psyllium (3.25 g), senna (0.74 g)	In the evening and/or before breakfast, 1 - 2 rounded teaspoonfuls in at least 8 oz. of cool beverage po.
PERI-COLACE	Irritant Laxative-Stool Softener	**Cpsl:** casanthranol (30 mg), docusate sodium (100 mg) **Syrup (per 15 mL):** casanthranol (30 mg), docusate sodium (60 mg), alcohol (10%)	1 - 2 cpsl hs po. 15 - 30 mL hs po.
PHRENILIN PHRENILIN FORTE	Analgesic	**Tab:** acetaminophen (325 mg), butalbital (50 mg) **Cpsl:** acetaminophen (650 mg), butalbital (50 mg)	1 - 2 tab q 4 h po, prn. 1 cpsl q 4 h po, prn.
POLY-PRED	Antibacterial-Corticosteroid	**Ophth Suspension (per mL):** neomycin sulfate (equal to 3.5 mg of neomycin base), polymyxin B sulfate (10,000 Units), prednisolone acetate (0.5%)	1 or 2 drops q 3 - 4 h into affected eye(s). Acute infections may require dosing q 30 minutes, initially.

POLYSPORIN	Antibacterial	**Ophth Oint (per g):** polymyxin B sulfate (10,000 Units), bacitracin zinc (500 Units) **Powder & Oint (per g):** polymyxin B sulfate (10,000 Units), bacitracin zinc (500 units)	Apply to eye(s) q 3 - 4 h. Apply topically 1 - 3 times daily.
POLYTRIM	Antibacterial	**Ophth Solution (per mL):** trimethoprim sulfate (equal to 1 mg of trimethoprim base), polymyxin B sulfate (10,000 Units)	1 drop into affected eye(s) q 3 h (maximum of 6 doses per day) for 7 - 10 days.
PRED-G	Antibacterial-Corticosteroid	**Ophth Suspension:** gentamicin sulfate (0.3%), prednisolone acetate (1.0%) **Ophth Oint:** gentamicin sulfate (0.3%), prednisolone acetate (0.6%)	1 drop into affected eye(s) bid to qid. During the initial 24 to 48 h, dosage may be raised up to 1 drop every hour. Apply a small amount (1/2 in.) to the conjunctival sac 1 - 3 times daily.
PREMPHASE	Estrogen-Progestin	**Tab (maroon):** conjugated estrogens (0.625 mg); **Tab (light-blue):** conjugated estrogens (0.625 mg), medroxyprogesterone acetate (5 mg)	1 maroon tab daily po for 28 days; 1 light-blue tab daily po on Days 15 through 28.
PREMPRO 0.625/2.5	Estrogen-Progestin	**Tab:** conjugated estrogens (0.625 mg), medroxyprogesterone acetate (2.5 mg)	1 tab daily po.
PREMPRO 0.625/5	Estrogen-Progestin	**Tab:** conjugated estrogens (0.625 mg), medroxyprogesterone acetate (5 mg)	1 tab daily po.
PREPARATION H	Antihemorrhoidal	**Ointment:** petrolatum (71.9%), mineral oil (14%), shark liver oil (3%), phenylephrine HCl (0.25%)	Apply to the affected area up to qid, especially at night, in the morning, or after each bowel movement.
		Cream: petrolatum (18%), glycerin (12%), shark liver oil (3%), phenylephrine HCl (0.25%)	Apply externally to the affected area up to qid, especially at night, in the morning, or after each bowel movement.
		Rectal Suppositories: cocoa butter (79%), shark liver oil (3%)	Insert 1 into the rectum up to 6 times daily, especially at night, in the morning, or after each bowel movement.

TRADE NAME	THERAPEUTIC CATEGORY	DOSAGE FORMS AND COMPOSITION	COMMON ADULT DOSAGE
PRIMATENE	Decongestant-Expectorant	Tab: ephedrine HCl (12.5 mg), guaifenesin (200 mg)	2 tab q 4 h po.
PRIMAXIN I.M.	Antibacterial	Powd for Inj: imipenem (500 mg), cilastatin sodium (500 mg) Powd for Inj: imipenem (750 mg), cilastatin sodium (750 mg)	Lower Respiratory Tract, Skin & Skin Structure, and Gynecologic Infections: 500 or 750 mg (of imipenem) q 12 h IM. Intra-Abdominal Infections: 750 mg q 12 h IM.
PRIMAXIN I.V.	Antibacterial	Powd for Inj: imipenem (250 mg), cilastatin sodium (250 mg) Powd for Inj: imipenem (500 mg), cilastatin sodium (500 mg)	Administer by IV infusion. Each 250 or 500 mg dose (of imipenem) should be given over 20 - 30 min. Each 1000 mg dose should be infused over 40 - 60 min. Infections: Mild: 250 - 500 mg q 6 h. Moderate: 500 - 1000 mg q 6 to 8 h. Severe, Life-Threatening: 500 mg q 6 h to 1000 mg q 6 to 8 h. Urinary Tract (Uncomplicated): 250 mg q 6 h. Urinary Tract (Complicated): 500 mg q 6 h.
PRINZIDE 10-12.5 PRINZIDE 20-12.5 PRINZIDE 20-25	Antihypertensive	Tab: lisinopril (10 mg), hydrochlorothiazide (12.5 mg) Tab: lisinopril (20 mg), hydrochlorothiazide (12.5 mg) Tab: lisinopril (20 mg), hydrochlorothiazide (25 mg)	1 - 2 tab once daily po. 1 - 2 tab once daily po. 1 - 2 tab once daily po.
PROCTOCREAM-HC	Local Anesthetic-Corticosteroid	Cream: pramoxine HCl (1%), hydrocortisone acetate (1%)	Apply to the affected area as a thin film tid - qid.
PROCTOFOAM-HC	Local Anesthetic-Corticosteroid	Aerosol: pramoxine HCl (1%), hydrocortisone acetate (1%)	Apply to the affected area tid to qid.

QUADRINAL	Drug for COPD	**Tab:** theophylline calcium salicylate (130 mg; equivalent to 65 mg of theophylline base), ephedrine HCl (24 mg), potassium iodide (320 mg), phenobarbital (24 mg)	1 tab tid - qid po; if needed, an additional tab hs for nighttime relief.
QUELIDRINE	Decongestant-Expectorant-Antitussive-Antihistamine	**Syrup (per 5 mL):** ephedrine HCl (5 mg), phenylephrine HCl (5 mg), ammonium chloride (40 mg), ipecac fluidextract (0.005 mL), dextromethorphan HBr (10 mg), chlorpheniramine maleate (2 mg), alcohol (2%)	5 mL 1 to 4 times daily po.
QUIBRON QUIBRON-300	Drug for COPD	**Cpsl:** theophylline (150 mg), guaifenesin (90 mg) **Cpsl:** theophylline (300 mg), guaifenesin (180 mg)	Dose based on theophylline; see Oral Theophylline Doses Table, p. 312.
R & C	Pediculicide	**Shampoo:** pyrethrins (0.30%), piperonyl butoxide technical (3%)	Apply to dry hair and scalp or other affected areas. Use enough to completely wet area being treated; massage in. Allow the product to remain for 10 min. Rinse and towel dry. Repeat in 7 - 10 days if reinfestation occurs.
RID	Pediculicide	**Shampoo:** pyrethrum extract (0.33%), piperonyl butoxide (4%), related compounds (0.8%)	Same dosage and directions as for R & C Shampoo above.
RID MOUSSE	Pediculicide	**Mousse:** pyrethrum extract (0.33%), piperonyl butoxide (4%)	Same dosage and directions as for R & C Shampoo above.
RIFAMATE	Tuberculostatic	**Cpsl:** rifampin (300 mg), isoniazid (150 mg)	2 cpsl daily po, 1 hour before or 2 hours after a meal.
RIFATER	Tuberculostatic	**Tab:** rifampin (120 mg), isoniazid (50 mg), pyrazinamide (300 mg)	**Over 15 yrs and:** **≤ 44 kg:** 4 tab po once daily. **44-54 kg:** 5 tab po once daily. **≥ 55 kg:** 6 tab po once daily. Give on an empty stomach with a full glass of water.

253

TRADE NAME	THERAPEUTIC CATEGORY	DOSAGE FORMS AND COMPOSITION	COMMON ADULT DOSAGE
ROBITUSSIN COLD & CONGESTION	Decongestant-Antitussive-Expectorant	**Cplt & Softgel:** pseudoephedrine HCl (30 mg), dextromethorphan HBr (10 mg), guaifenesin (200 mg)	2 cplts (or softgels) q 4 h po.
ROBITUSSIN MAXIMUM STRENGTH COUGH & COLD LIQUID	Antitussive-Decongestant	**Syrup (per 5 mL):** dextromethorphan HBr (15 mg), pseudoephedrine HCl (30 mg)	10 mL q 6 h po.
ROBITUSSIN MULTI-SYMPTOM COLD & FLU	Decongestant-Antitussive-Expectorant-Analgesic	**Softgel:** pseudoephedrine HCl (30 mg), dextromethorphan HBr (10 mg), guaifenesin (100 mg), acetaminophen (250 mg) **Cplt:** pseudoephedrine HCl (30 mg), dextromethorphan HBr (10 mg), guaifenesin (200 mg), acetaminophen (325 mg)	2 softgels q 4 h po. 2 cplts q 4 h po.
ROBITUSSIN SEVERE CONGESTION	Decongestant-Expectorant	**Softgel:** pseudoephedrine HCl (30 mg), guaifenesin (200 mg)	2 Softgels q 4 h po.
ROBITUSSIN-CF	Antitussive-Decongestant-Expectorant	**Syrup (per 5 mL):** dextromethorphan HBr (10 mg), pseudoephedrine HCl (30 mg), guaifenesin (100 mg)	10 mL q 4 h po.
ROBITUSSIN-DM	Antitussive-Expectorant	**Syrup (per 5 mL):** dextromethorphan HBr (10 mg), guaifenesin (100 mg)	10 mL q 4 h po.
ROBITUSSIN-PE	Decongestant-Expectorant	**Syrup (per 5 mL):** pseudoephedrine HCl (30 mg), guaifenesin (100 mg)	10 mL q 4 h po.
RONDEC	Decongestant-Antihistamine	**Syrup (per 5 mL):** pseudoephedrine HCl (45 mg), brompheniramine maleate (4 mg) **Tab:** pseudoephedrine HCl (60 mg), carbinoxamine maleate (4 mg)	5 mL qid po. 1 tab qid po.
RONDEC-DM	Decongestant-Antihistamine-Antitussive	**Syrup (per 5 mL):** pseudoephedrine HCl (45 mg), brompheniramine maleate (4 mg), dextromethorphan HBr (15 mg)	5 mL qid po.
RONDEC-TR		**Timed-Rel. Tab:** pseudoephedrine HCl (120 mg), carbinoxamine maleate (8 mg)	1 tab bid po.

ROXICET	Analgesic	**Tab:** oxycodone HCl (5 mg), acetaminophen (325 mg). **Solution (per 5 mL):** oxycodone HCl (5 mg), acetaminophen (325 mg), alcohol (0.4%)	1 tab q 6 h po, prn pain. 5 mL q 6 h po, prn pain.
ROXICET 5/500	Analgesic	**Cplt:** oxycodone HCl (5 mg), acetaminophen (500 mg)	1 cplt q 6 h po, prn pain.
ROXILOX	Analgesic	**Cpsl:** oxycodone HCl (5 mg), acetaminophen (500 mg)	1 cpsl q 6 h po, prn pain.
ROXIPRIN	Analgesic	**Tab:** oxycodone HCl (4.5 mg), oxycodone terephthalate (0.38 mg), aspirin (325 mg)	1 tab q 6 h po, prn pain.
RYNA	Decongestant-Antihistamine	**Liquid (per 5 mL):** pseudoephedrine HCl (30 mg), chlorpheniramine maleate (2 mg)	10 mL q 4 - 6 h po.
RYNA-12	Decongestant-Antihistamine	**Tab:** phenylephrine tannate (25 mg), pyrilamine tannate (60 mg)	1 - 2 tabs q 12 h po.
RYNA-C (C-V)	Antitussive-Decongestant-Antihistamine	**Liquid (per 5 mL):** codeine phosphate (10 mg), pseudoephedrine HCl (30 mg), chlorpheniramine maleate (2 mg)	10 mL q 6 h po.
RYNATAN	Decongestant-Antihistamine	**Tab:** pseudoephedrine sulfate (120 mg), azatadine maleate (1 mg)	1 tab q 12 h po.
RYNATUSS	Decongestant-Antihistamine-Antitussive	**Tab:** phenylephrine tannate (10 mg), ephedrine tannate (10 mg), chlorpheniramine tannate (5 mg), carbetapentane tannate (60 mg)	1 - 2 tab q 12 h po.
SEMPREX-D	Decongestant-Antihistamine	**Cpsl:** pseudoephedrine HCl (60 mg), acrivastine (8 mg)	1 cpsl qid po.

TRADE NAME	THERAPEUTIC CATEGORY	DOSAGE FORMS AND COMPOSITION	COMMON ADULT DOSAGE
SEPTRA	Antibacterial	**Susp (per 5 mL):** sulfamethoxazole (200 mg), trimethoprim (40 mg) **Tab:** sulfamethoxazole (400 mg), trimethoprim (80 mg)	**Urinary Tract Infections:** 1 SEPTRA DS tab, 2 SEPTRA tab or 20 mL of Suspension q 12 h po for 10 - 14 days.
SEPTRA DS		**Tab:** sulfamethoxazole (800 mg), trimethoprim (160 mg)	**Shigellosis:** 1 SEPTRA DS tab, 2 SEPTRA tab or 20 mL of Suspension for 5 days. **Acute Exacerbations of Chronic Bronchitis:** 1 SEPTRA DS tab, 2 SEPTRA tab or 20 mL of Susp. q 12 h po for 14 days. ***P. carinii* Pneumonia Treatment:** 20 mg/kg trimethoprim and 100 mg/kg sulfamethoxazole per 24 h in equally divided doses q 6 h for 14 days. ***P. carinii* Pneumonia Prophylax.:** 1 SEPTRA DS tab, 2 SEPTRA tab or 20 mL of Suspension q 24 h po. **Travelers' Diarrhea:** 1 SEPTRA DS tab, 2 SEPTRA tab or 20 mL of Suspension q 12 h po for 5 days.
SEPTRA I.V. INFUSION	Antibacterial	**Inj (per 5 mL):** sulfamethoxazole (400 mg), trimethoprim (80 mg)	**Severe Urinary Tract Infections and Shigellosis:** 8 - 10 mg/kg daily (based on trimethoprim) in 2 - 4 equally divided doses q 6, 8 or 12 h by IV infusion for up to 14 days for UTI and 5 days for shigellosis. ***P. carinii* Pneumonia:** 15 - 20 mg/kg daily (based on trimethoprim) in 3 - 4 equally divided doses q 6 - 8 h by IV infusion for up to 14 days.

SER-AP-ES	Antihypertensive	**Tab:** reserpine (0.1 mg), hydralazine HCl (25 mg), hydrochlorothiazide (15 mg)	1-2 tab tid po.
SINEMET 10-100	Antiparkinsonian	**Tab:** carbidopa (10 mg), levodopa (100 mg)	The optimum daily dosage of SINEMET must be determined by careful titration in each patient. **Usual Initial Dosage:** 1 tab of SINEMET 25-100 tid po. If SINEMET 10-100 is used, the initial dosage may be 1 tab tid or qid po. The dosage of either preparation may be increased by 1 tab every day or every other day, prn, until 8 tab/day is reached.
SINEMET 25-100		**Tab:** carbidopa (25 mg), levodopa (100 mg)	**Maintenance:** At least 70 to 100 mg of carbidopa/day should be provided. When a greater proportion of carbidopa is required, 1 tab of SINEMET 25-100 may be substituted for each SINEMET 10-100.
SINEMET 25-250	Antiparkinsonian	**Tab:** carbidopa (25 mg), levodopa (250 mg)	**Maintenance Only:** At least 70 to 100 mg of carbidopa/day should be provided. When a larger proportion of levodopa is required, SINEMET 25-250 may be substituted for either of the above two products.
SINE-OFF NO DROWSINESS FORMULA	Decongestant-Analgesic	**Cplt:** pseudoephedrine HCl (30 mg), acetaminophen (500 mg)	2 cplt q 6 h po.
SINE-OFF SINUS MEDICINE	Decongestant-Antihistamine-Analgesic	**Tab:** pseudoephedrine HCl (30 mg), chlorpheniramine maleate (2 mg), acetaminophen (500 mg)	2 tab q 6 h po. up to 8 tab per day.

TRADE NAME	THERAPEUTIC CATEGORY	DOSAGE FORMS AND COMPOSITION	COMMON ADULT DOSAGE
SINUTAB NON-DRYING	Decongestant-Expectorant	Liquid Cpsl: pseudoephedrine HCl (30 mg), guaifenesin (200 mg)	2 cpsl q 4 h po, not to exceed 8 cpsl in 24 h.
SINUTAB SINUS ALLERGY MEDICATION, MAXIMUM STRENGTH	Decongestant-Antihistamine-Analgesic	Cplt & Tab: pseudoephedrine HCl (30 mg), chlorpheniramine maleate (2 mg), acetaminophen (500 mg)	2 cplt (or tab) q 6 h po.
SINUTAB SINUS, MAXIMUM STRENGTH WITHOUT DROWSINESS	Decongestant-Analgesic	Cplt & Tab: pseudoephedrine HCl (30 mg), acetaminophen (500 mg)	2 cplt (or tab) q 6 h po.
SLO-PHYLLIN GG	Drug for COPD	Syrup (per 15 mL): theophylline anhydrous (150 mg), guaifenesin (90 mg) Cpsl: theophylline anhydrous (150 mg), guaifenesin (90 mg)	Dose based on theophylline; see Oral Theophylline Doses Table, p. 312. Initially 16 mg/kg/day po, up to 400 mg/day in 3 - 4 divided doses q 6 - 8 h. At 3 day intervals, incr. if needed in 25% increments as tolerated.
SLOW FE WITH FOLIC ACID	Hematinic	Slow-Rel. Tab: dried ferrous sulfate (160 mg), folic acid (400 µg)	1 or 2 tab once daily po.
SOMA COMPOUND	Skeletal Muscle Relaxant-Analgesic	Tab: carisoprodol (200 mg), aspirin (325 mg)	1 - 2 tab qid po.
SOMA COMPOUND W/ CODEINE (C-III)	Skeletal Muscle Relaxant-Analgesic	Tab: carisoprodol (200 mg), aspirin (325 mg), codeine phosphate (16 mg)	1 - 2 tab qid po.
SUDAFED COLD & COUGH	Decongestant-Antitussive-Expectorant	Liquid Cpsl: pseudoephedrine HCl (60 mg), dextromethorphan HBr (10 mg), guaifenesin (100 mg)	2 cpsl q 4 h po.
SUDAFED COLD & SINUS	Decongestant-Analgesic	Liquid Cpsl: pseudoephedrine HCl (30 mg), acetaminophen (325 mg)	2 cpsl q 4 - 6 h po.
SULFACET-R MVL	Anti-Acne Agent	Lotion: sulfacetamide sodium (10%), sulfur (5%)	Apply a thin film to affected areas 1 to 3 times daily.

258

SYNALGOS-DC (C-III)	Analgesic	**Cpsl:** dihydrocodeine bitartrate (16 mg), aspirin (356.4 mg), caffeine (30 mg)	2 cpsl q 4 h po, prn pain.
SYNERCID	Antibacterial	**Powd for Inj:** quinupristin (150 mg), dalfopristin (350 mg)	**Vancomycin-resistant *E. faecium* Bacteremia:** 7.5 mg/kg q 8 h by IV infusion (over 60 min.). Duration of therapy dependent on site of infection and severity. **Complicated Skin and Skin-Structure Infections:** 7.5 mg/kg q 12 h by IV infusion (over 60 min.) for at least 7 days.
TALACEN (C-IV)	Analgesic	**Tab:** pentazocine HCl (equal to 25 mg pentazocine base), acetaminophen (650 mg)	1 tab q 4 h po, prn pain.
TALWIN COMPOUND (C-IV)	Analgesic	**Cplt:** pentazocine HCl (equal to 12.5 mg pentazocine base), aspirin (325 mg)	2 cplt tid or qid po, prn pain.
TALWIN NX	Analgesic	**Tab:** pentazocine HCl (equal to 50 mg pentazocine base), naloxone HCl (0.5 mg)	1 tab q 3 - 4 h po.
TARKA 2/180	Antihypertensive	**Tab:** trandolapril (2 mg), verapamil HCl ER (180 mg)	1 tab daily po.
TARKA 1/240		**Tab:** trandolapril (1 mg), verapamil HCl ER (240 mg)	1 tab daily po.
TARKA 2/240		**Tab:** trandolapril (2 mg), verapamil HCl ER (240 mg)	1 tab daily po.
TARKA 4/240		**Tab:** trandolapril (4 mg), verapamil HCl ER (240 mg) (ER = Extended-Release formulation)	1 tab daily po.
TAVIST SINUS	Decongestant-Analgesic	**Tab:** pseudoephedrine HCl (30 mg), acetaminophen (500 mg)	2 cplt q 6 h po.
TECZEM	Antihypertensive	**Extended-Rel. Tab:** enalapril maleate (5 mg), diltiazem malate (180 mg)	1 tab daily po.
TENORETIC 50	Antihypertensive	**Tab:** atenolol (50 mg), chlorthalidone (25 mg)	1 tab daily po.
TENORETIC 100		**Tab:** atenolol (100 mg), chlorthalidone (25 mg)	1 tab daily po.

259

TRADE NAME	THERAPEUTIC CATEGORY	DOSAGE FORMS AND COMPOSITION	COMMON ADULT DOSAGE
TEVETEN HCT 600 mg/12.5 mg TEVETEN HCT 600 mg/25 mg	Antihypertensive	**Tab:** eprosartan mesylate (600 mg), hydrochlorothiazide (12.5 mg) **Tab:** eprosartan mesylate (600 mg), hydrochlorothiazide (25 mg)	1 600/12.5 tab once daily po. After 2 - 3 weeks, the dosage may be increased to 1 600/25 tab once daily po. May add eprosartan 300 mg (TEVETEN) once daily in the PM if additional blood pressure control is needed at the trough.
THYROLAR 1/4	Thyroid Hormone	**Tab:** levothyroxine sodium (12.5 μg), liothyronine sodium (3.1 μg)	**Initial:** Usually 50 μg of levo-thyroxine po or its isocaloric
THYROLAR 1/2		**Tab:** levothyroxine sodium (25 μg), liothyronine sodium (6.25 μg)	**Initial:** Usually 50 μg of levo-thyroxine po or its isocaloric equivalent (THYROLAR 1/2),
THYROLAR 1		**Tab:** levothyroxine sodium (50 μg), liothyronine sodium (12.5 μg)	with increments of 25 μg q 2 to 3 weeks.
THYROLAR 2		**Tab:** levothyroxine sodium (100 μg), liothyronine sodium (25 μg)	**Maintenance:** Usually 100 - 200 μg/day po (THYROLAR 1 or THYROLAR 2).
THYROLAR 3		**Tab:** levothyroxine sodium (150 μg), liothyronine sodium (37.5 μg)	
TIMENTIN	Antibacterial	**Powd for Inj:** 3.1 g (3 g ticarcillin, 0.1 g clavulanic acid) **Inj:** 3.1 g (3 g ticarcillin, 0.2 g clavulanic acid)/100 mL	**Systemic and Urinary Tract Infections and ≥ 60 kg:** 3.1 g q 4 - 6 h by IV infusion. **Gynecologic Infections:** **Moderate and ≥ 60 kg:** 200 mg/kg/day in divided doses q 6 h by IV infusion. **Severe and ≥ 60 kg:** 300 mg/kg/day in divided doses q 4 h by IV infusion. **Adults < 60 kg:** 200 - 300 mg/kg/day in divided doses q 4 - 6 h by IV infusion.
TIMOLIDE 10-25	Antihypertensive	**Tab:** timolol maleate (10 mg), hydrochlorothiazide (25 mg)	1 tab bid po or 2 tab once daily.

TITRALAC PLUS	Antacid-Antigas Drug	**Chewable Tab:** calcium carbonate (420 mg), simethicone (21 mg)	Chew 2 tab q 2 - 3 h.
TOBRADEX	Antibacterial-Corticosteroid	**Ophth Suspension:** tobramycin (0.3%), dexamethasone (0.1%)	1 or 2 drops into affected eye(s) q 4 - 6 h. During the initial 24 to 48 h, the dosage may be raised to 1 or 2 drops q 2 h.
		Ophth Oint: tobramycin (0.3%), dexamethasone (0.1%)	Apply a small amount (1/2 in.) to the conjunctival sac tid or qid.
TRIAMINIC CHEST CONGESTION	Decongestant-Expectorant	**Liquid (per 5 mL):** pseudoephedrine HCl (15 mg), guaifenesin (50 mg)	20 mL q 4 - 6 h po.
TRIAMINIC COLD & ALLERGY	Decongestant-Antihistamine	**Liquid (per 5 mL):** pseudoephedrine HCl (15 mg), chlorpheniramine maleate (1 mg)	20 mL q 6 h po.
		Softchew Tab: pseudoephedrine HCl (15 mg), chlorpheniramine maleate (1 mg)	Chew 4 tabs q 4 - 6 h.
TRIAMINIC COLD & COUGH	Decongestant-Antihistamine-Antitussive	**Liquid (per 5 mL):** pseudoephedrine HCl (15 mg), chlorpheniramine maleate (1 mg), dextromethorphan HBr (5 mg)	20 mL q 6 h po.
		Softchew Tab: pseudoephedrine HCl (15 mg), chlorpheniramine maleate (1 mg), dextromethorphan HBr (5 mg)	Chew 4 tabs q 4 - 6 h.
TRIAMINIC COLD & NIGHT TIME COUGH	Decongestant-Antihistamine-Antitussive	**Liquid (per 5 mL):** pseudoephedrine HCl (15 mg), chlorpheniramine maleate (1 mg), dextromethorphan HBr (7.5 mg)	20 mL q 6 h po.
TRIAMINIC COLD, COUGH & FEVER	Decongestant-Antihistamine-Antitussive-Antipyretic	**Liquid (per 5 mL):** pseudoephedrine HCl (15 mg), chlorpheniramine maleate (1 mg), dextromethorphan HBr (7.5 mg), acetaminophen (160 mg)	20 mL q 6 h po.
TRIAMINIC COUGH	Decongestant-Antitussive	**Liquid (per 5 mL):** pseudoephedrine HBr (5 mg), dextromethorphan HBr (5 mg)	20 mL q 6 h po.
TRIAMINIC COUGH & CONGESTION	Decongestant-Antitussive	**Liquid (per 5 mL):** pseudoephedrine HCl (15 mg), dextromethorphan HBr (7.5 mg)	20 mL q 6 h po.

TRADE NAME	THERAPEUTIC CATEGORY	DOSAGE FORMS AND COMPOSITION	COMMON ADULT DOSAGE
TRIAMINIC COUGH & SORE THROAT	Decongestant-Antitussive-Analgesic	**Liquid (per 5 mL):** pseudoephedrine HCl (15 mg), dextromethorphan HBr (7.5 mg), acetaminophen (160 mg). **Softchew Tab:** pseudoephedrine HCl (15 mg), dextromethorphan HBr (5 mg), acetaminophen (160 mg)	20 mL q 6 h po. Chew 4 tabs q 4 - 6 h.
TRIAMINIC NIGHT TIME	Decongestant-Antihistamine-Antitussive	**Liquid (per 5 mL):** pseudoephedrine HCl (15 mg), chlorpheniramine maleate (1 mg), dextromethorphan HBr (7.5 mg)	20 mL q 6 h po.
TRIAVIL 2-10 TRIAVIL 2-25 TRIAVIL 4-10 TRIAVIL 4-25	Antipsychotic-Antidepressant	**Tab:** perphenazine (2 mg), amitriptyline HCl (10 mg) **Tab:** perphenazine (2 mg), amitriptyline HCl (25 mg) **Tab:** perphenazine (4 mg), amitriptyline HCl (10 mg) **Tab:** perphenazine (4 mg), amitriptyline HCl (25 mg)	**Psychoneuroses:** 1 tab TRIAVIL 2-25 or TRIAVIL 4-25 tid - qid po.
TRI-LEVLEN	Oral Contraceptive (Combination Triphasic)	**Tab:** 6 tabs: ethinyl estradiol (30 μg), levonorgestrel (0.05 mg); 5 tabs: ethinyl estradiol (40 μg), levonorgestrel (0.075 mg); 10 tabs: ethinyl estradiol (30 μg), levonorgestrel (0.125 mg) in 21-Day and 28-Day Compacts (contains 7 inert tabs)	21-Day regimen po or 28-Day regimen po.
TRILISATE	Non-Opioid Analgesic, Antipyretic, Antiinflammatory	**Tab:** choline magnesium salicylate (500 mg as: choline salicylate (293 mg) and magnesium salicylate (362 mg)) **Tab:** choline magnesium salicylate (750 mg as: choline salicylate (440 mg) and magnesium salicylate (544 mg)) **Tab:** choline magnesium salicylate (1000 mg as: choline salicylate (587 mg) and magnesium salicylate (725 mg)) **Liquid (per 5 mL):** choline magnesium salicylate (500 mg as: choline salicylate (293 mg) and magnesium salicylate (362 mg))	**Pain & Fever:** 1000 - 1500 mg bid po. **Inflammation:** 1500 mg bid po or 3000 mg once daily hs po.
TRINALIN REPETABS	Decongestant-Antihistamine	**Long-Acting Tab:** pseudoephedrine sulfate (120 mg), azatadine maleate (1 mg)	1 tab bid po.
TRI-NORINYL	Oral Contraceptive (Combination Triphasic)	**Tab:** 7 tabs: ethinyl estradiol (35 μg), norethindrone (0.5 mg); 9 tabs: ethinyl estradiol (35 μg), norethindrone (1 mg); 5 tabs: ethinyl estradiol (35 μg), norethindrone (0.5 mg) in 21-Day and 28-Day Wallettes (contains 7 inert tabs)	21-Day regimen po or 28-Day regimen po.

TRIPHASIL	Oral Contraceptive (Combination Triphasic)	**Tab:** 6 tabs: ethinyl estradiol (30 μg), levonorgestrel (0.05 mg); 5 tabs: ethinyl estradiol (40 μg), levonorgestrel (0.075 mg); 10 tabs: ethinyl estradiol (30 μg), levonorgestrel (0.125 mg) in 21-Day and 28-Day Pilpaks (contains 7 inert tabs)	21-Day regimen po or 28-Day regimen po.

TRIZIVIR	Antiviral	**Tab:** abacavir sulfate (300 mg), lamivudine (150 mg), zidovudine (300 mg)	**>40 kg:** 1 tab bid po.
TUINAL 100 MG (C-II)	Hypnotic	**Cpsl:** amobarbital sodium (50 mg), secobarbital sodium (50 mg)	1 cpsl po hs.
TUINAL 200 MG (C-II)		**Cpsl:** amobarbital sodium (100 mg), secobarbital sodium (100 mg)	1 cpsl po hs.
TUSSEND (C-III)	Decongestant-Antihistamine-Antitussive	**Syrup (per 5 mL):** pseudoephedrine HCl (30 mg), chlorpheniramine maleate (2 mg), hydrocodone bitartrate (2.5 mg), alcohol (5%)	10 mL q 4 - 6 h po.
TUSSIONEX (C-III)	Antihistamine-Antitussive	**Extended-Rel. Susp (per 5 mL):** chlorpheniramine polistirex (8 mg), hydrocodone polistirex (10 mg)	5 mL q 12 h po.
TUSSI-ORGANIDIN NR (C-V)	Antitussive-Expectorant	**Liquid (per 5 mL):** codeine phosphate (10 mg), guaifenesin (100 mg)	10 mL q 4 h po.
TUSSI-ORGANIDIN DM NR	Antitussive-Expectorant	**Liquid (per 5 mL):** dextromethorphan HBr (10 mg), guaifenesin (100 mg)	10 mL q 4 h po.
TUSSIZONE-12 RF	Antitussive-Antihistamine	**Tab:** carbetapentane tannate (60 mg), chlorpheniramine tannate (5 mg)	1 - 2 tab q 12 h po.
TYLENOL ALLERGY SINUS	Analgesic-Antihistamine-Decongestant	**Cplt, Gelcap & Geltab:** acetaminophen (500 mg), chlorpheniramine maleate (2 mg), pseudoephedrine HCl (30 mg)	2 cplt (or gelcap or geltab) q 4 - 6 h po. Do not exceed 8 cplt in 24 h.
TYLENOL ALLERGY SINUS NIGHTTIME	Analgesic-Decongestant-Sedative	**Cplt:** acetaminophen (500 mg), pseudoephedrine HCl (30 mg), diphenhydramine HCl (25 mg)	2 cplt hs po. May repeat q 4 - 6 h. Maximum: 8 cplt in 24 h.
TYLENOL COLD COMPLETE FORMULA	Analgesic-Antihistamine-Decongestant-Antitussive	**Cplt:** acetaminophen (325 mg), chlorpheniramine maleate (2 mg), pseudoephedrine HCl (30 mg), dextromethorphan HBr (15 mg)	2 cplt q 6 h po. Do not exceed 8 cplt in 24 h.

TRADE NAME	THERAPEUTIC CATEGORY	DOSAGE FORMS AND COMPOSITION	COMMON ADULT DOSAGE
TYLENOL COLD NON-DROWSY	Analgesic-Antitussive-Decongestant	Cplt & Gelcap: acetaminophen (325 mg), dextromethorphan HBr (15 mg), pseudoephedrine HCl (30 mg)	2 cplt (or gelcap) q 6 h po. Do not exceed 8 cplt in 24 h.
TYLENOL COLD SEVERE CONGESTION NON-DROWSY	Analgesic-Antitussive-Decongestant-Expectorant	Cplt: acetaminophen (325 mg), dextromethorphan HBr (15 mg), pseudoephedrine HCl (30 mg), guaifenesin (200 mg)	2 cplt (or gelcap) q 6 - 8 h po. Do not exceed 8 cplt in 24 h.
TYLENOL FLU NIGHTTIME	Analgesic-Decongestant-Sedative	Gelcap: acetaminophen (500 mg), pseudoephedrine HCl (30 mg), diphenhydramine HCl (25 mg) Liquid (per 15 mL): acetaminophen (500 mg), pseudo-ephedrine (30 mg), diphenhydramine HCl (25 mg)	2 gelcap hs po. May repeat q 6 h. Max: 8 gelcap in 24 h. 30 mL hs po. May repeat q 6 h.
TYLENOL FLU NON-DROWSY	Analgesic-Antitussive-Decongestant	Gelcap: acetaminophen (500 mg), dextromethorphan HBr (15 mg), pseudoephedrine HCl (30 mg)	2 gelcap q 6 h po. Do not exceed 8 gelcap in 24 h.
TYLENOL PM	Analgesic-Sedative	Cplt, Gelcap & Geltab: acetaminophen (500 mg), diphenhydramine HCl (25 mg)	2 cplt (or gelcap or geltab) hs po.
TYLENOL SEVERE ALLERGY	Analgesic-Antihistamine	Cplt: acetaminophen (500 mg), diphenhydramine HCl (12.5 mg)	2 cplt q 4 - 6 h po. Do not exceed 8 cplt in 24 h.
TYLENOL SINUS NIGHTTIME	Analgesic-Decongestant-Sedative	Cplt: acetaminophen (500 mg), pseudoephedrine HCl (30 mg), doxylamine succinate (6.25 mg)	2 cplt hs po. May repeat q 4 - 6 h. Maximum: 8 cplt in 24 h.
TYLENOL SINUS NON-DROWSY	Analgesic-Decongestant	Cplt, Tab, Gelcap & Geltab: acetaminophen (500 mg), pseudoephedrine HCl (30 mg)	2 cplt (or others) q 4 - 6 h po. Do not exceed 8 cplt in 24 h.
TYLENOL W/CODEINE (C-V)	Analgesic	Elixir (per 5 mL): acetaminophen (120 mg), codeine phosphate (12 mg), alcohol (7%)	15 mL q 4 h po, prn pain.
TYLENOL W/CODEINE #2 (C-III) #3 (C-III) #4 (C-III)	Analgesic	Tab: acetaminophen (300 mg), codeine phosphate (15 mg) Tab: acetaminophen (300 mg), codeine phosphate (30 mg) Tab: acetaminophen (300 mg), codeine phosphate (60 mg)	2 - 3 tab q 4 h po, prn pain. 1 - 2 tab q 4 h po, prn pain. 1 tab q 4 h po, prn pain.
TYLOX (C-II)	Analgesic	Cpsl: oxycodone HCl (5 mg), acetaminophen (500 mg)	1 cpsl q 6 h po, prn pain.

264

TYMPAGESIC	Analgesic (Topical)-Otic Decongestant	**Otic Solution (per mL):** benzocaine (5%), antipyrine (5%), phenylephrine HCl (0.25%)	Instill in ear canal until filled, then insert a cotton pledget moistened with solution into meatus. Repeat q 2 - 4 h.
ULTRACET	Analgesic	**Tab:** tramadol HCl (37.5 mg), acetaminophen (325 mg)	2 tabs q 4 - 6 h po.
UNASYN	Antibacterial	**Powd for Inj:** 1.5 g (1 g ampicillin sodium, 0.5 g sulbactam sodium) **Powd for Inj:** 3.0 g (2 g ampicillin sodium, 1 g sulbactam sodium)	1.5 - 3.0 g q 6 h by deep IM inj, by slow IV injection (over at least 10 - 15 min), or by IV infusion (diluted with 50 - 100 mL of a compatible diluent and given over 15 - 30 mins).
UNIRETIC 7.5/12.5	Antihypertensive	**Tab:** moexipril HCl (7.5 mg), hydrochlorothiazide (12.5 mg)	1 tab once daily po at least 1 h before a meal.
UNIRETIC 15/25		**Tab:** moexipril HCl (15 mg), hydrochlorothiazide (25 mg)	1 tab once daily po at least 1 h before a meal.
UNISOM WITH PAIN RELIEF	Analgesic-Sedative	**Tab:** acetaminophen (650 mg), diphenhydramine HCl (50 mg)	1 tab po, 30 minutes before retiring.
URISED	Urinary Analgesic	**Tab:** methenamine (40.8 mg), phenyl salicylate (18.1 mg), methylene blue (5.4 mg), benzoic acid (4.5 mg), atropine sulfate (0.03 mg), hyoscyamine (0.03 mg)	2 tab qid po.
VANOXIDE-HC	Anti-Acne Agent	**Lotion (per g):** benzoyl peroxide (50 mg), hydrocortisone acetate (5 mg)	Gently massage a thin film into affected skin areas 1 to 3 times daily.
VANQUISH	Analgesic	**Cplt:** aspirin (227 mg), acetaminophen (194 mg), caffeine (33 mg)	2 cplt q 4 h po. Maximum: 12 cplt in 24 h.
VASERETIC 5-12.5 VASERETIC 10-25	Antihypertensive	**Tab:** enalapril maleate (5 mg), hydrochlorothiazide (12.5 mg) **Tab:** enalapril maleate (10 mg), hydrochlorothiazide (25 mg)	1 - 2 tab once daily po. 1 - 2 tab once daily po.
VASOCIDIN	Antibacterial-Corticosteroid	**Ophth Solution:** sulfacetamide sodium (10%), prednisolone acetate (0.25%)	2 drops into affected eye(s) q 4 h. Prolong dosing interval as the condition improves.

265

TRADE NAME	THERAPEUTIC CATEGORY	DOSAGE FORMS AND COMPOSITION	COMMON ADULT DOSAGE
VICODIN (C-III) VICODIN ES (C-III)	Analgesic	**Tab:** hydrocodone bitartrate (5 mg), acetaminophen (500 mg) **Tab:** hydrocodone bitartrate (7.5 mg), acetaminophen (750 mg)	1 - 2 tab q 4 - 6 h po, prn pain. 1 tab q 4 - 6 h po, prn pain.
VICODIN HP		**Tab:** hydrocodone bitartrate (10 mg), acetaminophen (660 mg)	1 tab q 4 - 6 h po, prn pain.
VICODIN TUSS (C-III)	Antitussive-Expectorant	**Syrup (per 5 mL):** hydrocodone bitartrate (5 mg), guaifenesin (100 mg)	5 mL po after meals and hs (not less than 4 hours apart).
VICOPROFEN	Analgesic	**Tab:** hydrocodone bitartrate (7.5 mg), ibuprofen (200 mg)	1 tab q 4 - 6 h po, prn pain.
VOSOL HC	Antibacterial-Corticosteroid	**Otic Solution:** acetic acid (2%), hydrocortisone (1%)	Carefully remove all cerumen & debris. Insert a wick saturated with the solution into the ear canal. Keep in for at least 24 h and keep moist by adding 3 to 5 drops of solution q 4 - 6 h.
WIGRAINE	Antimigraine Agent	**Rectal Suppos:** ergotamine tartrate (2 mg), caffeine (100 mg)	Insert 1 rectally at the first sign of a migraine attack. Maximum: 2 suppositories for an individual attack.
		Tab: ergotamine tartrate (1 mg), caffeine (100 mg)	2 tab po at the first sign of a migraine attack; followed by 1 tab q 30 minutes, prn, up to 6 tabs per attack. Maximum of 10 tabs per week.
WYGESIC (C-IV)	Analgesic	**Tab:** propoxyphene HCl (65 mg), acetaminophen (650 mg)	1 tab q 4 h po, prn pain.
YASMIN	Oral Contraceptive (Combination Monophasic)	**Tab:** ethinyl estradiol (30 μg), drospirenone (3 mg) in 28-Day Packs (contains 7 inert tabs)	28-Day regimen po.
ZESTORETIC 10-12.5 ZESTORETIC 20-12.5 ZESTORETIC 20-25	Antihypertensive	**Tab:** lisinopril (10 mg), hydrochlorothiazide (12.5 mg) **Tab:** lisinopril (20 mg), hydrochlorothiazide (12.5 mg) **Tab:** lisinopril (20 mg), hydrochlorothiazide (25 mg)	1 - 2 tab once daily po. 1 - 2 tab once daily po. 1 - 2 tab once daily po.

ZIAC	Antihypertensive	**Tab:** bisoprolol fumarate (2.5 mg), hydrochlorothiazide (6.25 mg) **Tab:** bisoprolol fumarate (5 mg), hydrochlorothiazide (6.25 mg) **Tab:** bisoprolol fumarate (10 mg), hydrochlorothiazide (6.25 mg)	Initially, one 2.5/6.25 mg tab once daily po. Adjust dosage at 14 day intervals. Maximum: two 10/ 6.25 mg tabs once daily po.
ZOSYN	Antibacterial	**Powd for Inj:** 2.25 g (2 g piperacillin, 0.25 g tazobactam) **Powd for Inj:** 3.375 g (3 g piperacillin, 0.375 g tazobactam) **Powd for Inj:** 4.5 g (4 g piperacillin, 0.5 g tazobactam)	**Usual Dosage:** 12 g/1.5 g daily by IV infusion (over 30 min), given as 3.375 g q 6 h. **Nosocomial Pneumonia:** 3.375 g q 4 h by IV infusion (over 30 min) plus an aminoglycoside.
ZOVIA 1/35E	Oral Contraceptive (Combination Monophasic)	**Tab:** ethynodiol diacetate (1 mg), ethinyl estradiol (35 µg) in 21-Day and 28-Day Dispensers (contains 7 inert tabs)	21-Day regimen po or 28-Day regimen po.
ZOVIA 1/50E		**Tab:** ethynodiol diacetate (1 mg), ethinyl estradiol (50 µg) in 21-Day and 28-Day Dispensers (contains 7 inert tabs)	21-Day regimen po or 28-Day regimen po.
ZYDONE (C-III)	Analgesic	**Cpsl:** hydrocodone bitartrate (5 mg), acetaminophen (500 mg)	1 - 2 cpsl q 4 - 6 h po, prn pain.

C-II: Controlled Substance, Schedule II
C-III: Controlled Substance, Schedule III
C-IV: Controlled Substance, Schedule IV
C-V: Controlled Substance, Schedule V

267

Notes

DRUG

LEVELS

(Therapeutic, Toxic and Lethal)

Indicated by a (*) in the SELECTED INDIVIDUAL DRUG
PREPARATIONS Section (pp. 29 to 220).

Drug	Therapeutic Level	Toxic Level	Lethal Level
Acebutolol Hydrochloride	Peak plasma level: 0.74 µg/mL (with a 400 mg po dose). Mean steady-state plasma levels: 0.68 µg/mL (range, 0.33 to 1.24) (with 900 to 2000 mg daily po doses).	Toxicities reported with plasma levels of 15 µg/mL.	A fatality reported with a postmortem blood level of 21.5 µg/mL and a liver level of 127.8 µg/mL.
Acetaminophen	Plasma levels: 10 to 20 µg/mL.	Serum levels: > 300 µg/mL.	
Acetazolamide	Blood levels: 5 to 10 ng/mL.	Toxicities reported with serum levels between 26.48 µg/mL and 76.5 µg/mL and a whole blood level of 38.8 µg/mL.	
Acetohexamide	Serum level: 42 µg/mL (after chronic oral dosing with 500 mg).		
Acyclovir Acyclovir Sodium	Plasma acyclovir levels are dose dependent. Doses of 750 mg/m² /day have produced a plasma level of 10.3 µg/mL while doses of 2700 to 3000 mg/m²/day peaked at 36.3 µg/mL. Steady-state peak and trough concentrations ranging from 5.5 to 13.8 µg/mL and 0.2 to 1.0 µg/mL, respectively, were achieved in adults who received 5 mg/kg or approximately 250 mg/m² over 1 h by constant rate IV infusion every 8 hours.	Toxicities reported with a serum level of 190 µmoles/L and peak serum levels ranging from 90 to 470 µmoles/L.	
Albuterol Sulfate	Following 3 days of oral dosing (4 mg 5 times daily), pre-dose mean serum level was 8 ng/mL and the 4-hour post-dose level was 12 ng/mL.	Toxicity was reported with a plasma level of 160 µg/mL, 6 hours after ingestion.	
Alfentanil Hydrochloride	Plasma levels: 100 to 200 ng/mL (superficial surgery anesthesia) and 310 to 340 ng/mL (abdominal surgery anesthesia).	Toxicity reported with a blood level of 79 ng/mL.	
Allopurinol			A fatality was reported with a blood level of 230.8 µg/mL.

Alprazolam (C-IV)	Plasma levels: 20 to 40 ng/mL.	Plasma level: 350 ng/mL.
Amantadine Hydrochloride	Plasma levels: 0.3 to 0.6 μg/mL.	Plasma levels: >1 μg/mL.	Fatalities reported with a serum level of 23.4 μg/mL and plasma level of 1 μg/mL and greater.
Amikacin Sulfate	Peak serum levels: 20 - 35 μg/mL. Trough serum levels: less than or equal to 10 μg/mL.	Peak serum levels: >35 μg/mL. Trough serum levels: >5 μg/mL.
Aminocaproic Acid	Plasma level: 130 μg/mL.	
Aminosalicylic Acid	Serum levels: 20 to 60 μg/mL.	
Amiodarone Hydrochloride	Plasma levels: 0.6 to 2.5 μg/mL (amiodarone). No therapeutic range is established for the desethylamiodarone metabolite.	Toxicities reported with plasma levels ranging from 2.5 to 6.7 μg/mL for amiodarone and 1.0 to 1.5 μg/mL for desethylamiodarone. Plasma levels may not accurately predict toxicity.
Amitriptyline Hydrochloride	Plasma levels: 60 to 220 ng/mL.	Toxicities sometimes observed with plasma levels below 500 ng/mL. Serious symptoms are usually seen with levels greater than 1000 ng/mL.	Fatal tricyclic antidepressant levels reported from forensic studies have ranged from 1100 to 21800 ng/mL. A reported fatality had a blood level of 820 ng/mL, a urine level of 2580 ng/mL and a vitreous humor level of 6050 ng/mL.
Amlodipine Besylate	Serum levels: 10 to 15 ng/mL.	Toxicity reported with a peak serum level of 185 ng/mL.	One death reported had a postmortem blood level of 2.7 μg/mL.
Amoxapine	Serum levels: 10 to 100 ng/mL.	Toxicities reported with serum levels ranging from 650 to 2500 ng/mL.	Fatalities reported with blood levels ranging from 260 to 7100 ng/mL.
Amoxicillin	Peak serum level: 9 μg/mL.	
Amphetamine Sulfate (C-II)	Plasma level: 30 to 40 ng/mL.	

271

Drug	Therapeutic Level	Toxic Level	Lethal Level
Amphotericin B	Susceptible fungi are usually inhibited or killed by serum concentrations less than 10 µg/mL.	Toxic levels are unknown.	
Amphotericin B Cholesteryl	Susceptible fungi are usually inhibited or killed by amphotericin B serum concentrations less than 10 µg/mL.	Toxic levels are unknown.	
Amphotericin B Desoxycholate	Susceptible fungi are usually inhibited or killed by amphotericin B serum concentrations less than 10 µg/mL.	Toxic levels are unknown.	
Amphotericin B Lipid Complex	Susceptible fungi are usually inhibited or killed by amphotericin B serum concentrations less than 10 µg/mL.	Toxic levels are unknown.	
Amphotericin B Liposomal	Susceptible fungi are usually inhibited or killed by amphotericin B serum concentrations less than 10 µg/mL.	Toxic levels are unknown.	
Ampicillin Anhydrous	Peak po serum level: 4 µg/mL.		
Ampicillin Sodium	Peak IV serum level: 58 µg/mL.		
Ampicillin Trihydrate	Peak po serum level: 4 µg/mL.		
Aspirin	Serum levels: 150 to 300 µg/mL.	Serum levels: > 200 µg/mL.	
Atenolol	Plasma levels: 0.1 µg/mL to achieve a 15% reduction in exercise heart rate; 1.0 µg/mL to achieve a 30% reduction in exercise heart rate.	Toxicity reported with a blood level of 250 µg/mL.	
Atovaquone	Plasma level: 10 to 20 µg/mL.		
Atracurium Besylate	Plasma levels: 0.5 ± 0.1 µg/mL to achieve 50% depression of twitch tension; 1.2 ± 0.2 µg/mL to achieve 95% depression of twitch tension.		No lethal levels have been established; however, any level above the therapeutic range may be sufficient to cause respiratory paralysis, hypoxia, and death if respiratory assistance is not available.

272

Atropine Sulfate	Serum level: 200 ng/mL (with a 1 mg IV dose).	Toxicities reported with serum levels ranging from 7.5 to 130 ng/mL.
Auranofin	Plasma levels: 0.5 to 0.7 μg/mL.	
Azithromycin Dihydrate	Peak plasma level: 0.4 μg/mL (with a 500 mg loading dose); steady state peak plasma level: 0.24 μg/mL.	
Aztreonam	Peak serum levels: 164 μg/mL (with a 1 g dose) and 225 μg/mL (with a 2 g dose).	
Baclofen	Plasma level: 0.1 to 0.4 μg/mL.	Toxicities reported with a serum level of 17 μg/mL and a urine level of 760 μg/mL.
Benzonatate	No data are available.	A fatality was reported with a blood level of 35 μg/mL, a brain level of 22 μg /g, and a kidney level of 1.5 μg/g.
Benzphetamine HCl (C-III)	No data are available.	A fatality was reported with a postmortem blood level of 13.9 μg/mL.
Benztropine Mesylate	Plasma level: 6.7 ng/mL (after a 2 mg dose). Plasma steady-state levels: 80 to 125 ng/mL (after daily 4 mg po doses).	Toxicities reported with a peak serum level of 100 ng/mL and serum levels greater than 9 ng/mL.
Bepridil Hydrochloride	Serum levels: 1000 to 2000 ng/mL.	Not established.
Betaxolol Hydrochloride	Plasma levels: 20 to 50 ng/mL.	
Biperiden Hydrochloride	Plasma levels: 3.9 to 6.3 ng/mL (with a 4 mg dose).	Fatalities reported with blood levels of 200 to 1100 ng/mL.
Biperiden Lactate	Plasma levels: 3 to 13 ng/mL (with a 4 mg IV dose).	Fatalities reported with blood levels of 250 to 660 ng/mL.

Drug	Therapeutic Level	Toxic Level	Lethal Level
Bisacodyl		Toxicity reported in which the bisacodyl diphenol (bisacodyl metabolite) serum level was 1.05 µg/mL while the peak bisacodyl diphenol urine concentration was 91.2 µg/mL.	
Bretylium Tosylate		Toxic effects are not correlated with plasma concentrations; however, toxicities have been reported with plasma levels ranging from 8.8 to 17 µg/mL.	
Brompheniramine Maleate	Steady-state plasma levels: 18 ng/mL (trough) to 220 ng/mL (peak) after a 2 mg oral dose q 4 hours for 7 days.		
Buprenorphine HCl (C-V)	Plasma level: 0.5 ng/mL (with a 0.3 mg IV dose).		
Bupropion Hydrochloride	Serum levels: 0.025 to 0.2 µg/mL.	Toxicities reported with serum levels ranging from 220 ng/mL to 440 ng/mL.	One fatality was associated with a postmortem blood level of 700 ng/mL.
Buspirone Hydrochloride	A single 20 mg dose resulted in a mean maximum plasma level of 1.15 ng/mL (range, 0.49 to 3.07) at 0.5 to 1.0 hours with an additional second peak averaging 0.47 ng/mL (range, 0.21 to 1.03) between 2 and 4 hours after administration.		
Butorphanol Tartrate (C-IV)	Peak serum levels: 1.1 to 1.7 ng/mL (after 1 mg IV) and 1.3 to 2.2. ng/mL (after 2 mg IM).		
Caffeine	Peak plasma levels: 2.0 to 4.0 µg/mL (with a 120 mg po dose).	Toxicities reported with serum levels ranging from 40 to 400 µg/mL.	Fatalities reported with postmortem blood levels in excess of 80 µg/mL.
Calcitriol	Serum levels: 10 to 20 pg/mL.		
Calcium Carbonate	Serum levels: 90 to 104 µg/mL.	> 120 µg/mL.	

274

Captopril	Plasma levels: 0.5 to 1.3 µg/mL.	Toxicities reported with plasma levels ranging from 6 to 20 µg/mL.	A fatality was reported with a postmortem blood level of 60.4 µg/mL.
Carbamazepine	Plasma levels: 6 to12 µg/mL.	Toxicities reported with serum levels > 12 µg/mL.	A fatality was reported with a serum level of 54 µg/mL.
Carboplatin	A target AUC of 4 to 6 mg/mL/min.		No minimum lethal dose has been reported.
Carisoprodol	Average peak plasma level: 2.1 µg/mL (with a 350 mg po dose).	Toxicities reported with serum levels ranging from 6.5 to 39.3 µg/mL.	Lethal doses have not been established.
Cefaclor	Peak serum levels: 10 to 15 µg/mL.		
Cefadroxil Monohydrate	Peak serum levels: 12 to 16 µg/mL.		
Cefazolin Sodium	Peak serum levels: 80 to 110 µg/mL.		
Cefdinir	Peak serum level: 2.9 µg/mL (with a 600 mg po dose).		
Cefepime Hydrochloride	Peak serum level: 79 µg/mL.		
Cefixime	Peak serum level: 4.9 µg/mL.		
Cefonicid Sodium	Peak serum level: 220 µg/mL.		
Cefoperazone Sodium	Peak serum level: 125 µg/mL.		
Cefotaxime Sodium	Peak serum level: 40 µg/mL.		
Cefotetan Disodium	Peak serum levels: 140 to 180 µg/mL.		
Cefoxitin Sodium	Peak serum levels: 30 to 50 µg/mL.		
Cefpodoxime Proxetil	Peak serum level: 23 µg/mL.		
Cefprozil	Peak serum level: 10.5 µg/mL.		

Drug	Therapeutic Level	Toxic Level	Lethal Level
Ceftazidime	Peak serum level: 55 μg/mL.	Toxicities reported with serum levels ranging from 253 to 402 μg/mL.	
Ceftazidime Sodium			
Ceftibuten	Peak serum levels: 60 to 77 μg/mL.		
Cefizoxime Sodium	Peak serum levels: 75 to 90 μg/mL.		
Ceftriaxone Sodium	Peak serum level: 145 μg/mL.		
Cefuroxime Axetil	Peak serum level: 3.6 μg/mL.		
Cefuroxime Sodium	Peak serum level: 140 μg/mL.		
Cephalexin	Peak serum levels: 10 to 20 μg/mL.		
Cephalexin Hydrochloride	Peak serum levels: 10 to 20 μg/mL.		
Cephapirin Sodium	Peak serum levels: 10 to 20 μg/mL.		
Cephradine	Peak serum levels: 10 to 20 μg/mL (po); 15 to 30 μg/mL (IV).		
Cetirizine Hydrochloride	Peak plasma levels: 0.19 to 1.45 μg/mL (with a 10 mg po dose).	A toxicity reported with a blood level of 2.4 μg/mL.	
Chloral Hydrate (C-IV)	Plasma levels: 10 to 20 μg/mL (as the trichloroethanol metabolite).	100 μg/mL (as the trichloroethanol metabolite).	250 μg/mL (as the trichloroethanol metabolite).
Chloramphenicol	Plasma levels: 10 to 25 μg/mL.	Toxicities reported with plasma levels ranging from 50 to 200 μg/mL.	A fatality reported with a serum level of 277 μg/mL.
Chloramphenicol Sodium Succinate			
Chlordiazepoxide HCl (C-IV)	Plasma levels: 300 to 700 ng/mL.		
Chloroquine Hydrochloride	Plasma levels: 20 to 40 ng/mL.	Toxicities reported with serum levels ranging from 1.6 to 5 μg/mL.	Fatalities reported with blood levels ranging from 8 to 36 μg/mL.
Chloroquine Phosphate	Plasma levels: 20 to 40 ng/mL.	Toxicities reported with serum levels ranging from 1.6 to 5 μg/mL.	Fatalities reported with blood levels ranging from 8 to 36 μg/mL.

Chlorothiazide	Peak plasma levels: 0.4 to 0.9 μg/mL (with a 500 mg po dose).	
Chlorothiazide Sodium	Peak serum levels: 39 to 200 μg/mL (with a 500 mg IV dose).	
Chlorpheniramine Maleate	Plasma levels: 4 to 17 ng/mL.	
Chlorpromazine	Plasma levels: 100 to 300 ng/mL.	Plasma levels: 750 to 1000 ng/mL.
Chlorpropamide	Plasma peak level: 29 μg/mL (with a 250 mg po dose).	Serum levels > 400 μg/mL in the non-diabetic subject.
Cidofovir	Peak serum levels average 26.1 ± 3.2 μg/mL (after a 5 mg/kg IV infusion with concomitant probenecid and hydration).	
Cimetidine	Peak plasma levels: 0.3 to 4.4 μg/mL (with po doses from 200 to 800 mg).	Toxicities reported with serum levels as high as 57 μg/mL and trough levels exceeding 1.25 μg/mL.	No documented fatalities exist.
Ciprofloxacin	Peak serum levels: 4 to 6 μg/mL.	Toxic serum/plasma concentrations have not been established.
Cisplatin		Toxicity reported with a mean total platinum plasma level of 6.2 μg/mL.
Citalopram Hydrobromide	Peak plasma levels: 42 to 52 ng/mL (after a single 50 mg po dose). Mean steady-state plasma levels: 45 ng/mL (with 30 mg daily doses); 79 ng/mL (with 40 mg daily doses); 107 ng/mL (with 50 mg daily doses).		Fatalities reported with postmortem femoral blood levels of 4.8 to 6.1 μg/mL.
Clarithromycin	Steady-state peak plasma concentrations: 2 to 3 μg/mL (with a 500mg po dose).	

Drug	Therapeutic Level	Toxic Level	Lethal Level
Clindamycin Hydrochloride Clindamycin Palmitate HCl	Peak plasma concentrations: 2 to 3 μg/mL (with a 150 mg po dose).		
Clindamycin Phosphate	Peak plasma concentrations: 6 to 9 μg/mL (with 300 to 600 mg IM doses).		
Clofazimine	Peak serum concentrations: 0.5 to 2 μg/mL.		
Clomipramine Hydrochloride	Peak plasma levels: 75 to 150 ng/mL.	Toxicities reported with plasma levels above 300 ng/mL.	Fatal levels reported from forensic studies have ranged from 1.1 to 21.8 μg/mL.
Clonazepam (C-IV)	Plasma levels: 5 to 70 ng/mL.		
Clonidine Hydrochloride	Plasma levels: 0.2 to 2 ng/mL.	Plasma levels: 1 ng/mL.	A fatality reported with a postmortem blood level of 23 μg/mL.
Clorazepate Dipotassium (C-IV)	Plasma peak levels: 160 ng/mL (as nordiazepam with a 15 mg po dose).	Toxicities reported with serum levels (of nordiazepam) ranging from 700 to 5100 ng/mL.	
Cloxacillin Sodium	Plasma concentrations: 0.1 to 3 μg/mL.		
Clozapine	Serum levels: 70 to 400 ng/mL.	Toxicities reported with serum levels between 2.9 and 4.4 μg/mL.	Fatalities reported with blood levels between 1.9 and 9.4 μg/mL, and urine levels of 11.3 μg/mL.
Codeine Phosphate (C-II)	Plasma levels: 30 to 130 ng/mL.	Toxicities reported with serum levels between 1.4 and 5.6 μg/mL.	Fatalities reported with mean blood levels of 2.8 μg/mL (range, 1.0 to 8.8 μg/mL).
Colchicine	Peak plasma levels: 4.0 to 7.6 ng/mL (with a 1 mg po dose).	Toxicity has been associated with blood levels greater than 5 ng/mL.	A fatality reported with postmortem blood levels of 0.3 to 0.4 micromoles/L.
Cyclizine Hydrochloride	Peak blood level: 69 ng/mL (with a 50 mg po dose).		A fatality reported with a blood level of 80 μg/mL.
Cyclobenzaprine Hydrochloride	Blood levels: 10 to 40 ng/mL.		Fatalities reported with blood levels of 250 to 300 ng/mL.

Cyclosporine	Trough blood levels: 250 to 800 ng/mL (RIA). Trough plasma levels: 50 to 300 ng/mL (RIA).	Toxicities reported with plasma levels between 50 and 6700 ng/mL and blood levels of about 1800 ng/mL.	
Cytarabine, Conventional	Serum levels: 50 to 100 μg/mL.		
Dapsone		Toxicities reported with blood levels ranging from 22.3 to 120 μg/mL.	
Desipramine Hydrochloride	Plasma levels: 40 to 160 ng/mL.	Toxicity has been associated with plasma levels above 300 ng/mL.	Fatalities reported with blood levels from 3 to 22 μg/mL.
Dextroamphetamine Sulfate (C-II)	Peak blood levels: 35 ng/mL (with a 10 mg po dose).		
Dextromethorphan Hydrobromide	Peak serum levels: 0.1 to 2 ng/mL (with a 20 mg po dose).	Toxicities reported with serum levels of 100 ng/mL.	Fatalities reported with blood levels ranging from 3.3 to 9.2 μg/mL.
Diazepam (C-IV)	Plasma levels: 300 to 400 ng/mL (antianxiety); >600 ng/mL (anticonvulsant).		Fatalities reported with blood levels between 4 and 64.0 μg/mL.
Diazoxide	Plasma level: 35 μg/mL produces a 20% reduction in mean arterial pressure.		
Diclofenac Potassium	Peak plasma levels: 0.75 to 2.0 μg/mL (with a 50 mg dose).		
Diclofenac Sodium	Peak plasma levels: 0.75 to 2.0 μg/mL (with a 50 mg dose).	Toxicity reported with a serum level of 60 μg/mL.	
Dicloxacillin Sodium	Plasma levels: 0.05 to 0.8 μg/mL.		
Dicyclomine Hydrochloride	Plasma levels: 20 to 60 ng/mL.		
Didanosine	Peak serum levels: 1.1 ± 0.7 μg/mL (with a 375 mg po dose of the powder for solution).		The minimum lethal human dose has not been determined.
Diethylpropion HCl (C-IV)	Mean plasma level: 7 ng/mL (with a 75 mg po dose).		

Drug	Therapeutic Level	Toxic Level	Lethal Level
Diflunisal	Mean peak plasma levels: 62 µg/mL (range, 6.8 to 95 µg/mL) (with a 500 mg dose); 99 µg/mL (with a 750 mg dose). Trough steady state levels: 85 to 130 µg/mL (with chronic dosing of 500 mg twice daily).	Toxicities reported with plasma levels of 260 to 500 µg/mL.	One fatality reported with a postmortem blood level of 260 µg/mL.
Digoxin	Serum levels: 0.5 to 2.0 ng/mL.	Toxicities reported with serum levels greater than 2.0 ng/mL.	Fatalities reported with blood levels of 20 ng/mL.
Diltiazem Hydrochloride	Serum levels: 50 to 200 ng/mL.	Toxicities reported with serum levels of 114 ng/mL to 6.1 µg/mL.	Reported lethal levels have ranged from 6.7 to 33 µg/mL.
Diphenhydramine Hydrochloride	Mean plasma levels: >25 ng/mL (antihistaminic effect); 30 to 40 ng/mL (drowsiness).	Plasma levels: >60 ng/mL.	Fatalities reported with blood levels of 8 to 30 µg/mL.
Disopyramide Phosphate	Plasma levels: 2 to 6 µg/mL.	Toxicities reported with plasma levels ranging from 3.6 to 10 µg/mL.	Fatalities reported with plasma levels of approx. 16 µg/mL and whole blood levels ranging from 27 to 146 µg/mL.
Disulfiram	Blood levels: 2 to 10 µg/mL.	Toxicities reported with blood levels of approx. 17.4 µg/mL.	Fatalities reported with metabolite levels of 31 µg/mL (diethyldithiocarbamate) and 8 µg/mL (diethylamine).
Divalproex Sodium	Serum levels: 50 to 120 µg/mL.	Serum levels: >100 to 150 µg/mL.	
Dobutamine Hydrochloride	Plasma levels: >35 µg/mL (threshold change in cardiac output); >50 µg/mL (threshold change in heart rate).		
Doxazosin Mesylate	Plasma levels: 2.2 ± 0.5 ng/mL.		

Doxepin Hydrochloride	Plasma levels: 5 to 115 ng/mL (doxepin alone); 30 to 150 ng/mL (doxepin + desmethyldoxepin).	Toxicities reported with serum levels of 110 to 430 ng/mL (doxepin only).	Fatalities reported with blood levels of 0.7 to 29 µg/mL (doxepin only).
Doxycycline [Salts]	Maximum plasma level: 3 µg/mL. (2 hours after a 200 mg dose) and plasma level is maintained above 1 µg/mL for 8 to 12 hours.		
Doxylamine Succinate	Mean plasma levels: 100 ng/mL (range, 70 to 140 ng/mL).	One toxicity reported with a plasma level of 7.5 µg/mL.	Fatalities reported with postmortem blood levels of 0.7 to 12 µg/mL.
Dyphylline	Peak serum levels: 6.5 µg/mL (with a 5 mg/kg po dose) and 12 µg/mL (with a 15 mg/kg po dose).	The relationship between serum levels and the appearance of toxicity is not known. Peak serum levels of 19 to 30 µg/mL have been tolerated without adverse effects.	
Edrophonium Chloride	Plasma levels: < 0.15 µg/mL.		
Enalapril Maleate	Peak serum levels (enalapril): 20 to 95 ng/mL (with a 10 mg po dose). Peak serum levels (enalaprilat): 30 to 160 ng/mL (with chronic po dosing of 10 mg of enalapril).		
Enoxacin	Peak serum level: 5.5 µg/mL.	Toxic serum/plasma concentrations have not been established.	
Entacapone		Toxicity reported with peak plasma levels averaging 2.0 µg/mL.	
Ephedrine Sulfate	Serum levels: 0.04 to 0.08 µg/mL.	One toxicity reported with a serum level of 23 µg/mL.	Fatalities reported with blood levels of 3.5 to 21 µg/mL.
Ergotamine Tartrate	Serum levels: 200 pg/mL or greater may be therapeutic.	Serum levels: >1.8 ng/mL.	

281

Drug	Therapeutic Level	Toxic Level	Lethal Level
Erythromycin	Peak plasma levels: 0.3 to 0.5 μg/mL (with a 250 mg po dose) and 0.3 to 1.9 μg/mL (with a 500 mg po dose).		
Erythromycin Estolate	Peak plasma levels: 1.5 μg/mL (with a 250 mg po dose)and 4 μg/mL (with a 500 mg po dose).		
Erythromycin Ethylsuccinate	Peak plasma level: 1.5 μg/mL (with a 500 mg po dose).		
Erythromycin Gluceptate	Peak plasma level: approximately 10 μg/mL (with a 500 to 1000 mg IV dose).		
Erythromycin Lactobionate	Peak plasma level: approximately 10 μg/mL (with a 500 to 1000 mg IV dose).		
Erythromycin Stearate	Peak plasma levels: 0.3 to 0.5 μg/mL (with a 250 mg po dose) and 0.3 to 1.9 μg/mL (with a 500 mg dose).		
Esmolol Hydrochloride	Plasma levels: about 1 to 1.5 μg/mL.		
Estazolam (C-IV)	Mean peak plasma level: 55 ng/mL (range, 42 to 70 ng/mL) (with a 1 mg po dose).		
Estradiol	Serum levels for relief of menopausal symptoms: apparent over 40 ng/mL.; 80% relief with 68 ng/mL; 100% relief with 122 ng/mL. Serum levels for prevention of osteoporosis: 60 ng/mL.	Not determined.	
Estradiol Cypionate Estradiol Hemihydrate Estradiol Valereate	[See Estradiol above]	Not determined.	

Estrogens, Conjugated	[See Estradiol above]	Not determined.
Estrogens, A Synthetic Conjugated		
Estrogens, Esterified	[See Estradiol above]	Not determined.
Estropipate	Mean serum level: 34 ng/mL (with a 0.6 mg po dose and 42 ng/mL (with a 1.2 mg po dose).	Not determined.
Ethinyl Estradiol	[See Estradiol above]	Not determined.
Ethionamide	Peak serum levels: 1 to 5 μg/mL (with 250 to 500 mg po doses).	
Ethotoin	Steady state plasma levels: 5 to 14 μg/mL (with chronic po doses of 2 g/day).	
Etoposide	Serum levels at steady state are variable. One study reported serum levels of 2.7 μg/mL (with doses between 75 and 200 mg/m² as a 72 hour infusion).	Serum levels at steady state are variable. One study reported severe hematologic toxicity with serum levels of 4.7 μg/mL (with doses between 75 and 200 mg/m² as a 72 hour infusion).
Famciclovir	Peak serum levels (as the penciclovir metabolite): 0.84 ± 0.22 μg/mL (with a 125 mg po dose) and 3.34 ± 0.58 μg/mL (with a 500 mg po dose).	
Famotidine	Plasma levels: 20 to 150 μg/mL.	
Felbamate	Serum levels: 2.7 to 4.1 μg/mL (with a 200 mg po dose); 24 to 31 μg/mL (with chronic doses of 800 mg daily); 18 to 52 μg/mL (with chronic doses of 2300 mg daily). Mean plasma levels: 63 ± 18 μg/mL (with chronic doses of 3600 mg daily).	Toxicities reported with plasma levels ranging from 12 to 200 μg/mL (several hours post-ingestion).

283

Drug	Therapeutic Level	Toxic Level	Lethal Level
Fenoprofen Calcium	Mean peak plasma levels: 27 µg/mL (range, 23 to 31 µg/mL (with a 250 mg po dose).	One toxicity reported with a blood level of 711 µg/mL.	
Fentanyl (C-II) Fentanyl Citrate (C-II)	Plasma levels: 1 ng/mL (postoperative analgesia) and 3 ng/mL (intraoperative analgesia). Peak plasma levels of 3.0 ng/mL (with oral transmucosal) and 1.6 ng/mL (with oral solution) IV use: 10 fold increase in peak plasma levels.		Fatalities reported with serum levels between 2.5 and 17.7 ng/mL and whole blood levels between 4.9 and 27.5 ng/mL.
Ferrous Gluconate (11.6% iron) Ferrous Sulfate (20% iron)	Serum iron levels: 0.65 to 1.70 µg/dL (for adult males) and 0.50 to 1.70 µg/dL (for adult females).	Toxicities reported with serum iron levels ranging from 3.0 to 23.85 µg/dL.	
Fexofenadine Hydrochloride	Mean peak plasma level: 210 ng/mL (with an 80 mg po dose).		
Flecainide Acetate	Serum levels: 175 to 870 ng/mL.	Toxicities reported with serum levels ranging from 200 to 2500 ng/mL.	Fatalities reported with serum levels of 3300 ng/mL and whole blood levels ranging from 16.3 to 100 µg/mL.
Fluconazole	Peak plasma levels: 4 to 8 µg/mL (with repetitive100 mg po doses).	Toxicities reported with serum levels ranging from 6.5 to 15.1 µg/mL.	
Flucytosine	Plasma levels: 35 to 70 µg/mL.	Plasma levels: >100 µg/mL.	
Flumazenil	Plasma levels: >5 ng/mL. Studies suggest that 10 to 20 ng/mL will reverse benzodiazepine-induced CNS depression.		
Fluorouracil	Mean plasma level: 13 µg/mL (range, 6.5 to 30 µg/mL) (with approx. 4 mg/kg IV dose).		

Fluoxetine Hydrochloride	Peak plasma levels: 15 to 55 ng/mL (with a 40 mg po dose). Steady state plasma levels: 103 to 282 ng/mL of fluoxetine and 47 to 181 ng/mL of norfluoxetine (with a 60 mg po dose).	A toxicity reported with a serum level of 1956 ng/mL.	Fatalities reported with plasma levels between 1.9 and 4.6 $\mu g/ML$ and whole blood levels of 0.8 to 6.0 $\mu g/mL$.
Fluphenazine Decanoate	Peak plasma levels: 2.0 to 20 ng/mL (with a 25 mg IM dose); declining to 0.5 ng/mL by 12 to 24 hours. Steady-state plasma levels: 0.9 to 3.5 ng/mL (with chronic 12.5 mg IM doses); 4.7 to 7.3 ng/mL (with chronic 25 mg doses); 5.1 to 16.8 ng/mL (with chronic 50 mg doses).		
Fluphenazine Hydrochloride	Peak plasma levels: 0.26 to 1.1 ng/mL (with a 5 mg po dose).		
Flurazepam Hydrochloride (C-IV)	Plasma peak levels: 2.1 ng/mL (with a 30 mg po dose).		A fatality reported with a blood level of 5.5 $\mu g/mL$.
Flurbiprofen	Plasma levels: 4 to 14 $\mu g/mL$.		
Fluvoxamine Maleate	Peak plasma levels: 8.4 to 28 ng/mL (with a 50 mg po dose).	Toxicity reported with a serum level of 1.5 $\mu g/mL$.	
Fosphenytoin Sodium	Fosphenytoin serum level monitoring is not clinically useful. Phenytoin serum levels correlate with efficacy and toxicity. Serum levels (phenytoin): 10 to 20 $\mu g/mL$.	Serum levels (phenytoin): >20 $\mu g/mL$.	
Furosemide	Serum levels do not reflect diuretic activity.	Serum levels: >25 $\mu g/mL$.	
Gabapentin	Not established. Reported therapeutic serum levels range from 2.0 to 8.0 $\mu g/mL$.	Toxicities reported with serum levels ranging from 16.4 to 60 $\mu g/mL$.	

285

Drug	Therapeutic Level	Toxic Level	Lethal Level
Gentamicin Sulfate	Peak serum levels: 6 to 12 μg/mL. Trough levels: less than or equal to 2.0 μg/mL.	Peak serum level: > 12 μg/mL. Trough serum level: > 2 μg/mL.	
Glyburide	Serum Levels: 40 to 50 ng/mL.		
Guaifenesin	Peak blood levels: 1.4 μg/mL (with a 600 mg po dose).		
Guanethidine Monosulfate	Adrenergic blockade occurs with a minimum plasma level of 8 ng/mL.		
Haloperidol	Plasma levels: 4 to 20 ng/mL.		
Heparin Sodium	Plasma levels of 0.4 units/mL have resulted in APTT of 11 to 57/seconds.		
Hydralazine Hydrochloride	Plasma levels: 90 to 130 ng/mL.		
Hydrochlorothiazide	Mean peak plasma levels: 140 ng/mL (with a 25 mg po dose); 260 ng/mL (with a 50 mg po dose); 375 ng/mL (with a 75 mg po dose). Mean plasma levels: 17 ng/mL (with chronic 25 mg po doses) and 34 ng/mL (with chronic 75 mg po doses).		
Hydromorphone HCl (C-II)	Plasma levels: 1 to 32 ng/mL.		Fatalities reported with postmortem blood levels of 20 to 1200 ng/mL.
Hydroxyzine Hydrochloride	Serum levels: 6 to 42 ng/mL.		One fatality reported with a blood level of 1.1 μg/mL.
Ibuprofen	Plasma levels: 20 to 30 μg/mL.	Toxicities reported with plasma levels ranging from 80 to 360 μg/mL.	Fatalities reported with blood levels ranging from 81 to 440 μg/mL.

Imipramine Hydrochloride	Plasma levels: 150 to 250 ng/mL (imipramine + desipramine metabolite).	Toxicities reported with plasma levels of 400 ng/mL (imipramine + desipramine).	Fatalities reported with blood levels between 6.0 and 8.5 μg/mL (imipramine) and 0.5 to 7.8 μg/mL (desipramine metabolite).
Inamrinone Lactate	Steady state plasma level: about 3 μg/mL.	Toxic plasma levels have not been established.	
Indomethacin	Plasma levels: 0.3 to 3 μg/mL (po dose).	Plasma levels: > 5 μg/mL.	
Insulin Insulin Glargine Insulin Lispro	Diabetics vary widely in their response to insulin, and serum levels are not normally monitored clinically.		
Interferon alfa-2a	Peak serum levels following a single dose of 36 million units: 10,400 to 17,470 pg/mL (with a 40 minute IV infusion); 1668 to 2372 pg/mL (with an IM dose); 1253 pg/mL (with a SC dose).	Toxic serum levels have not been determined.	
Isoniazid	Peak serum levels: 3 to 5 μg/mL (with a 300 mg po dose).	Toxicities reported with blood levels greater than 10 μg/mL.	Fatalities reported with postmortem blood levels of 43 to 168 μg/mL.
Isoproterenol Hydrochloride	Peak plasma level: 0.4 ng/mL (with a 4.4 μg/70 kg IV dose).		
Isosorbide Dinitrate	Peak plasma levels : 3.1 to 8.9 ng/mL (with a 5 mg po dose).		
Ivermectin	Serum levels: 4 to 5 ng/mL at 4 hours (with a 30 μg/kg dose); 9 to 13 ng/mL at 4 hours (with a 50 μg/kg dose). A 150 mg/kg single oral dose resulted in mean serum levels of 16.4 ng/mL (at 24 hours) and 6.6 ng/mL (at 48 hours).		

287

Drug	Therapeutic Level	Toxic Level	Lethal Level
Ketoconazole	Peak plasma levels: 2 to 6 μg/mL (in 2 to 4 hours).		
Ketoprofen	Peak plasma levels: 1.9 to 8.4 μg/mL (with a 50 mg po dose) and 4.1 to 11.3 μg/mL (with a 100 mg po dose).	Toxicity reported with a serum level of over 1100 μg/mL (3 to 4 hours after ingestion).	
Ketorolac Tromethamine	Peak plasma levels: 0.87 μg/mL (with a 10 mg po dose); 1.0 to 1.4 μg/mL (with a 15 mg IM dose) and 2.2 to 3.0 μg/mL (with a 30 mg IM dose).	Plasma levels: >5 μg/mL.	
Labetalol Hydrochloride	Mean steady state serum levels: 36 to 183 ng/mL (with chronic 200 mg daily po doses) and 84 to 205 ng/mL (with chronic 400 mg daily po doses).	Serum levels: >500 ng/mL.	
Lamotrigine	A target plasma therapeutic range has not been established. Putative therapeutic plasma levels are estimated to be in the range of 1 to 3 μg/mL. Mean plasma concentrations were reported to be 3.2 and 3.0 μg/mL at 2 and 6.5 hours, respectively, following 300 mg doses in healthy volunteers.	Toxicities reported with serum levels of 6.4 to 52.5 μg/mL.	

Levofloxacin	Peak serum levels: 0.7 $\mu g/mL$ (with a 500 mg po dose) and; 6.4 $\mu g/mL$ (with a 500 mg IV dose).	Toxic serum levels have not been established.
Levonorgestrel	Maximum plasma levels: 3 to 5 ng/mL (after po use) and 0.2 ng/mL (minimum effective concentration for a SC implant).	
Levorphanol Tartrate (C-II)	Plasma levels: 2 to 6 ng/mL (after a 2 mg IV dose).	A fatality reported at a postmortem blood level of 800 ng/mL (after a 30 mg po dose).
Levothyroxine Sodium	Correlation of serum values and clinical symptoms is poor.	High levels of T4 do not necessarily assure toxicity. A toxicity reported had free T4 serum levels ranging from >130 ng/mL (on Day 6) to 12 ng/mL (on Day 12).
Lidocaine Hydrochloride	Plasma levels:1.5 to 5 $\mu g/mL$.	Toxicities reported with plasma levels of 5 to 10 $\mu g/mL$. Fatalities have occurred at plasma levels > 15 $\mu g/mL$.
Lindane	Serum levels: <2 ng/mL.	Toxic blood levels: 500 ng/mL. One toxicity reported with a serum level of 42.7 ng/mL.
Liothyronine Sodium	Correlation of serum values and clinical symptoms is poor.	High levels of T3 do not necessarily assure toxicity.
Lisinopril	Plasma levels: 20 to 70 ng/mL.	One toxicity reported with plasma levels ranging from 200 to 500 ng/mL.

289

Drug	Therapeutic Level	Toxic Level	Lethal Level
Lithium Carbonate Lithium Citrate	Serum levels: 0.6 to 1.2 mEq/L.	Toxicity does not necessarily correspond with serum levels in an acute lithium overdose and any of the signs and symptoms may occur first. Toxicities reported with serum levels of 6.8 mEq/L and whole blood levels ranging from 1.5 to 4 mEq/L.	Fatalities reported with serum levels > 3 to 4 mEq/L and whole blood levels of about 2.0 mEq/L.
Lomefloxacin Hydrochloride	Peak serum level: 25 μg/mL (with a 400 mg po dose).	Toxic serum levels have not been established.	
Loracarbef	Peak serum level: 6.8 μg/mL (with a 200 mg po dose).		
Loratadine	Peak plasma level: 4.7 ng/mL (with a 10 mg po dose).		
Lorazepam	Plasma levels: 9 to 18 ng/mL (with a 2 mg po dose).		
Loxapine Hydrochloride	Serum levels: 10 to 210 ng/mL.	Toxicity reported with serum levels of above 200 ng/mL.	Fatalities reported with blood levels of 2 to 3 μg/mL.
Maprotiline Hydrochloride	Mean steady state serum level: 350 ng/mL (range, 150 to 700 ng/mL) (with chronic 150 mg po doses).	Toxicities reported with serum levels of 237 to 317 ng/mL and plasma levels of 450 to 800 ng/mL.	Fatalities reported with blood levels of 1300 ng/mL.
Mebendazole		Serum levels have yet to be correlated with toxic effects; however, toxicities reported with serum levels of 239 ng/mL.	
Meclizine Hydrochloride		A toxicity reported with a serum level of 10 ng/mL.	
Medroxyprogesterone Acetate	Serum levels: > 0.1 ng/mL (for inhibition of ovulation and tumor response).		

Mefenamic Acid	Mean peak plasma level: 10 µg/mL (with a 1000 mg po dose).	Toxicities reported with plasma levels of 11 to 150 µg/mL.	
Meperidine Hydrochloride (C-II)	Plasma levels: 0.4 to 0.7 µg/mL.		Fatalities reported with blood levels ranging from 1 to 20 µg/mL.
Mephobarbital (C-IV)	Mean plasma levels: 2.5 to 3.5 µg/mL (with a daily po dose of 800 mg).		
Meprobamate (C-IV)	Plasma levels: 5 to 20 µg/mL.	Toxicities reported with plasma levels above 70 µg/mL.	Fatalities reported with blood levels above 120 µg/mL.
Meropenem	Peak serum level: 55 µg/mL.		
Mesoridazine Besylate	Mean plasma level: 0.51 µg/mL (range, 0.10 to 1.1) (with a 2 µg/kg IM dose).		Fatalities reported with blood levels of 16 µg/mL, plasma levels of 3 µg/mL, and serum levels of 4 µg/mL.
Metformin Hydrochloride	Plasma levels: 236 to 718 ng/mL.	Toxicities reported with plasma levels of 45 to 70 µg/mL.	
Methadone Hydrochloride (C-II)	Plasma levels: < 100 ng/mL (in non-tolerant patients) and 500 to 1000 ng/mL (in tolerant subjects).		Fatalities reported with blood levels ranging from 400 to 1800 ng/mL.
Methamphetamine HCl (C-II)	Plasma levels: 20 to 30 ng/mL.		Blood levels: 1.5 to 2.0 µg/mL.
Methimazole	Serum levels: <0.2 µg/mL inhibits iodide organification.		
Methocarbamol	Mean peak plasma level: 41 µg/mL (with a 4000 mg daily po dose).		Lethal levels have not been established; however, fatalities reported with blood levels between 250 and 525 µg/mL.
Methotrexate Sodium	Initial serum levels: 10 to 1000 µmol/L (after an IV dose of 1 to 15 g/m²).		Toxicities reported with serum levels above 1×10^{-8} Molar; blood levels ranging from 1.2 to 575 µmol/L.

Drug	Therapeutic Level	Toxic Level	Lethal Level
Methsuximide	Mean plasma level: 6.8 µg/mL (with a 1200 mg daily po dose).	Toxicities reported with plasma levels above 18 µg/mL of methsuximide and 40 µg/mL of normethsuximide metabolite.	
Methyldopa	There is no correlation between serum levels and therapeutic effect. Reported serum levels are between 2 and 3 µg/mL with po doses of 250 to 750 mg daily.		Fatalities reported with serum levels of 7.2 to 9.4 µg/mL.
Methyldopate Hydrochloride	There is no correlation between serum levels and therapeutic effect. Reported serum levels are between 1 and 2 µg/mL with IV injection of 250 mg.		
Methylergonovine		Toxicity may not easily be correlated to the serum level and quantitative blood levels are not clinically useful. Reported toxicities yielded serum levels ranging from 0.07 to 1.9 ng/mL.	
Methylphenidate HCl (C-II)	Plasma levels: 5 to 40 ng/mL.		
Metoprolol Tartrate	Blood levels: 60 to 100 ng/mL. Plasma levels: 20 to 35 ng/mL.	A toxicity reported with a plasma level of 5.3 µg/mL.	Fatalities reported with blood levels between 20 and 75 µg/mL.
Metronidazole	Plasma levels: 3 to 6 µg/mL.		
Mexiletine Hydrochloride	Plasma levels: 0.5 to 2 µg/mL.		
Midazolam Hydrochloride (C-1V)	Plasma levels: 50 ± 20 ng/mL.		Fatality reported with a postmortem blood level of 2.4 µg/mL.
Minoxidil	Mean serum levels: 32.8 ng/mL (with a 2.5 mg po dose) and 59.2 ng/mL (with a 5 mg po dose); 1.1 ng/mL (with 1% used topically) and 1.7 ng/mL (with 2% used topically).	A toxicity reported with a serum level of 3.1 µg/mL.	

Mirtazapine	Therapeutic serum levels have not been well established; however, reported mean serum levels of approximately 70 ng/mL were derived from steady state blood levels of patients maintained on 60 mg daily in studies.	Toxicities reported with plasma levels ranging from 368 to 2300 ng/mL.
Modafinil	Mean plasma level: 4.8 μg/mL (at 2 hours) (with a 200 mg po dose).	
Molindone Hydrochloride	Serum levels: 44 to 374 ng/mL.	Toxic levels are controversial and not well documented. Toxicities reported with serum levels ranging from 152 to 374 ng/mL. One fatality reported with a blood level of 9.3 μg/mL.
Montelukast Sodium	Plasma levels: > 5 ng/mL.	
Moricizine Hydrochloride	Correlation between serum levels and therapeutic effect is not well established; however, serum levels of 0.2 to 3.6 μg/mL have been suggested.	
Morphine Sulfate (C-II)	Plasma levels: 65 ± 80 ng/mL.	Fatalities reported with blood levels of 200 to 2300 ng/mL.
Nabumetone	Little or no parent drug is found in plasma after po administration. Peak levels of the active metabolite, 6-methoxy-2-naphthylacetic acid, average 22 μg/mL after a single 1000 mg po dose and 34 μg/mL after chronic po dosing.	
Nadolol	Serum levels: 100 to 340 ng/mL.	A toxicity reported with a serum level of 1300 ng/mL.
Nafcillin Sodium	Plasma levels: 0.06 to 2.0 μg/mL.	
Nalbuphine Hydrochloride	Peak plasma levels: 38 to 59 ng/mL (after a 10 mg IM dose).	

293

Drug	Therapeutic Level	Toxic Level	Lethal Level
Nalidixic Acid	Plasma levels: 20 to 50 µg/mL.		
Naloxone Hydrochloride	Peak plasma level: 10 ng/mL (with a 0.4 mg IV dose).		
Naltrexone Hydrochloride	Peak plasma level: 9.0 ng/mL (with a 50 mg po dose).		
Naproxen	Serum levels: 400 to 900 µg/mL.	Toxicities reported with serum levels ranging from 400 to 13000 µg/mL.	
Nefazodone Hydrochloride	Mean peak plasma levels: 390 ng/mL (with a 200 mg po dose) and 2000 ng/mL (with chronic 200 mg po dose q 12 hours).		
Netilmicin Sulfate	Peak serum levels: 6 to 12 µg/mL. Trough serum levels: less than or equal to 2.0 µg/mL.	Peak serum levels: > 16 µg/mL. Trough serum levels: > 4 µg/mL.	
Nicardipine Hydrochloride	Steady state plasma levels: 36 ng/mL (with 20 mg po dosing); 88 ng/mL (with 30 mg po dosing); 133 ng/mL (with 40 mg po dosing).		
Nicotine	Serum levels: 4 to 440 ng/mL of nicotine and 35 to 250 ng/mL of the metabolite cotinine (with transdermal patch delivering 22 mg of nicotine per day).		A fatality reported with a blood level of 1.4 µg/mL of nicotine and 1.3 µg/mL of cotinine (from transdermal patch).
Nicotine Polacrilex	Plasma levels: 12 ng/mL (with chewing 2 mg doses) and 23 ng/mL (with chewing 4 mg doses).		
Nifedipine	Plasma levels: 45 ± 20 µg/mL.		
Nisoldipine	Mean peak plasma levels: 1.0, 1.4, and 2.5 ng/mL (with 10, 20, and 40 mg sustained release po doses, respectively).		

Nitroglycerin	Plasma levels: 1.2 to 11 ng/mL.	
Nizatidine	Mean plasma level: 60 ng/mL.	
Norethindrone	Serum level: 0.4 ng/mL (ovulation inhibition).	
Norethindrone Acetate	Serum level: 0.4 ng/mL (ovulation inhibition).	
Norfloxacin	Peak serum levels: 1.4 to 1.6 µg/mL (with a 400 mg po dose).	Toxic serum levels have not been established.
Nortriptyline Hydrochloride	Plasma levels: 100 to 260 ng/mL.	Toxicities reported with plasma levels above 300 ng/mL.
Ofloxacin	Peak serum levels: 3.5 to 5.3 µg/mL (with a 400 mg po dose).	Toxic serum levels have not been established. One toxicity reported with a 3 g overdose had serum levels of 39.3 µg/mL (at 15 minutes), 16.2 µg/mL (at 7 hours) and 2.7 µg/mL (at 24 hours).
Olanzapine	Serum levels: 9 to 23 ng/mL.	Toxicities reported with serum levels ranging from 11 to 640 ng/mL.
Omeprazole	Mean peak plasma level: 0.56 µg/mL (range, 0.22 to 1.15 µg/mL) (with a 30 mg po dose).	
Ondansetron Hydrochloride	Mean peak plasma level: 26 ng/mL (range, 22 to 32 ng/mL) (with an 8 mg po dose).	The minimum lethal human dose to this agent has not been delineated.
Orlistat	Plasma levels are reported to be greater than 4 ng/mL and less than 50 ng/mL.	
Orphenadrine Citrate	Serum levels: <0.2 µg/mL.	Toxicity begins at 2 to 3 µg/mL.
Oxacillin Sodium	Plasma levels: 0.4 to 6 µg/mL.	
Oxazepam (C-IV)	Mean peak serum levels: 310 ng/mL (with a 15 mg po dose).	

Drug	Therapeutic Level	Toxic Level	Lethal Level
Oxycodone Hydrochloride (C-II)	Mean peak plasma levels: 30 ng/mL (range, 13 to 46 ng/mL) (with a 10 mg po dose).		A fatality reported with a blood level of 5000 ng/mL.
Oxytetracycline	Peak plasma levels: 2 to 2.5 μg/mL.		
Pancuronium Bromide	Plasma levels: 0.25 ± 0.07 μg/ML and 0.4 μg/mL (50% and 95% decrease in twitch tension, respectively).		No lethal doses have been established; however, any dose above the therapeutic range may be sufficient to cause respiratory paralysis, hypoxia, and death if respiratory assistance is not available.
Papaverine Hydrochloride	Mean plasma levels: 120 to 245 ng/mL (with a 150 mg po dose).		
Paroxetine Hydrochloride	Peak steady state serum level: 60 ng/mL (with 30 mg daily po dose).	Toxicity reported with a serum level of 410 ng/mL.	Fatalities reported with postmortem blood levels of 1.4 to 3.8 μg/mL.
Pemoline (C-IV)	Plasma levels: 1 to 7 μg/mL.		
Penicillin G Benzathine	Peak serum levels: 0.063 μg/mL (with a 600,000 unit IM dose).		
Penicillin G Potassium	Peak serum levels: 1.5 to 2.7 μg/mL (with a 500 mg IV dose).	Toxicity reported with a serum level of 433 μg/mL (2 hours after the IV injection of 10 million units (6 grams).	
Penicillin G Procaine	Peak serum level: 0.9 μg/mL (with a 300,000 unit IM dose).		
Penicillin V Potassium	Peak serum levels: 3 to 8 μg/mL (with a 500 mg po dose).		
Pentazocine Lactate (C-IV)	Peak plasma levels: 140 to 160 ng/mL. Plasma levels in surgical patients: 200 to 1000 ng/mL (5 to 10 min after IV injection).	Plasma levels: 0.8 to 38 μg/mL.	Fatal blood levels: 1 to 10 μg/mL.

Drug	Therapeutic levels	Toxicities	Fatalities
Pentobarbital Sodium (C-II)	Peak serum levels: 1.2 to 3.1 µg/mL (with a 100 mg po dose) and 3 µg/mL (with a 100 mg IV dose).	Toxicities reported with plasma levels of greater than 13 to 28 µg/mL.	Fatalities reported with blood levels of 10 to 50 µg/mL.
Pentoxifylline	Serum levels: 0.1 to 0.4 µg/mL.	Toxicities reported with serum levels of 32 to 51 µg/mL.	
Perphenazine	Peak blood level: 7 ng/mL (with a 100 mg IM dose). Steady state plasma levels: 0.4 to 30 ng/mL (with 24 to 48 mg daily po doses).		
Phendimetrazine Tartrate (C-III)	Plasma levels: 50 to 90 ng/mL.		
Phenelzine Sulfate	Peak plasma level: 2.0 ng/mL (with a 30 mg po dose).		
Phenobarbital (C-IV)	Plasma levels: 10 to 30 µg/mL (for anticonvulsant therapy).	Plasma levels: >40 µg/mL.	Fatalities reported with blood levels between 65 and 170 µg/mL.
Phenobarbital Sodium (C-IV)			
Phentermine Hydrochloride (C-IV)	Plasma levels: 30 to 90 ng/mL.		
Phentermine Resin (C-IV)	Plasma levels: 30 to 90 ng/mL.		
Phenytoin	Serum levels (total phenytoin): 10 to 20 µg/mL.	Toxicities reported with serum levels greater than 30 µg/mL (total phenytoin) and 1.5 to >5 µg/mL (free phenytoin).	
Phenytoin Sodium	Serum levels (free phenytoin): 0.5 to 1.5 µg/mL.		
Pimozide	Steady state plasma levels: 1.7 to 3.0 ng/mL.	Reported toxicity was found to be a plasma concentration of 1.5 µg/mL.	
Pindolol	Mean plasma levels: 3.0 to 4.5 ng/mL.		

Drug	Therapeutic Level	Toxic Level	Lethal Level
Pipecuronium Bromide	Peak serum level: 244 µg/mL (with a 4 g IV dose).		No lethal doses have been established; however, any dose above the therapeutic range may be sufficient to cause respiratory paralysis, hypoxia, and death if respiratory assistance is not available.
Piperacillin Sodium	Serum levels: 1 to 5 µg/mL.		
Piroxicam		Toxicity reported with a peak serum level of 23.5 µg/mL.	
Potassium Chloride Potassium Gluconate	Serum levels: 3.5 to 5 mEq/L.	Toxicities reported with serum levels between 6.5 and > 8 mEq/L.	Fatalities reported with serum levels ranging from 10 to 12 mEq/L.
Prazosin Hydrochloride	Mean peak plasma levels: 36 mg/mL (range, 6 to 78 ng/mL) (with a 5 mg po dose).	Toxicities reported with serum levels between 50 and 900 ng/mL.	
Primidone	Plasma levels: 8 to 12 µg/mL.	Plasma levels: > 12 µg/mL.	
Procainamide Hydrochloride	Serum levels: 4 to 8 µg/mL.	Serum levels: > 16 µg/mL.	A fatality reported with a postmortem blood level of 114 µg/mL.
Prochlorperazine Edisylate	Plasma levels: 6 to 22 µg/mL (with a 12.5 mg IV dose).		
Prochlorperazine Maleate	Peak plasma level: 0.8 µg/mL (with a 12.5 mg po dose). Mean plasma level: 3.4 µg/mL (range, 1.6 to 7.6) (with a 25 mg po dose).		
Procyclidine Hydrochloride	Steady state plasma levels: 0.15 to 0.63 µg/mL (with 10 to 30 mg daily po doses).		Fatalities reported with postmortem blood levels of 0.4 to 7.8 µg/mL.
Progesterone	Serum levels: 15 ng/mL or greater.		

Promethazine Hydrochloride	Peak plasma levels: 11 to 23 ng/mL.	Toxicities reported at plasma levels of approximately 50 ng/mL.	Fatalities reported at postmortem blood levels of 2.4 to 12 µg/mL.
Propafenone Hydrochloride	Serum levels: 200 to 450 ng/mL.	Toxicities commonly reported at serum levels above 900 µg/mL.	
Propoxyphene HCl (C-IV)	Peak serum levels: 0.2 to 0.5 µg/mL.	Toxicities reported with serum levels ranging from 0.7 to 2 µg/mL.	Fatalities reported with postmortem blood levels between 1.0 and 17 µg/mL.
Propoxyphene Napsylate (C-IV)			
Propranolol Hydrochloride	Steady state peak plasma levels: 10 to 335 ng/mL (with po daily doses from 40 to 320 mg, respectively).	Toxicity reported with serum levels of 2.2 to 4.5 µg/mL.	Fatalities reported with postmortem blood levels of 14 to 16 µg/mL.
Propylhexadrine	Serum levels: approx. 10 ng/mL.		Fatalities reported with blood levels of 3.75 and 36 µg/mL.
Propylthiouracil	Peak serum levels: >4 µg/mL (for antithyroid activity); 3 µg/mL (to reduce organification by 50%); 0.8 µg/mL (to reduce peripheral T4 conversion activity by 50%).		
Protriptyline Hydrochloride	Steady state plasma levels: 22 to 165 ng/mL (with 20 mg daily po doses) and 115 to 375 ng/mL (with 40 mg daily po doses).		
Pseudoephedrine Hydrochloride	Mean peak plasma levels: 210 ng/mL (with a 60 mg po dose) and 770 ng/mL (with a 180 mg po dose).	Toxicity reported with a serum level of 1.4 µg/mL (60 hours after chronic daily doses of 240 mg were discontinued).	Fatalities reported with postmortem blood levels of 19 and 66 µg/mL.
Pseudoephedrine Sulfate			
Pyridostigmine Bromide	Plasma levels: 50 to 100 ng/mL.	Toxicity reported at plasma levels >100 ng/mL.	
Quazepam (C-IV)	Mean steady state plasma level: 110 ng/mL (with daily 15 mg po doses).		

Drug	Therapeutic Level	Toxic Level	Lethal Level
Quetiapine Fumarate	Mean peak serum level: 278 ng/mL (range, 140 to 365 ng/mL) (with a 75 mg dose). Mean steady state serum level: 400 ng/mL (range, 195 to 630 ng/mL) (with chronic daily po doses of 450 mg).	A toxicity reported with a serum level of 13 µg/mL.	
Quinapril Hydrochloride	Mean plasma level: 1.5 ng/mL.		
Quinidine (salts)	Plasma levels: 2 to 6 µg/mL.	Toxicities reported with serum levels between 9.7 and 28 µg/mL.	A fatality reported with a postmortem blood level of 45 µg/mL.
Quinine Sulfate	Plasma levels: <0.3 µg/mL (from drinking tonic water) and 1.9 to 2.8 µg/mL (with a 650 mg po dose).	Toxicities reported with plasma levels between 6.8 and 26 µg/mL.	Fatalities reported with postmortem blood levels between 6 and 24 µg/mL.
Ramipril	Plasma levels: 4.7 to 8.8 ng/mL.		
Ranitidine Hydrochloride	Plasma levels: 0.1 to 0.2 µg/mL (with a 70 mg IV dose). Peak plasma levels: 0.84 µg/mL (with a 250 mg po dose) and 1.4 µg/mL (with a 400 mg po dose).		
Rifabutin	Mean peak plasma levels: 375 ± 267 ng/mL (with a 300 mg po dose).		
Rifampin	Peak plasma levels: 7 to 12 µg/mL (with a single 10 mg/kg dose).	Toxicities reported with plasma levels ranging from 204 to 400 µg/mL.	
Risperidone	Steady state plasma levels: 4 to 8 ng/mL.	Toxicity reported with a serum level of 1070 ng/mL.	One fatality reported with a postmortem blood level of 1800 ng/mL.
Scopolamine	Mean plasma level: 130 pg/mL (range, 80 to 240 pg/mL) (with a 0.5 mg transdermal patch).	Toxicity reported with a plasma level of 890 pg/mL.	One fatality reported with a postmortem blood level of 1890 ng/mL.

Drug	Therapeutic/Peak Levels	Toxicities	Fatalities
Secobarbital Sodium (C-II)	Mean peak blood level: 2.0 µg/mL (range, 1.8 to 2.2 µg/mL) diminishing to 1.3 µg/mL after 20 hours.	Toxicities reported with blood levels ranging from 18 to 24 µg/mL.	A fatality reported with a blood level of 11.5 µg/mL.
Selegiline Hydrochloride	Mean peak plasma level: 0.9 ng/mL (with a 10 mg po dose).		
Sertraline Hydrochloride	Serum levels: 30 to 200 ng/mL.	Toxicities reported with mean peak plasma levels ranging from 55 to 253 ng/mL and serum levels ranging from < 10 ng/mL to > 1000 ng/mL.	Fatalities reported with serum levels of 1.5 µg/ML and postmortem blood levels of 620 ng/mL.
Sibutramine	Mean peak plasma level: 4.0 ng/mL (range, 3.2 to 4.8) as the norsibutramine metabolite (with a 15 mg po dose of sibutramine).		
Sildenafil Citrate	Peak plasma level: 260 ng/mL (one subject given a 50 mg po dose).		
Sodium Nitroprusside	Serum level: 5.0 to 29 µg/mL (as the thiocyanate metabolite), depending on the nitroprusside infusion rate and length of therapy.	Blood cyanide and serum thiocyanate levels are toxic if they are > 500 ng/mL and > 100 µg/mL, respectively.	
Sotalol Hydrochloride	Serum levels: 1.25 to 3 µg/mL.	Toxicities reported with serum levels of 5 µg/ML and above.	Fatalities reported with postmortem blood levels of 40 µg/mL.
Sparfloxacin	Peak serum levels: 0.62 to 0.71 µg/mL (with a 200 mg po dose) and 0.56 to 1.60 µg/mL (with a 400 mg po dose).	Toxic serum levels have not been established.	
Streptomycin Sulfate	Peak serum levels: 15 to 30 µg/mL. Trough serum levels: less than or equal to 5 µg/mL.	Peak serum levels: > 50 µg/mL.	
Sulfamethoxazole	Peak serum levels: about 100 µg/mL.		

301

Drug	Therapeutic Level	Toxic Level	Lethal Level
Sulfasalazine		Serum levels: >50 μg/mL (as the sulfapyridine metabolite).	
Sulfisoxazole	Peak plasma levels: 110 to 250 μg/mL.		
Sulindac	Peak plasma levels: 4 to 5 μg/mL (with a 200 mg po dose).	Toxicities reported with plasma levels ranging from 1 to 50.8 μg/mL.	One fatality reported with a blood level of 130 μg/mL.
Sumatriptan Succinate	Mean peak plasma levels: 42 ng/mL (range, 24 to 65 ng/mL (with a 3 mg SC dose) and 95 ng/mL (range, 52 to 222 ng/mL) (with a 200 mg po dose).		
Tacrine Hydrochloride	Serum level: 7 to 16 ng/mL.	Toxicities reported with serum levels ranging from 16 to 96 ng/mL.	
Tacrolimus	Therapeutic range note clearly defined. Whole blood trough levels: 10 to 20 μg/mL are often considered therapeutic.	Toxicities reported with peak serum/plasma levels of 8.5 and 11.4 ng/mL.	
Temazepam (C-IV)	Mean peak plasma level: 870 ng/mL (range, 500 to 1100 ng/mL) (with a 30 mg po dose).	Toxicities reported with serum levels of 0.75 μg/ML and above.	Fatalities reported with postmortem blood levels of 3.8 to 9.0 μg/mL.
Terbutaline Sulfate	Plasma levels: 2 to 6 ng/mL.	Toxicities reported with plasma levels ranging from 34 to 200 ng/mL.	
Tetracycline Hydrochloride	Peak plasma levels: 2 to 2.5 μg/mL.	Plasma levels: >20 μg/mL.	Fatalities reported with postmortem blood levels between 60 and 250 μg/mL.
Theophylline, Anhydrous	Plasma levels: 8 to 20 μg/mL.		
Thiabendazole		Toxicity reported with a serum level of 239 ng/mL.	
Thioridazine	Mean steady state serum level: 0.64 μg/mL (range, 0.14 to 2.6 μg/mL).	Toxicities reported with serum levels ranging from 2.4 to 11.8 μg/mL.	
Thioridazine Hydrochloride			Fatalities reported with blood levels of 0.8 to 13 μg/mL.

Thiothixine	Serum levels: 2 to 15 ng/mL.	Toxicity reported with a serum level of 520 ng/mL.	
Thiothixene Hydrochloride			
Tiagabine Hydrochloride	Therapeutic range has not been established. A target serum level of 0.1 μg/mL has been suggested.	Toxicities reported with a plasma level of 3.1 μg/ML and a serum level of 710 ng/mL.	
Ticarcillin Disodium	Peak serum level: 324 μg/mL (with a 3 g IV dose).		
Timolol Maleate	Mean steady state plasma level: 110 ng/mL (range, 40 to 230 ng/mL) (with chronic po 45 mg daily doses).		
Tobramycin Sulfate	Peak serum levels: 5 to 8 μg/mL. Trough serum levels: 1 to 2 μg/mL.	Peak serum levels: 10 to 15 μg/mL. Trough serum levels: >2 to 4 μg/mL.	
Tocainide Hydrochloride	Plasma levels: 3 to 9 μg/mL.	Plasma levels: >10 μg/mL.	A fatality reported with a blood level of 74 μg/mL.
Tolbutamide	Plasma levels: 80 to 240 μg/mL.		A fatality reported with a blood level of 640 μg/mL.
Tolcapone	Peak plasma levels: 3 to 6 μg/mL.	Toxicity reported with a peak plasma level of 30 μg/mL.	
Tolmetin Sodium	Mean peak blood level: 39 μg/mL (range, 32 to 49 μg/mL) (with a 300 mg po dose).		
Tramadol Hydrochloride	Mean serum levels: 100 ng/mL (at 45 minutes following a 100 mg po dose) is considered to be the threshold value for analgesic efficacy; 613 ng/mL (at 15 minutes) and 409 ng/mL (at 2 hours).	Toxicities reported with serum levels >20 μg/mL.	Fatalities reported with postmortem blood levels between 13 and 38 μg/mL.

Drug	Therapeutic Level	Toxic Level	Lethal Level
Tranylcypromine Sulfate	Blood level: 0.1 μg/mL.		Fatalities reported with blood levels ranging from 0.25 to 9.1 μg/mL.
Trazodone Hydrochloride	Mean steady state plasma level: 1.5 μg/mL (range, 0.24 to 4.89) (with chronic po doses of 150 to 500 mg daily).	Toxicities reported with plasma levels ranging from 4.2 to 19 μg/mL.	Fatalities reported with postmortem blood levels above 9 μg/mL.
Tretinoin	Peak serum level: 294 μg/mL.		
Triazolam (C-IV)	Serum levels: 4.3 ± 0.4 ng/mL.	Toxicities reported with serum levels ranging from 7.9 to 31 ng/mL.	
Trifluoperazine Hydrochloride	Mean peak plasma level: 1.4 μg/mL (range, 0.5 to 3.1 μg/mL) (with a 5 mg po dose).		Fatalities reported with blood levels above 60 μg/mL.
Trihexyphenidyl Hydrochloride	Peak plasma levels: 31 ng/mL (at 2 hours) and 15 ng/mL (at 4 ours) (with a 5 mg po dose).		
Trimethobenzamide Hydrochloride	Peak serum levels: 4.5 μg/mL (with a 200 mg IM dose tid) and 3.1 μg/mL (with a 250 mg po dose tid).		Fatality reported with a blood level of 155 μg/mL.
Trimethoprim	Serum level: 1 μg/mL (with a 100 mg po dose).		
Trimethoprim Hydrochloride			
Trimipramine Maleate	Mean steady state serum level: 86 ng/mL (range, 11 to 241 ng/mL) (with chronic po doses of 75 to 150 mg daily).	Toxicities reported with serum levels ranging from 300 to 1000 ng/mL.	Fatalities reported with blood levels ranging from 0.4 to 12 μg/mL.
Trovafloxacin Mesylate	Peak serum levels: 1.1 μg/mL (with a 100 mg po dose) and 3.3 μg/mL (with a 300 mg po dose).		

Tubocurarine Chloride	Plasma levels: 0.6 ± 0.2 µg/ML and 1.2 µg/mL (for 50% and 95% reduction in skeletal muscle twitch tension, respectively).	No lethal doses have been established; however, any dose above the therapeutic range may be sufficient to cause respiratory paralysis, hypoxia, and death if respiratory assistance is not available.
Valproic Acid	Serum levels: 50 to 120 µg/mL.	Serum levels: > 100 to 150 µg/mL.	A fatality reported with a postmortem blood level of 1050 µg/mL.
Vancomycin Hydrochloride	Target trough levels: 5 to 15 µg/mL.	Plasma levels: 35 to 150 µg/mL.	
Vecuronium Bromide	Plasma levels: 0.20 µg/ML and 0.37 µg/mL (for 50% and 95% reduction of skeletal muscle twitch tension, respectively).		No lethal doses have been established; however, any dose above the therapeutic range may be sufficient to cause respiratory paralysis, hypoxia, and death if respiratory assistance is not available.
Venlafaxine	Mean peak serum levels: 37 to 53 ng/mL (with a 25 mg po dose); 102 to 167 ng/mL (with a 75 mg po dose); 163 to 393 ng/mL (with a 150 mg po dose).	Toxicities reported with peak plasma levels ranging from 1.2 to 2.35 µg/mL.	A fatality reported with a peak plasma level of 89 µg/mL.
Verapamil Hydrochloride	Serum levels: 50 to 400 ng/mL.	Toxicities reported with serum levels of > 360 ng/mL.	Fatalities reported with postmortem blood levels of 0.9 to 85 µg/mL.
Vincristine Sulfate		Toxicities reported with plasma levels ranging from 1.8 to 10.9 ng/mL at 1 hour, a mean steady state concentration of 1.7 ng/mL and less than 0.25 ng/mL within 24 hours of discontinuation of the infusion.	
Warfarin Sodium	Serum levels: 0.5 to 3 µg/mL (total warfarin) and 5 to 23 ng/mL (free warfarin).	Toxicities reported with plasma levels ranging from 1 to 11.3 µg/mL (total warfarin).	

Drug	Therapeutic Level	Toxic Level	Lethal Level
Zafirlukast	Plasma levels: > 5 ng/mL.		
Zidovudine	Serum levels are not established. Peak serum level reported: approximately 0.9 μg/mL (with a 200 mg po dose).	Toxicities reported with serum levels ranging from 24 to 49 μg/mL.	
Zileuton	Peak plasma level: 2.1 μg/mL (with a 600 mg po dose).		
Zolmitriptan	Mean steady state plasma level: 10 ng/mL (range, 6.7 to 18 ng/mL) (with chronic 5 mg po doses).		
Zolpidem Tartrate (C-IV)	Mean peak plasma levels: 59 ng/mL (range, 29 to 113 ng/mL) (with a 5 mg po dose) and 121 ng/mL (range, 58 to 272 ng/mL) (with a 10 mg po dose).	Toxicities reported with plasma levels greater than 500 ng/mL.	Fatalities reported with postmortem blood levels ranging from 1.6 to 7.7 μg/mL.
Zonisamide	Plasma levels: 10 to 30 μg/mL.	Toxicities reported with plasma levels ranging from 30 to 100 μg/mL.	

References:

Anderson, P.O., J.E. Knoben, and W.G. Troutman: Handbook of Clinical Drug Data, Ninth Edition, Appleton & Lange, Stamford, 1999.

Baselt, R.: Disposition of Toxic Drugs and Chemicals in Man, Fifth Edition, Chemical Toxicology Institute, Foster City, 2000.

Hardman, J.G., Limbird, L.E. (Eds): Goodman and Gilman's The Pharmacological Basis of Therapeutics, Ninth Edition, McGraw-Hill, New York, 1996.

Poisindex Toxicologic Substance Identification. Micromedex Healthcare Series, Volume 109, Micromedex, Inc., 1974 - 2001.

SPECIAL

DOSAGE

TABLES

DIGOXIN DOSES

I. RAPID DIGITALIZATION WITH A LOADING DOSE -

In most patients with heart failure and normal sinus rhythm, a therapeutic effect with minimum risk of toxicity should occur with peak body digoxin stores of 8 to 12 μg/kg. For adequate control of ventricular rate in patients with atrial flutter or fibrillation, larger digoxin body stores (10 to 15 μg/kg) are often required. In patients with renal insufficiency, the projected peak body stores of digoxin should be conservative (6 to 10 μg/kg) due to altered distribution and elimination.

The loading dose should be based on the projected peak body stores and administered in several portions; approximately half the total is usually given as the first dose.

FOR ORAL DOSING -

Preparation	In previously undigitalized patients, a single initial oral dose of the following produces a detectable effect in 0.5 to 2 hours that becomes maximal in 2 to 6 hours	The following additional doses may be given cautiously at 6 to 8 hour intervals until clinical evidence of an adequate effect is noted	The usual amount of each preparation that a 70 kg patient requires to achieve 8 to 15 μg/kg peak body stores is
LANOXIN Tablets	0.5 - 0.75 mg po	0.125 - 0.375 mg po	0.75 - 1.25 mg po
LANOXIN ELIXIR PEDIATRIC	0.5 - 0.75 mg po	0.125 - 0.375 mg po	0.75 - 1.25 mg po
LANOXICAPS Capsules	0.4 - 0.6 mg po	0.1 - 0.3 mg po	0.6 - 1.0 mg po

FOR INTRAVENOUS DOSING -

Preparation	In previously undigitalized patients, a single initial intravenous dose of the following produces a detectable effect in 5 to 30 minutes that becomes maximal in 1 to 4 hours	The following additional doses may be given cautiously at 4 to 8 hour intervals until clinical evidence of an adequate effect is noted	The usual amount of LANOXIN Injection that a 70 kg patient requires to achieve 8 to 15 μg/kg peak body stores is
LANOXIN Injection	0.4 - 0.6 mg IV	0.1 - 0.3 mg IV	0.6 - 1.0 mg IV

The maintenance dose should be based upon the percentage of the peak body stores lost each day through elimination. The following formula has wide clinical use:

$$\text{Maintenance Dose} = \text{Peak Body Stores (i.e., Loading Dose)} \times \%\ \text{Daily Loss}/100$$

where: % Daily Loss = 14 + Creatinine Clearance (corrected to 70 kg body weight or 1.73 m² surface area)/5

A common practice involves the use of LANOXIN Injection to achieve rapid digitalization, with conversion to LANOXIN Tablets, LANOXIN ELIXIR PEDIATRIC, or LANOXICAPS Capsules for maintenance therapy. If patients are switched from an IV to an oral digoxin preparation, allowances must be made for difference in bioavailability when calculating maintenance doses (see inset Table below).

PRODUCT	ABSOLUTE BIOAVAILABILITY	EQUIVALENT DOSES (IN MG)			
LANOXIN Tablets	60 to 80%	0.125	0.25	0.5	
LANOXIN ELIXIR PEDIATRIC	70 to 85%	0.125	0.25	0.5	
LANOXIN Injection / IM	70 to 85%	0.125	0.25	0.5	
LANOXIN Injection / IV	100%	0.1	0.2	0.4	
LANOXICAPS Capsules	90 to 100%	0.1	0.2	0.4	

309

II. GRADUAL DIGITALIZATION WITH A MAINTENANCE DOSE -

The following Table provides average LANOXIN Tablet daily maintenance dose requirements for patients with heart failure based upon lean body weight and renal function:

USUAL LANOXIN DAILY MAINTENANCE DOSE REQUIREMENTS (in mcg) FOR ESTIMATED PEAK BODY STORES OF 10 μg/kg

		Lean Body Weight (kg / lbs)						Number of Days Before Steady-State is Achieved
		50 / 110	60 / 132	70 / 154	80 / 176	90 / 198	100 / 220	
Corrected Creatinine Clearance (mL/min per 70 kg)	0	62.5	125	125	125	187.5	187.5	22
	10	125	125	125	187.5	187.5	187.5	19
	20	125	125	187.5	187.5	187.5	250	16
	30	125	187.5	187.5	187.5	250	250	14
	40	125	187.5	187.5	250	250	250	13
	50	187.5	187.5	250	250	250	250	12
	60	187.5	187.5	250	250	250	375	11
	70	187.5	250	250	250	250	375	10
	80	187.5	250	250	250	375	375	9
	90	187.5	250	250	250	375	500	8
	100	250	250	250	375	375	500	7

The following Table provides average **LANOXICAP Capsule** daily maintenance dose requirements for patients with heart failure based upon lean body weight and renal function:

USUAL LANOXICAP DAILY MAINTENANCE DOSE REQUIREMENTS (in mcg) FOR ESTIMATED PEAK BODY STORES OF 10 µg/kg

		Lean Body Weight (kg / lbs)						
		50 / 110	60 / 132	70 / 154	80 / 176	90 / 198	100 / 220	
Corrected Creatinine Clearance (mL/min per 70 kg)	0	50	100	100	100	150	150	22
	10	100	100	100	150	150	150	19
	20	100	100	150	150	150	200	16
	30	100	150	150	150	200	200	14
	40	100	150	150	200	200	250	13
	50	150	150	200	200	250	250	12
	60	150	150	200	250	250	300	11
	70	150	200	200	250	250	300	10
	80	150	200	250	250	300	300	9
	90	150	200	250	250	300	350	8
	100	200	200	250	300	300	350	7
								Number of Days Before Steady-State is Achieved

ORAL THEOPHYLLINE DOSES

I. **IMMEDIATE-RELEASE PREPARATIONS** (e.g., ELIXOPHYLLIN Elixir and Capsules, ELIXOPHYLLIN-GG Liquid, ELIXOPHYLLIN-KI Elixir, QUIBRON and QUIBRON-300 Capsules, SLO-PHYLLIN Syrup and Tablets, SLO-PHYLLIN GG Capsules and Syrup, and THEOLAIR Liquid and Tablets). -

Acute Symptoms of Bronchospasm Requiring Rapid Attainment of Theophylline Serum Levels for Bronchodilation -

Otherwise healthy nonsmoking adults: 5 mg/kg po (oral loading dose); then, 3 mg/kg q 8 h po (maintenance doses).

Older patients and those with cor pulmonale: 5 mg/kg po (oral loading dose); then, 2 mg/kg q 8 h po (maintenance doses).

Patients with congestive heart failure: 5 mg/kg po (oral loading dose); then, 1 - 2 mg/kg q 12 h po (maintenance doses).

Chronic Therapy -

Initial Dose: 16 mg/kg/24 h or 400 mg/24 h (whichever is less) in divided doses q 6 - 8 h po.

Increasing Dose: The initial dosage may be increased in approximately 25% increments at 3 day intervals, as long as the drug is tolerated, until the clinical response is satisfactory, or the maximum dose is reached.

Maximum Dose: 13 mg/kg/day po or 900 mg/day, whichever is less

CHECK SERUM CONCENTRATION BETWEEN 1 AND 2 HOURS AFTER A DOSE WHEN NONE HAVE BEEN MISSED OR ADDED FOR AT LEAST 3 DAYS. If serum theophylline concentration is between 10 and 20 µg/mL, maintain dose, if tolerated. RECHECK THEOPHYLLINE CONCENTRATION AT 6- TO 12-MONTH INTERVALS.

II.   SUSTAINED-RELEASE PREPARATIONS -

A.   **RESPBID Sustained-Release Tablets, SLO-BID Extended-Release Capsules, SLO-PHYLLIN Extended-Release Capsules, THEOLAIR-SR Sustained-Release Tablets and T-PHYL Controlled-Release Tablets -**

Initial Therapy: 16 mg/kg/24 h or 400 mg/24 h (whichever is less) in 2 or 3 divided doses at 8 or 12 h intervals po.

Maintenance Therapy: The initial dosage may be increased in approximately 25% increments at 3-day intervals, as long as the drug is tolerated, until the clinical response is satisfactory, or the maximum dose is reached.

Maximum Dose: 13 mg/kg/day po or 900 mg/day, whichever is less

CHECK SERUM CONCENTRATION BETWEEN 5 AND 10 HOURS AFTER A DOSE WHEN NONE HAVE BEEN MISSED OR ADDED FOR AT LEAST 3 DAYS. If serum theophylline concentration is between 10 and 20 µg/mL, maintain dose, if tolerated.   RECHECK THEOPHYLLINE CONCENTRATION AT 6- TO 12-MONTH INTERVALS.

B.   **THEO-DUR Extended-Release Tablets -**

Initial Therapy: 200 mg q 12 h po

Maintenance Therapy: The dose may be increased in approximately 25% increments at 3 day intervals, as long as the drug is tolerated, until the clinical response is satisfactory, or the maximum dose is reached.

Maximum Doses: 35 - 70 kg: 300 mg q 12 h po.   Over 70 kg: 450 mg q 12 h po.

CHECK SERUM CONCENTRATION AT APPROXIMATELY 8 HOURS AFTER A DOSE WHEN NONE HAVE BEEN MISSED OR ADDED FOR AT LEAST 3 DAYS. If serum theophylline concentration is between 10 and 20 µg/mL, maintain dose, if tolerated.   RECHECK THEOPHYLLINE CONCENTRATION AT 6- TO 12-MONTH INTERVALS.

313

C. **THEO-24 Extended-Release Capsules -**

Initial Therapy: 200 mg q 12 h po

Maintenance Therapy: If serum levels cannot be measured and the response is unsatisfactory, after 3 days the dose may be increased by 100 mg increments. Reevaluated after 3 days.

Maximum Dose: 13 mg/kg/day po   or 900 mg/day, whichever is less

CHECK PEAK SERUM CONCENTRATION (12 HOURS AFTER THE MORNING DOSE) AND TROUGH LEVEL (24 HOURS AFTER THE MORNING DOSE) WHEN NO DOSES HAVE BEEN MISSED OR ADDED FOR AT LEAST 3 DAYS. If serum theophylline concentration is between 10 and 20 μg/mL, maintain dose, if tolerated. RECHECK THEOPHYLLINE CONCENTRATION AT 6- TO 12-MONTH INTERVALS.

MISCELLANEOUS

TABLES

COMPARISON OF VARIOUS TYPES OF INSULIN

GENERIC NAME	TRADE NAME	SOURCE OF INSULIN (SPECIES)	ONSET OF ACTION (HOURS)	PEAK ACTIVITY (HOURS)	DURATION OF ACTION (HOURS)	HOW SUPPLIED
Insulin Injection (Regular)	REGULAR ILETIN II	Purified Pork	0.5 - 1	2.5 - 4	6 - 8	Inj: 100 units/mL
	HUMULIN R	Human[a]				Inj: 100 units/mL
	NOVOLIN R	Human[b]				Inj: 100 units/mL
	VELOSULIN BR	Human[b]				Inj: 100 units/mL
	NOVOLIN R PENFILL	Human[b]				Cartridge: 100 units/mL
	NOVOLIN R PREFILLED	Human[b]				Inj: 100 units/mL
Insulin Aspart	NOVOLOG	Human[a]	0.25	1 - 3	3 - 5	Inj: 100 units/mL
Insulin Lispro	HUMALOG	Human[a]	0.25	1 - 1.5	3.5 - 4.5	Inj: 100 units/mL Cartridge: 1.5 mL Prefilled Pen: 3 mL

			Onset	Peak	Duration	
Isophane Insulin Suspension (NPH)			1 - 2	6 - 12	18 - 26	
	NPH ILETIN II	Purified Pork				**Inj:** 100 units/mL
	HUMULIN N	Human[a]				**Inj:** 100 units/mL
	NOVOLIN N	Human[b]				**Inj:** 100 units/mL
	NOVOLIN N PENFILL	Human[b]				**Cartridge:** 100 units/mL
	NOVOLIN N PREFILLED	Human[b]				**Inj:** 100 units/mL
Insulin Zinc Suspension (Lente)			1 - 3	6 - 12	18 - 26	
	LENTE ILETIN II	Purified Pork				**Inj:** 100 units/mL
	HUMULIN L	Human[a]				**Inj:** 100 units/mL
	NOVOLIN L	Human[b]				**Inj:** 100 units/mL
Extended Insulin Zinc Suspension (Ultralente)			4 - 8	10 - 18	24 - 36	
	HUMULIN U	Human[a]				**Inj:** 100 units/mL

GENERIC NAME	TRADE NAME	SOURCE OF INSULIN (SPECIES)	ONSET OF ACTION (HOURS)	PEAK ACTIVITY (HOURS)	DURATION OF ACTION (HOURS)	HOW SUPPLIED
70% Isophane Insulin Suspension + 30% Regular Insulin Injection			0.5	2 - 12	up to 24	
	HUMULIN 70/30	Human[a]				**Inj:** 100 units/mL
	NOVOLIN 70/30	Human[b]				**Inj:** 100 units/mL
	NOVOLIN 70/30 PENFILL	Human[b]				**Cartridge:** 100 units/mL
	NOVOLIN 70/30 PREFILLED	Human[b]				**Inj:** 100 units/mL
50% Isophane Insulin Suspension + 50% Regular Insulin Injection			0.5	2 - 5	up to 24	
	HUMULIN 50/50	Human[a]				**Inj:** 100 units/mL

50% Insulin Lispro Protamine Suspension + 50% Insulin Lispro	HUMALOG MIX 50/50	Human[a]	0.25	0.5 - 1.5	up to 18	**Inj:** 100 units/mL
75% Insulin Lispro Protamine Suspension + 25% Insulin Lispro	HUMALOG MIX 75/25	Human[a]	0.25	0.5 - 1.5	up to 24	**Inj:** 100 units/mL

[a] Produced from proinsulin synthesized by bacteria using recombinant DNA technology.

[b] Produced from baker's yeast using recombinant DNA technology.

Notes

PRESCRIPTION WRITING

INTRODUCTION

A **prescription** is an order for a specific medication for a specified patient at a particular time. It is the way in which a physician (or another health care professional) communicates a patient's selected drug therapy to the pharmacist and instructs the patient on how to use the prescribed medication. The prescription order may be given by a physician, dentist, veterinarian, physician assistant, nurse practitioner, or any other legally-recognized medical practitioner; the order may be written and signed or it may be oral, in which case the pharmacist is required to transcribe it into written form and obtain the prescriber's signature, if necessary, at a later time.

The transfer of the therapeutic information from prescriber to pharmacist to patient must be clear. With all of the many drug products available to the prescriber, it is easy to understand how drug strengths, dosage forms, and dosage regimens can be confused. Many drug names may also look alike (especially when written hastily) or may sound alike (when garbled over the telephone). Furthermore, numerous studies have indicated that many patients do not use their prescription medication properly; the patient often fails to take the drug or uses the medication either in an incorrect dose, at an improper time, or for the wrong condition. Most errors can be traced to the prescription order or the failure of the prescriber to adequately communicate this information to the patient.

In order that these types of errors be avoided and the patient gain the maximum benefit from the prescribed drugs, it is important for the prescriber to understand the basic principles of prescription writing.

COMPOSITION OF THE PRESCRIPTION ORDER

A complete prescription order is composed of eight parts and follows a standardized format which facilitates its interpretation by the pharmacist. The eight major parts of a prescription order include:

1. The date prescribed
2. The name, address, and age of the patient
3. The superscription
4. The inscription
5. The subscription
6. The signa
7. The renewal information
8. The name of the prescriber

Figure 1 illustrates a sample precompounded prescription order with the eight major elements numbered for reference purposes.

1. **The Date Prescribed** - The date on which a prescription was issued is important since a patient may not always have a prescription filled on the day it was written; days, weeks, months, or on occasion, years may pass before a patient presents the prescription to the pharmacist. Medications are intended for a patient at a particular time; the date prescribed may reveal that the presented prescription was not filled when written and now, for example, months later, the patient has "symptoms which are exactly the same as the last time" and is attempting to self-diagnose and self-medicate. Furthermore, drugs controlled by special laws and regulations, e.g., the Controlled Substances Act of 1970, cannot be dispensed or renewed more than six months from the date prescribed. Therefore, the date prescribed provides an accurate record of when a prescription was originally issued to the patient.

TELEPHONE (215) 555-2474

John V. Smith, M.D.
Paula A. Doe, M.D.

3002 BROAD STREET ANYTOWN, ANYSTATE 00000

1 DATE 4/10/02 AGE 53

2 NAME Jeff Kraus
ADDRESS 100 Pleasant Street

3 ℞ Coreg 3.125 mg.
#60

4

5 Sig: 1 tab po
bid

6

Dr. John V. Smith Dr.

8 Do Not Substitute Substitution Permissible

7 Renew: 0 1 2 3 4 5 DEA #

FIGURE 1. A Sample Precompounded Prescription Order

2. **The Name, Address, and Age of the Patient** - This information serves to identify for whom the prescribed medication is intended. The full name of the patient may help to prevent a mixup of drugs within a household when, for example, a parent and child have the same name. If the patient's first name is not known or omitted, the use of the titles Mr., Mrs., Ms. or Miss is appropriate. Information regarding the patient's age should also be indicated, e.g., "adult," "child," or in the case of a young child, the exact age; this allows the pharmacist to monitor the prescribed dosage, especially since the pharmacokinetics of many drugs differ markedly in newborn, pediatric, adult, and geriatric patient populations.

3. **The Superscription** - This portion of the prescription refers to the symbol R_x, a contraction of the Latin verb *recipe*, meaning "take thou." It serves to introduce the drug(s) prescribed and the directions for use.

4. **The Inscription** - The name, strength and quantity of the desired drug is enclosed within this section of the prescription. Although drugs may be prescribed by any known name, i.e., chemical name, trivial name, nonproprietary name (more commonly referred to as the generic name) and manufacturer's proprietary (trade) name, most drugs are prescribed either by the trade name or by the generic name. Chemical and trivial names of drugs are generally not suitable for this purpose and are seldom used. When the trade name is written, the prescription must be filled with product of the specified manufacturer, unless the prescriber and patient approved substitution with another brand. If the generic name is employed, the pharmacist can select from any of the available drug preparations. When two or more drugs are written on the same prescription for compounding purposes, the name and quantity of each should be listed on a separate line directly below the preceding one. To avoid confusion, the salt of a particular medicament should be clearly indicated if more than one is available, e.g., codeine **sulfate** or codeine **phosphate**. The quantities of the ingredients may be written in either the apothecary or metric system. The latter is more popular; it is used exclusively by official pharmaceutical reference texts, and in most cases, in medical schools, hospitals, and other health agencies.

The apothecary system is an older and less popular method of measurement; however, prescriptions are still written in this system and texts may, on occasion, report drug doses in apothecary units. For example, 1 fluid-ounce (apothecary) equals approximately 30 mL (metric) and 1 pint equals 473 mL.

Regardless of which system is employed on the prescription, most patients are more comfortable with household measures, especially with liquid medications. Although the sizes of the household teaspoon and tablespoon vary considerably, the standard household teaspoon should be regarded as containing 5 mL and the tablespoon, 15 mL. Standard disposable plastic teaspoons, tablespoons and graduated two fluid-ounce cups are available in an attempt to reduce liquid dose variability, and the use of these should be encouraged.

5. **The Subscription** - Directions to the pharmacist from the prescriber comprise this section of the prescription; these state the specific dosage form to be dispensed or the desired method of preparation. The subscription is usually a short phrase or sentence such as "Dispense 30 capsules" or "Dispense 90 mL" for a precompounded prescription or "Mix and prepare 10 suppositories" for an extemporaneous preparation.

6. **The Signa** - The directions to the patient are given in this part of the prescription and are usually introduced by the latin *Signa* or *Sig.*, meaning "mark thou". These directions should be as clear and as complete as possible, so that the patient may easily follow the desired dosage schedule and receive the maximum benefit from the medication. Instructions should be provided as to the route of administration, the amount of drug to be taken, and the time and frequency of the dose. Phrases such as "take as directed" and "use as required" are not satisfactory instructions and should be avoided whenever possible.

Latin, often considered to be the language of the medical profession, was used extensively in writing prescription orders until the early part of the 20th century. Although prescription orders in the United States today are almost always written in English, many Latin words and phrases have been retained and are commonly used (as abbreviations) in the Signa. Some of the more commonly-employed Latin terms and abbreviations are given in Table 1. Thus the Signa: "Caps 1 q.i.d. p.c. + H.S. c milk" translates to: "One capsule 4 times daily after meals and at bedtime with milk".

7. **The Renewal Information** - The wishes of the prescriber with regard to refilling the medication should be indicated on every prescription, and if renewals are authorized, the number of times should be designated. Prescription orders for drugs that bear the legend: "Caution: Federal law prohibits dispensing without prescription" may not be renewed without the expressed consent of the prescriber. Prescriptions for drugs covered under Schedule III or IV of the Controlled Substances Act of 1970 may be renewed, if so authorized, not more than five times within six months of date of issue; drugs within Schedule II may not be renewed.

8. **The Name of the Prescriber** - Although in most cases the name and address of the prescriber are printed on the prescription blank, the signature of the prescriber affixed to the bottom completes and validates the prescription order. For prescriptions written on hospital prescription blanks, the prescriber must print (or stamp) his/her name on the document, as well as sign it. This is a safe-guard in case a question arises concerning any aspect of the prescription order, the printed name will make it easier to identify and contact the prescriber. On oral prescriptions, the pharmacist adds the prescriber's name to the prescription; however, Federal law requires that prescriptions for Schedule II drugs be validated by the full signature of the prescriber and his/her registered Drug Enforcement Administration (DEA) number. The prescriber's registered DEA number must appear on all prescriptions for drug covered under the Controlled Substances Act (see below).

CLASSES OF PRESCRIPTION ORDERS

Prescription orders may be divided into two general classes based on the availability of the medication. A **precompounded** prescription order requests a drug or a drug mixture prepared and supplied by a pharmaceutical company; prescriptions of this class require no pharmaceutical alteration by the pharmacist. The prescription order shown in Figure 1 is a precompounded prescription. An **extemporaneous** or **compounded** prescription order is one in which the drugs, doses and dosage form, as selected by the prescriber, must be prepared by the pharmacist. Figure 2 shows an example of an extemporaneous prescription order. Most prescriptions written today are of the precompounded type; however extemporaneous prescription orders are not uncommon, especially with liquid, cream and ointment preparations.

CONTROLLED SUBSTANCES ACT

The legal aspects of prescription writing and dispensing are incorporated in various federal, state and local laws, which the medical practitioner must understand and observe; the strictest law regardless of governmental level, always takes precedence unless Federal Law is preemptive. In 1970, the Comprehensive Drug Abuse Prevention and Control Act, commonly called the Controlled Substances Act, was signed into law. This act imposes even more stringent controls on the distribution and use of all stimulant and depressant drugs and substances with the potential for abuse as designated by the Drug Enforcement Administration (DEA), U.S. Department of Justice. This act divides drugs with abuse potential into five categories or schedules as follows:

Schedule I (C-I) — Drugs in this schedule have a high potential for abuse and no currently accepted medical use in the United States. Examples of such drugs include cocaine base ("crack"), heroin, marijuana, peyote, mescaline, some tetrahydrocannabinols, LSD, and various opioid derivatives.

324

TABLE 1. COMMON LATIN ABBREVIATIONS

WORD OR PHRASE	ABBREVIATION	MEANING
Ad	Ad	Up to
Ana	aa	Of each
Ante cibos	a.c.	Before meals
Aqua	Aq.	Water
Aures utrae	a.u.	Each ear
Aurio dextra	a.d.	Right ear
Aurio laeva	a.l.	Left ear
Bis in die	b.i.d.	Twice a day
Capsula	Caps.	Capsule
Compositus	Comps.	Compounded
Cum	c	With
Et	Et	And
Gutta	Gtt.	A drop, drops
Hora somni	H.S.	At bedtime
Non repetatur	Non rep.	Do not repeat
Oculo utro	O.U.	Each eye
Oculus dexter	O.D.	Right eye
Oculus sinister	O.S.	Left eye
Per os	p.o.	By mouth
Post cibos	p.c.	After meals
Pro re nata	p.r.n.	When necessary
Quaque	q.	Each, every
Quantum satis	Q.S.	As much as is sufficient
Quarter in die	q.i.d.	Four times daily
Semis	ss	A half
Sine	s	Without
Statim	Stat.	Immediately
Tabella	tab	Tablet
Ter in die	t.i.d.	Three times daily
Ut dictum	Ut Dict.	As directed

TELEPHONE (215) 555-2474

John V. Smith, M.D.
Paula A. Doe, M.D.

3002 BROAD STREET   ANYTOWN, ANYSTATE 00000

DATE 3/22/02   AGE 56
NAME Sarah Lewis
ADDRESS 890 Main Blvd.

℞ Triancisolone Cream
0.5%   10 g
Water   6 ml
Hydrophilic Ointment
q s ad 30 g
Sig: Apply to affected
area BID

Dr. John V. Smith Dr. _____
Do Not Substitute   Substitution
                           Permissible

Renew: 0 1 2 3 4 5   DEA # _____

FIGURE 2.   A Sample Extemporaneous Prescription Order

326

Substances listed in this schedule are not for prescription use; they may be obtained for chemical analysis, research, or instruction purposes by submitting an application and a protocol of the proposed use to the DEA.

Schedule II (C-II) — The drugs in this schedule have a high abuse potential with severe psychological or physical dependence liability. Schedule II controlled substances consist of certain opioid drugs, preparations containing amphetamines or methamphetamines as the single active ingredient or in combination with each other, and certain sedatives. Examples of opioids included in this schedule are opium, morphine sulfate, codeine sulfate, codeine phosphate, alfentanil hydrochloride (ALFENTA), fentanil (DURAGESIC), fentanyl citrate (FENTANYL ORALET), hydromorphone hydrochloride (DILAUDID, DILAUDID-HP), methadone hydrochloride (DOLOPHINE HYDROCHLORIDE), meperidine hydrochloride (DEMEROL), oxycodone hydrochloride (ROXICODONE, OXYCONTIN; and in the PERCODAN, PERCODAN-DEMI, various PERCOCET preparations, ROXICET, ROXICET 5/500, ROXILOX, ROXIPRIN, and TYLOX), oxycodone terephthalate (in PERCODAN, PERCODAN-DEMI), and oxymorphone hydrochloride (NUMORPHAN). Also included are stimulants, e.g., cocaine hydrochloride, amphetamine asparate and saccharate (in ADDERALL preparations), dextroamphetamine sulfate (DEXEDRINE) and saccharate (in ADDERALL), methamphetamine hydrochloride (DESOXYN), methylphenidate hydrochloride (RITALIN, RITALIN LA, RITALIN SR, METHYLIN, METHYLIN ER, CONCERTA), dexmethylphenidate (FOCALIN) and depressants, e.g., pentobarbital sodium (NEMBUTAL SODIUM), and amobarbital sodium and secobarbital sodium (in TUINAL 100 and TUINAL 200).

Schedule III (C-III) — The drugs in this schedule have a potential for abuse that is less than for those drugs in Schedules I and II. The use or abuse of these drugs may lead to low or moderate physical dependence or high psychological dependence. Included in this schedule are: analgesic mixtures containing limited amounts of codeine phosphate (e.g., EMPIRIN W/CODEINE, FIORICET W/CODEINE, FIORINAL W/CODEINE, SOMA COMPOUND W/CODEINE, and TYLENOL W/CODEINE), hydrocodone bitartrate (e.g., various ANEXSIA combinations, BANCAP HC, DURATUSS HD, HYDROCET, the various LORTAB preparations, LORTAB ASA, VICODIN, VICODIN ES, and VICODIN HP), or dihydrocodeine bitartrate (SYNALGOS-DC); or cough mixtures containing hydrocodone bitartrate (e.g., HYCODAN, HYCOTUSS EXPECTORANT, and TUSSEND), or hydrocodone polistirex (e.g., TUSSIONEX). Also included in this schedule are certain anabolic steroids (e.g., nandrolone decanoate (DECA-DURABOLIN), oxandrolone (OXANDRIN), testosterone and its cypionate and enanthate salts).

Schedule IV (C-IV) — The drugs in this category have the potential for limited physical or psychological dependence and include phenobarbital, phenobarbital sodium, paraldehyde, chloral hydrate, meprobamate (MILTOWN), alprazolam (XANAX), chlordiazepoxide hydrochloride (LIBRIUM), diazepam (VALIUM), clorazepate dipotassium (TRANXENE-T TAB, TRANXENE-SD), flurazepam hydrochloride (DALMANE), oxazepam (SERAX), clonazepam (KLONOPIN), lorazepam (ATIVAN), quazepam (DORAL), the hydrochloride and napsylate salts of propoxyphene (DARVON and DARVON-N) and butorphanol tartrate (STADOL, STADOL NS). Certain other mixtures are included; for example, the antidiarrheal MOTOFEN and the analgesics DARVON COMPOUND-65, DARVOCET-N 50, DARVOCET-N 100, TALACEN, TALWIN COMPOUND, and WYGESIC.

Schedule V (C-V) — Schedule V drugs have a potential for abuse that is less than those listed in Schedule IV. These consist of preparations containing moderate quantities of certain opioids for use in pain (i.e., buprenorphine hydrochloride (BUPRENEX)) or as antidiarrheals (e.g., diphenoxylate hydrochloride (in LOMOTIL)), or as antitussives (such as codeine-containing cough mixtures. Some of the latter may be dispensed without a prescription order, in certain States, provided that specified dispensing criteria are met by the pharmacist.

Everyone involved in the manufacture, importing, exporting, distribution or dispensing of any controlled drug must register annually with the DEA. Health care practitioners must be registered before he/she can administer or dispense any of the drugs listed in the DEA schedules. Furthermore, the physician's DEA registration number must be noted on every prescription for controlled substances.

Notes

331

335

337

340

341

345

Methylphenidate Hydrochloride: 144-145, 292, 327
Methylprednisolone: 145
Methylprednisolone Acetate: 145
Methylprednisolone Sodium Succinate: 145
Methyltestosterone: 145, 238
Methysergide Maleate: 145
METIMYD: 244
Metipranolol Hydrochloride: 145
Metoclopramide Hydrochloride: 146
Metolazone: 146
Metoprolol Succinate: 146
Metoprolol Tartrate: 146-147, 242, 292
METROCREAM: 147
METROGEL: 147
METROGEL VAGINAL: 147
Metronidazole: 147, 292
Metronidazole Hydrochloride: 148
Metyrosine: 148
MEVACOR: 138
Mexiletine Hydrochloride: 148, 292
MEXITIL: 148
MIACALCIN: 53
MICATIN: 148
MICARDIS: 202
MICARDIS HCT 40/12.5: 244
MICARDIS HCT 80/12.5: 244
Miconazole Nitrate: 148
MICRO-K EXTENCAPS: 178
MICRO-K LS: 178
MICRONASE: 114
MICROZIDE: 117
MIDAMOR: 36
Midazolam Hydrochloride: 148, 292
Midodrine Hydrochloride: 149
MIDRIN: 245
Miglitol: 149
MILK OF MAGNESIA: 139
MILK OF MAGNESIA CONCENTRATED: 139
Milrinone Lactate: 149
MILTOWN: 141, 327
Mineralocorticoid: 24
Mineral Oil: 149, 226, 240, 251
MINIPRESS: 179
MINITRAN: 161
MINIZIDE 1: 245
MINIZIDE 2: 245
MINIZIDE 5: 245
MINOCIN IV: 149
Minocycline Hydrochloride: 149
Minoxidil: 149, 292
MINTEZOL: 205
MIRALAX: 177
MIRAPEX: 179

MIRCETTE: 245
MIRENA: 133
Mirtazapine: 149, 293
Misoprostol: 149, 226
MITROLAN: 55
MIVACRON: 150
Mivacurium Chloride: 150
MOBAN: 150
MOBIC: 141
Modafinil: 150, 293
MODICON: 245
MODURETIC: 245
Moexipril Hydrochloride: 150, 265
Molindone Hydrochloride: 150, 293
MOMENTUM: 139
Mometasone Furoate: 150
MONISTAT 3: 148
MONISTAT 7: 148
MONISTAT-DERM: 148
MONOCID: 60
MONOKET: 126
MONOPRIL: 111
Montelukast Sodium: 150, 293
MONUROL: 111
Moricizine Hydrochloride: 150, 293
Morphine Sulfate: 151, 293, 327
MOTOFEN: 245, 327
MOTRIN: 120
MOTRIN IB: 120
MOTRIN MIGRAINE PAIN: 120
MOTRIN SINUS / HEADACHE: 245
Moxifloxacin Hydrochloride: 152
MS CONTIN: 151
MSIR: 151
Mucolytics: 24
MUCOMYST: 31
MUCOSIL: 31
Multiple Sclerosis Drugs: 24
Mupirocin: 152
Mupirocin Calcium: 152
MUSTARGEN: 139
MYAMBUTOL: 101
MYCELEX: 74
MYCELEX-3: 53
MYCELEX-7: 74
MYCOBUTIN: 189
Mycophenolate Mofetil: 152
MYCOSTATIN: 163
MYDRIACYL: 214
Mydriatics: 24
MYKROX: 146
MYLANTA AR ACID REDUCER: 103
MYLANTA GAS: 194
MYLANTA SOOTHING LOZENGES: 55

355

Notes

REQUEST FOR INFORMATION

If you wish to be placed on a mailing list for information concerning new publications and updates, please fill out the form below and mail to:

MEDICAL SURVEILLANCE INC.
P.O. Box 480   Willow Grove, PA 19090

(PLEASE PRINT)

Name_____

Organization_____

Street Address_____

City_____State_____

Zip Code_____

Telephone Number (Optional)_____

FOR FURTHER INFORMATION CALL:
800 - 417-3189

E-Mail us at **medsurveillance@aol.com**

Visit Us on the **World Wide Web** at
medicalsurveillance.com

ORDER FORM

PHONE	FAX	VIA WEB SITE
1-800-417-3189	1-215-657-1475	MEDICALSURVEILLANCE.COM

E-MAIL	CHECKS OR MONEY ORDERS	MAIL
MEDSURVEILLANCE@AOL.COM	Make check payable to MSI and mail order form	P.O. Box 480 Willow Grove, Pa. 19090

Books	Price	Qty	Sub-Total
Handbook of Commonly Prescribed Drugs with Therapeutic, Toxic and Lethal Levels, 18th Edition (2003) ISBN # 0-942447-44-1	$ 25.50		
Handbook of Common Orthopaedic Fractures and Drugs, 1st Edition (2003) ISBN # 0-942447-43-3	$ 19.95		
Travelers Guide to International Drugs, **Western Hemisphere** (2001) ISBN # 942447-40-9	$ 14.00		
Travelers Guide to International Drugs, **European Volume I ** (2001) ISBN # 942447-39-5	$ 14.00		
Travelers Guide to International Drugs, **European Volume II ** (2001) ISBN # 942447-38-7	$ 14.00		
Travelers Guide to International Drugs, **Middle & Far East** (2001) ISBN # 0-942447-32-8	$ 14.00		
Handbook of Commonly Prescribed Pediatric Drugs, 6th Edition (1999) ISBN # 0-942447-27-1	$ 18.50		
Antimicrobial Therapy in Primary Care Medicine, 1st Edition (1997) ISBN # 0-942447-22-0	$ 17.00		
Drug Charts in Basic Pharmacology, 3rd Edition (2000) ISBN # 0-942447-37-9	$ 18.95		
Warning: Drugs in Sports, 1st Edition (1995) ISBN # 0-942447-16-6	$ 14.50		

Shipping and Handling Charges:			
Add $ 6.50 for orders between $10.00 - $49.99	**SUB-TOTAL**		
Add $ 9.00 for orders between $50.00 - $ 99.99	(*) Shipping & Handling		
Add $ 11.00 for orders between $100.00 – 149.99	PA Residents, Add 6% Sales Tax		
Add $ 13.00 for orders Greater then $ 150.00	**TOTAL**		

Bookstores subject to standard shipping and handling charges

Name: _____

Address: _____

City: _____ STATE: _____ ZIP: _____

E-Mail Address:_____

AMT. ENCLOSED _____ ☐ VISA ☐ M/C ☐ DISCOVER ☐ AMERICAN EXPRESS ☐ CHECK

CARD NUMBER: _____ EXP. DATE: _____

AUTHORIZED SIGNATURE _____ PHONE: _____

If you are paying by credit card, Call Toll Free or Fax

ORDER FORM

PHONE	FAX	VIA WEB SITE
1-800-417-3189	1-215-657-1475	MEDICALSURVEILLANCE.COM

E-MAIL	CHECKS OR MONEY ORDERS	MAIL
MEDSURVEILLANCE@AOL.COM	Make check payable to MSI and mail order form	P.O. Box 480 Willow Grove, Pa. 19090

Books	Price	Qty	Sub-Total
Handbook of Commonly Prescribed Drugs with Therapeutic, Toxic and Lethal Levels, 18th Edition (2003) ISBN # 0-942447-44-1	$ 25.50		
Handbook of Common Orthopaedic Fractures and Drugs, 1st Edition (2003) ISBN # 0-942447-43-3	$ 19.95		
Travelers Guide to International Drugs, **Western Hemisphere** (2001) ISBN # 942447-40-9	$ 14.00		
Travelers Guide to International Drugs, **European Volume I ** (2001) ISBN # 942447-39-5	$ 14.00		
Travelers Guide to International Drugs, **European Volume II ** (2001) ISBN # 942447-38-7	$ 14.00		
Travelers Guide to International Drugs, **Middle & Far East** (2001) ISBN # 0-942447-32-8	$ 14.00		
Handbook of Commonly Prescribed Pediatric Drugs, 6th Edition (1999) ISBN # 0-942447-27-1	$ 18.50		
Antimicrobial Therapy in Primary Care Medicine, 1st Edition (1997) ISBN # 0-942447-22-0	$ 17.00		
Drug Charts in Basic Pharmacology, 3rd Edition (2000) ISBN # 0-942447-37-9	$ 18.95		
Warning: Drugs in Sports, 1st Edition (1995) ISBN # 0-942447-16-6	$ 14.50		

Shipping and Handling Charges:				
Add $ 6.50 for orders between $10.00 - $49.99	**SUB-TOTAL**			
Add $ 9.00 for orders between $50.00 - $ 99.99	(*) Shipping & Handling			
Add $ 11.00 for orders between $100.00 – 149.99	PA Residents, Add 6% Sales Tax			
Add $ 13.00 for orders Greater then $ 150.00	**TOTAL**			

Bookstores subject to standard shipping and handling charges

Name: _____

Address: _____

City: _____ STATE: _____ ZIP: _____

E-Mail Address:_____

AMT. ENCLOSED _____ ☐ VISA ☐ M/C ☐ DISCOVER ☐ AMERICAN EXPRESS ☐ CHECK

CARD NUMBER: _____ EXP. DATE: _____

AUTHORIZED SIGNATURE _____ PHONE: _____

If you are paying by credit card, Call Toll Free or Fax

ORDER FORM

PHONE	FAX	VIA WEB SITE
1-800-417-3189	1-215-657-1475	MEDICALSURVEILLANCE.COM

E-MAIL	CHECKS OR MONEY ORDERS	MAIL
MEDSURVEILLANCE@AOL.COM	Make check payable to MSI and mail order form	P.O. Box 480 Willow Grove, Pa. 19090

Books	Price	Qty	Sub-Total
Handbook of Commonly Prescribed Drugs with Therapeutic, Toxic and Lethal Levels, 18th Edition (2003) ISBN # 0-942447-44-1	$ 25.50		
Handbook of Common Orthopaedic Fractures and Drugs, 1st Edition (2003) ISBN # 0-942447-43-3	$ 19.95		
Travelers Guide to International Drugs, **Western Hemisphere** (2001) ISBN # 942447-40-9	$ 14.00		
Travelers Guide to International Drugs, **European Volume I ** (2001) ISBN # 942447-39-5	$ 14.00		
Travelers Guide to International Drugs, **European Volume II ** (2001) ISBN # 942447-38-7	$ 14.00		
Travelers Guide to International Drugs, **Middle & Far East** (2001) ISBN # 0-942447-32-8	$ 14.00		
Handbook of Commonly Prescribed Pediatric Drugs, 6th Edition (1999) ISBN # 0-942447-27-1	$ 18.50		
Antimicrobial Therapy in Primary Care Medicine, 1st Edition (1997) ISBN # 0-942447-22-0	$ 17.00		
Drug Charts in Basic Pharmacology, 3rd Edition (2000) ISBN # 0-942447-37-9	$ 18.95		
Warning: Drugs in Sports, 1st Edition (1995) ISBN # 0-942447-16-6	$ 14.50		

Shipping and Handling Charges:				
Add $ 6.50 for orders between $ 10.00 - $49.99	**SUB-TOTAL**			
Add $ 9.00 for orders between $50.00 - $ 99.99	(*) Shipping & Handling			
Add $ 11.00 for orders between $100.00 – 149.99	PA Residents, Add 6% Sales Tax			
Add $ 13.00 for orders Greater then $ 150.00	**TOTAL**			

Bookstores subject to standard shipping and handling charges

Name: _____

Address: _____

City: _____ STATE: _____ ZIP: _____

E-Mail Address: _____

AMT. ENCLOSED _____ ☐ VISA ☐ M/C ☐ DISCOVER ☐ AMERICAN EXPRESS ☐ CHECK

CARD NUMBER: _____ EXP. DATE: _____

AUTHORIZED SIGNATURE _____ PHONE: _____

If you are paying by credit card, Call Toll Free or Fax

ORDER FORM

PHONE	FAX	VIA WEB SITE
1-800-417-3189	1-215-657-1475	MEDICALSURVEILLANCE.COM

E-MAIL	CHECKS OR MONEY ORDERS	MAIL
MEDSURVEILLANCE@AOL.COM	Make check payable to MSI and mail order form	P.O. Box 480 Willow Grove, Pa. 19090

Books	Price	Qty	Sub-Total
Handbook of Commonly Prescribed Drugs with Therapeutic, Toxic and Lethal Levels, 18th Edition (2003) ISBN # 0-942447-44-1	$ 25.50		
Handbook of Common Orthopaedic Fractures and Drugs, 1st Edition (2003) ISBN # 0-942447-43-3	$ 19.95		
Travelers Guide to International Drugs, **Western Hemisphere** (2001) ISBN # 942447-40-9	$ 14.00		
Travelers Guide to International Drugs, **European Volume I ** (2001) ISBN # 942447-39-5	$ 14.00		
Travelers Guide to International Drugs, **European Volume II ** (2001) ISBN # 942447-38-7	$ 14.00		
Travelers Guide to International Drugs, **Middle & Far East** (2001) ISBN # 0-942447-32-8	$ 14.00		
Handbook of Commonly Prescribed Pediatric Drugs, 6th Edition (1999) ISBN # 0-942447-27-1	$ 18.50		
Antimicrobial Therapy in Primary Care Medicine, 1st Edition (1997) ISBN # 0-942447-22-0	$ 17.00		
Drug Charts in Basic Pharmacology, 3rd Edition (2000) ISBN # 0-942447-37-9	$ 18.95		
Warning: Drugs in Sports, 1st Edition (1995) ISBN # 0-942447-16-6	$ 14.50		
Shipping and Handling Charges:			
Add $ 6.50 for orders between $10.00 - $49.99	SUB-TOTAL		
Add $ 9.00 for orders between $50.00 - $ 99.99	(*) Shipping & Handling		
Add $ 11.00 for orders between $100.00 – 149.99	PA Residents, Add 6% Sales Tax		
Add $ 13.00 for orders Greater then $ 150.00	TOTAL		

Bookstores subject to standard shipping and handling charges

Name: _____

Address: _____

City: _____ STATE: _____ ZIP: _____

E-Mail Address: _____

AMT. ENCLOSED _____ ☐ VISA ☐ M/C ☐ DISCOVER ☐ AMERICAN EXPRESS ☐ CHECK

CARD NUMBER: _____ EXP. DATE: _____

AUTHORIZED SIGNATURE _____ PHONE: _____

If you are paying by credit card, Call Toll Free or Fax

ORDER FORM

PHONE	FAX	VIA WEB SITE
1-800-417-3189	1-215-657-1475	MEDICALSURVEILLANCE.COM

E-MAIL	CHECKS OR MONEY ORDERS	MAIL
MEDSURVEILLANCE@AOL.COM	Make check payable to MSI and mail order form	P.O. Box 480 Willow Grove, Pa. 19090

Books	Price	Qty	Sub-Total
Handbook of Commonly Prescribed Drugs with Therapeutic, Toxic and Lethal Levels, 18th Edition (2003) ISBN # 0-942447-44-1	$ 25.50		
Handbook of Common Orthopaedic Fractures and Drugs, 1st Edition (2003) ISBN # 0-942447-43-3	$ 19.95		
Travelers Guide to International Drugs, **Western Hemisphere** (2001) ISBN # 942447-40-9	$ 14.00		
Travelers Guide to International Drugs, **European Volume I ** (2001) ISBN # 942447-39-5	$ 14.00		
Travelers Guide to International Drugs, **European Volume II ** (2001) ISBN # 942447-38-7	$ 14.00		
Travelers Guide to International Drugs, **Middle & Far East** (2001) ISBN # 0-942447-32-8	$ 14.00		
Handbook of Commonly Prescribed Pediatric Drugs, 6th Edition (1999) ISBN # 0-942447-27-1	$ 18.50		
Antimicrobial Therapy in Primary Care Medicine, 1st Edition (1997) ISBN # 0-942447-22-0	$ 17.00		
Drug Charts in Basic Pharmacology, 3rd Edition (2000) ISBN # 0-942447-37-9	$ 18.95		
Warning: Drugs in Sports, 1st Edition (1995) ISBN # 0-942447-16-6	$ 14.50		

Shipping and Handling Charges:		
Add $ 6.50 for orders between $10.00 - $49.99	**SUB-TOTAL**	
Add $ 9.00 for orders between $50.00 - $ 99.99	(*) Shipping & Handling	
Add $ 11.00 for orders between $100.00 – 149.99	PA Residents, Add 6% Sales Tax	
Add $ 13.00 for orders Greater then $ 150.00	**TOTAL**	

Bookstores subject to standard shipping and handling charges

Name: _____

Address: _____

City: _____ STATE: _____ ZIP: _____

E-Mail Address: _____

AMT. ENCLOSED _____ ☐ VISA ☐ M/C ☐ DISCOVER ☐ AMERICAN EXPRESS ☐ CHECK

CARD NUMBER: _____ EXP. DATE: _____

AUTHORIZED SIGNATURE _____ PHONE: _____

If you are paying by credit card, Call Toll Free or Fax

ORDER FORM

PHONE	FAX	VIA WEB SITE
1-800-417-3189	1-215-657-1475	MEDICALSURVEILLANCE.COM

E-MAIL	CHECKS OR MONEY ORDERS	MAIL
MEDSURVEILLANCE@AOL.COM	Make check payable to MSI and mail order form	P.O. Box 480 Willow Grove, Pa. 19090

Books	Price	Qty	Sub-Total
Handbook of Commonly Prescribed Drugs with Therapeutic, Toxic and Lethal Levels, 18th Edition (2003) ISBN # 0-942447-44-1	$ 25.50		
Handbook of Common Orthopaedic Fractures and Drugs, 1st Edition (2003) ISBN # 0-942447-43-3	$ 19.95		
Travelers Guide to International Drugs, **Western Hemisphere** (2001) ISBN # 942447-40-9	$ 14.00		
Travelers Guide to International Drugs, **European Volume I ** (2001) ISBN # 942447-39-5	$ 14.00		
Travelers Guide to International Drugs, **European Volume II ** (2001) ISBN # 0-942447-38-7	$ 14.00		
Travelers Guide to International Drugs, **Middle & Far East** (2001) ISBN # 0-942447-32-8	$ 14.00		
Handbook of Commonly Prescribed Pediatric Drugs, 6th Edition (1999) ISBN # 0-942447-27-1	$ 18.50		
Antimicrobial Therapy in Primary Care Medicine, 1st Edition (1997) ISBN # 0-942447-22-0	$ 17.00		
Drug Charts in Basic Pharmacology, 3rd Edition (2000) ISBN # 0-942447-37-9	$ 18.95		
Warning: Drugs in Sports, 1st Edition (1995) ISBN # 0-942447-16-6	$ 14.50		

Shipping and Handling Charges:			
Add $ 6.50 for orders between $10.00 - $49.99	**SUB-TOTAL**		
Add $ 9.00 for orders between $50.00 - $ 99.99	(*) Shipping & Handling		
Add $ 11.00 for orders between $100.00 – 149.99	PA Residents, Add 6% Sales Tax		
Add $ 13.00 for orders Greater then $ 150.00	**TOTAL**		

Bookstores subject to standard shipping and handling charges

Name: _____

Address: _____

City: _____ STATE: _____ ZIP: _____

E-Mail Address: _____

AMT. ENCLOSED _____ □ VISA □ M/C □ DISCOVER □ AMERICAN EXPRESS □ CHECK

CARD NUMBER: _____ EXP. DATE: _____

AUTHORIZED SIGNATURE _____ PHONE: _____

If you are paying by credit card, Call Toll Free or Fax

ORDER FORM

PHONE	FAX	VIA WEB SITE
1-800-417-3189	1-215-657-1475	MEDICALSURVEILLANCE.COM

E-MAIL	CHECKS OR MONEY ORDERS	MAIL
MEDSURVEILLANCE@AOL.COM	Make check payable to MSI and mail order form	P.O. Box 480 Willow Grove, Pa. 19090

Books	Price	Qty	Sub-Total
Handbook of Commonly Prescribed Drugs with Therapeutic, Toxic and Lethal Levels, 18th Edition (2003) ISBN # 0-942447-44-1	$ 25.50		
Handbook of Common Orthopaedic Fractures and Drugs, 1st Edition (2003) ISBN # 0-942447-43-3	$ 19.95		
Travelers Guide to International Drugs, **Western Hemisphere** (2001) ISBN # 942447-40-9	$ 14.00		
Travelers Guide to International Drugs, **European Volume I ** (2001) ISBN # 942447-39-5	$ 14.00		
Travelers Guide to International Drugs, **European Volume II ** (2001) ISBN # 942447-38-7	$ 14.00		
Travelers Guide to International Drugs, **Middle & Far East** (2001) ISBN # 0-942447-32-8	$ 14.00		
Handbook of Commonly Prescribed Pediatric Drugs, 6th Edition (1999) ISBN # 0-942447-27-1	$ 18.50		
Antimicrobial Therapy in Primary Care Medicine, 1st Edition (1997) ISBN # 0-942447-22-0	$ 17.00		
Drug Charts in Basic Pharmacology, 3rd Edition (2000) ISBN # 0-942447-37-9	$ 18.95		
Warning: Drugs in Sports, 1st Edition (1995) ISBN # 0-942447-16-6	$ 14.50		

Shipping and Handling Charges:				
Add $ 6.50 for orders between $10.00 - $49.99		**SUB-TOTAL**		
Add $ 9.00 for orders between $50.00 - $ 99.99		(*) Shipping & Handling		
Add $ 11.00 for orders between $100.00 – 149.99		PA Residents, Add 6% Sales Tax		
Add $ 13.00 for orders Greater then $ 150.00		**TOTAL**		

Bookstores subject to standard shipping and handling charges

Name: _____

Address: _____

City: _____ STATE: _____ ZIP: _____

E-Mail Address:_____

AMT. ENCLOSED _____ ☐ VISA ☐ M/C ☐ DISCOVER ☐ AMERICAN EXPRESS ☐ CHECK

CARD NUMBER: _____ EXP. DATE: _____

AUTHORIZED SIGNATURE _____ PHONE: _____

If you are paying by credit card, Call Toll Free or Fax